3000 800046 07765

St. Louis Community College

WITHDRAWN

St. Louis Community College

Forest Park
Florissant Valley
Meramec

Instructional Resources
St. Louis, Missouri

Stress, Culture, and Community

The Psychology and Philosophy of Stress

St. Louis Community College
at Meramec
LIBRARY

The Plenum Series on Stress and Coping

Series Editor:
Donald Meichenbaum, *University of Waterloo, Waterloo, Ontario, Canada*

Editorial Board: Bruce P. Dohrenwend, *Columbia University* •Marianne Frankenhauser, *University of Stockholm* • Norman Garmezy, *University of Minnesota* • Mardi J. Horowitz, *University of California Medical School, San Francisco* • Richard S. Lazarus, *University of California, Berkeley* • Michael Rutter, *University of London*• Dennis C. Turk, *University of Pittsburgh* • John P. Wilson, *Cleveland State University* • Camille Wortman, *University of Michigan*

A Continuation Order Plan is available for this series. A continuation order will bring delivery of each new volume immediately upon publication. Volumes are billed only upon actual shipment. For further information please contact the publisher.

Stress, Culture, and Community

The Psychology and Philosophy of Stress

Stevan E. Hobfoll

Kent State University
Kent, Ohio

PLENUM PRESS • NEW YORK AND LONDON

Library of Congress Cataloging-in-Publication Data

On file

Cover: Reproduction of "The Aran Fisherman's Drowned Child," by Frederick William Burton (1816 – 1900), courtesy of The National Gallery of Ireland.

ISBN 0-306-45942-6

© 1998 Plenum Press, New York
A Division of Plenum Publishing Corporation
233 Spring Street, New York, N.Y. 10013

http://www.plenum.com

All rights reserved

10 9 8 7 6 5 4 3 2 1

No part of this book may be reproduced, stored in a retrieval system, or transmitted in any form or by any means, electronic, mechanical, photocopying, microfilming, recording, or otherwise, without written permission from the Publisher

Printed in the United States of America

For my wife and hero Ivonne,
who gives me love and unassailable support

Preface

Stress, Culture, and Community is about how stress evolves and is resolved in the interplay between ourselves and our social connectedness within family, tribe, and culture. My approach is one that combines scientific inquiry with literary, social, religious, and historical analysis, because I believe that science exists within the greater context of culture and the meanings that culture imparts and the limitations that it imposes. As I sit down to write this Preface, I feel that I must offer the reader a number of admissions. I do not mean these to be disclaimers, because I take full responsibility for what I write in this book. I mean what I write, even the exaggerations. But perhaps with these cautionary notes you will understand more about things that lie behind my words. Although science pretends not to have hidden meanings and agendas, the point I raise in the very first chapter is that virtually all philosophers of science argue otherwise.

This is not a question of whether psychological science should abandon empirical research in favor of a qualitative, descriptive approach. Rather, it is a wake-up call that all approaches to science and knowledge have powerful inherent biases. The moment you look one place for answers, or explore by one method, you begin to ignore other possibilities. The selection of one set of research tools means that many types of information will remain hidden. These choices are not serendipity, either, but themselves reflect the culture and the segment of the culture that is entrusted with the mission of scientific discovery. Perry London in his landmark volume *The Modes and Morals of Psychotherapy* (1964), called psychology the *secular priesthood*, because in the latter half of the twentieth century, psychologists have replaced religious authority as the new meaning makers. In these words, he was also cautioning us not to take psychology's words lightly or without questioning, not to fall into the same traps that we had with religion. London, I believe, was a most insightful scholar.

I postponed writing this book for many years. Although I felt knowledgeable about the topic of stress, my main impediment was my awareness of how little I knew about philosophy. I felt ignorant and without credentials as a philosopher of science, let alone a describer of culture and context. Immersing myself in the study of philosophy, I came to realize that it was equally unlikely that a philosopher would know as much as I about the psychological study of stress. Yet philosophy has often delved into psychology and offered meaningful insights in the process. So I hope to offer you insight through a combination of good psychology and self-taught philosophy. I apologize in advance.

My next caution is that this book is not clearly placeable in any one discipline of the social or behavioral sciences. In some ways less difficult and in some ways more difficult than my venturing into philosophy was my decision to borrow from and integrate the work of the fields of sociology, anthropology, and psychiatry. We are taught in academia that these disciplinary boundaries are sacrosanct, and only recently has interdisciplinary work been taken seriously. The problem is, however, that each discipline inculcates the idea that one's own disciplinary approach is the correct one. At times, this is reflected in the mere disregard of the sister disciplines. They are hardly read in the formative years of training. Sociologists read little psychology and vice-versa. Next, during professional careers, the sister disciplines are seldom mixed at scientific conferences or published together in scientific journals. There is an occasional invited speaker of eminence from another discipline, but even these types of events are rare. At those unique, small meetings, where a handful of well-known social scientists are invited from across disciplines, there have been some genuine attempts at cross-pollination. But again, those individuals tend to return to academic departments, with their thick dividing walls between disciplines. At best, the messages from other disciplines are used as vehicles for insights into one's own discipline, not as central, sustaining pillars of knowledge and discovery.

This book is very much about culture and the borders that exist between cultures, as well as their common elements. The appreciation of multiculturalism that is emerging in stress research reminds me of the neighborhood of my youth. Coming from a Chicago neighborhood of predominantly first-generation Americans, the vast apartment building mailboxes read with names like Giaconni, Pappandrikopolous, Lee, Gonzales, Kuwolski, Knutson, Beaudreau, Haucke, and O'Brian. Many of the names simply did not fit in the mailbox space provided. Children by the age of 12 skirting in and out of friends' houses were aware of dozens of cultures, had eaten all their foods, shared their holidays, and participated in their rites of passage.

Until the age of 18, I thought that religion was ethnically organized, because the neighborhood churches were. They were know as the Irish Church, the Greek Church, and the Italian Church. Of course, I was not far off, until you understand that I actually did not know that there were also Protestants in the world. I was basically dividing up Catholics. In other words, my ordering was pre-sixteenth century—except, of course, for the small group of poor Hasidic Jews, who dressed in a style of black garb that mimics seventeenth-century Polish nobles.

I also warn the reader about a number of clear biases in my thinking. First, for me, stress is real and really affects people's lives. It is born of objective circumstances, not perception. Stress emerges from context, and people's interpretation of their experience comes from context. Their perceptions are also important, but they are mainly shared perceptions because cultures and subcultures produce common narratives according to which experience is interpreted. We are not nearly so alone as individualized psychology and an idealized Northern European and Anglo-Saxon philosophy has promulgated.

My second bias is that science is meant to question. However, science tries to force us to question within acceptable borders. These borders are ever narrower. This is a crossroads that the sciences are being forced to consider in the face of postmodernism and beyond. The correct questions are often outside of the acceptable borders of inquiry.

My third bias is that my own cultural experience has taught me that we are all connected. I recognize individuality, of course, but the connections for me are primary. Psychology, in contrast, has made little of people's connections. For psychology, the individual is figure, and context is ground. I simply see things in reverse. I see us as interconnected by a common biology and by overlapping, if distinctive, cultures. This biology and these cultures create pathways by which stress is experienced and stress resistance is patterned. There are few individual pathways that have not been worn with former and fellow travelers.

My last bias comes out of a different area of my past. The women in my home participated equally as opinion makers, teachers, and guides of the family's and my direction. Hence, a world interpreted by men was always strange to me. My feminist leanings certainly emerge in this volume.

This book challenges many ideas in the field of stress, and builds on many others. On rereading it myself, I also came to understand that it also challenges a basic notion in psychology in general. Specifically, psychology has long rested on the assumption that people are ends oriented; that is, we seek reinforcement and avoid punishment. This book is about our striving to obtain, retain, foster, and protect resources—those things we value. However, we do so to preserve the means for sustaining ourselves, our families, and our cultures. There is an old adage, "Give a man a fish you feed him for a day. Teach a man to fish you feed him for a lifetime." Well, psychology has focused since the time of Skinner on the reinforcer—the given fish. This book, and the Conservation of Resources theory that I develop, focuses on the means of fishing. People are oriented not to seek reward, but to maintain a state in which rewards will be possible and in which punishments can be avoided or at least minimized. This is a fundamentally different approach, because it forces us to make "process" not "outcomes" the focus of study. Hence, psychological distress and physical illness are not as critical as the pathways we choose and the means we sustain in order to avoid these untoward ends. How do we function to avoid and minimize stress and its negative sequelae? This is the critical question. I embark on it with my biases exposed. I hope it will encourage the reader to also question and open new borders of exploration.

Acknowledgments

I am greatly indebted in so many ways for the help that I received in writing this book that it is difficult to know where to begin. Eliot Werner, Senior Editor at Plenum, was encouraging and helpful from the outset through the final stages, and Herman Makler was instrumental as production editor. Donald Meichenbaum, as Series Editor, not only provided the usual background guidance, but with his own profound knowledge of the stress field at both clinical and research levels was also instrumental in providing feedback and ideas. Two colleagues, Leonard Jason and Krzystof Kaniasty, read virtually the entire manuscript as I was writing and provided insightful ideas and serious criticisms that I had to address. I am greatly indebted to them for their contribution of time, energy, and thought.

A number of scholars read the completed work, or selected portions that fell into their particular area of expertise, and provided comments and criticism. They represent the fields of anthropology, philosophy, psychology, psychiatry, sociology, social epidemiology, and social work, and about as many countries. Their rich, diverse viewpoints greatly helped me expand the breadth of my own perspective. They are Michael Argyle, Paul Baltes, Marten deVries, Berkley Eddins, Esther Greenglass, Richard Hirschman, Howard Kaplan, Ralf Schwarzer, Johannes Siegrist, Zahava Solomon, Charles Spielberger, Mary Ann Stephens, and Shelley Taylor. Charlie Spielberger in particular has been a source of encouragement and guidance throughout my career and he remains the only person who marks up my work with copious corrections in red ink. His demands of me for excellence and exactitude, and his own unquenchable thirst for knowledge have shaped my intellectual growth. Jennifer Kay was extremely dedicated as my assistant and I am grateful to her for editorial assistance and referencing. Having to delve back into historical records, out-of-print publications, and microfilm was an arduous task that she did splendidly. Julie Trask was instrumental in manuscript preparation and obtaining the many copyright permissions. Sadhana Moneypenny frequently stepped in with clerical and computer assistance, and she had the uncanny ability to "find" material that I "lost" on the computer. Of course, these people are only responsible for what is positive in the volume; I am the sole arbiter of any errors, mistaken opinions and interpretations, and misjudgments.

Finally, I would like to thank my family. My parents always believed in me despite the obvious overwhelming data coming from years of school to the contrary. They often spent more time in my school than I did! My wife Ivonne, herself a psychologist, has always and continues to be unflinchingly supportive and her love is constant. My three children Ari, Sheera, and Jonathan are a source of strength and a place for frequent reality checks. I promised in writing this book not to work nights or weekends because "work won't love you back," and they held me to it in their own spirited ways.

Contents

Stress, Culture, and Community

The Psychology and Philosophy of Stress

1

The Social and Historical Context of Stress

No concept in the modern psychological, sociological, or psychiatric literature is more extensively studied than stress. The sheer amount of scientific literature is so extensive that it is no longer possible to conduct a comprehensive review. But the amount of research is only one facet of the attention given to stress. I submit that stress is also the social-psychological concept of greatest interest to Western society. Perhaps no other psychosocial topic is discussed more often in the lay press or kaffeeklatsches. We are consumed with the stress concept and we use it as a basic explanatory mechanism to describe the underpinnings of what we see as wrong with work, family life, and our society. Violence, marital discord, disease, mental illness, failed productivity, and juvenile delinquency are all depicted within a model that places stress as a central causative element.

Can we really have identified the basic ingredient of our social and psychological ills in one fell swoop? Have twentieth-century psychology and sociology been so successful that now our only task is to disentangle the mystery of stress? Have we isolated the basic building block of people's malaise, malady, and mania, or have we found a "whipping boy" so that our noble fears have a scapegoat to draw attention from them? This chapter attempts to delve into the philosophy of the psychosocial study of stress so that we can have a deeper and more inclusive sense of the substance of our inquiry. By understanding the historical, religious, and philosophical roots of stress, I hope to lead us to a clearer view of the science of stress research—

where the study of stress has gone, and possible directions for its future examination.

Stress is hardly a new term. It has been used in medicine for centuries (Hinkle, 1977). Robert Burton, in 1624, wrote of the sources of disease and melancholy (depression) in particular, emphasizing social stress as one of the greatest causes of malady.

> Dearths, tempests, plagues, our astrologers foretell us; Earthquakes, inundations, ruins of houses, consuming fires, come little by little, or make some noise beforehand; but the knaveries, impostures, injuries and villainies of men no art can avoid. We can keep our professed enemies from our cities, by gates, walls and towers, defend ourselves from thieves and robbers by watchfulness and weapons; but this malice of men, and their pernicious endeavours, no caution can divert, no vigilancy foresee, we have so many secret plots and devices to mischief one another. (p. 84)

The essence of what we mean by stress is found in an ancient form in one of the most poignant stories of the Bible. The Book of Job is the tale of a man of enormous wealth and righteous character. Satan challenged this righteousness, claiming it was based on Job's good fortune, and not his faith. So God was forced to test Job by taking all he prized.

> There came a messenger onto Job, and said "the oxen were plowing, and the asses feeding beside them; and the Sabeans made a raid, and took them away.... A fire ... hath burned up all thy sheep and the servants.... The Chaldeans set themselves ... and fell upon thy camels, and have taken them away.... Thy sons and thy daughters were eating and drinking wine in their elder brother's house; and, behold, there came a great wind ... and smote the four corners of the house, and it fell upon the young people, and they are dead."

When this did not break Job's faith,

> So Satan went forth from the presence of the Lord, and smote Job with sore boils from the sole of his foot even unto his crown. [And Job was so utterly transformed that his three best friends] knew him not. (Job 1:13–2:13)

The list of Job's losses could have been transcribed directly from the Hebrew to create the stressful life event lists used in stress research today. It was Job's faith, his sense of the meaning of his place before his God, that saw him through his travails until all he had was restored twofold.

It would seem that our attraction to Job's saga is our identification with the basic message. We live a life in which troubles are inevitable. We know that as Job knew ... *But man is born unto trouble, as* [certainly as] *the sparks fly upward* (Job 5:7). The question becomes what influence will our stress have, knowing that it will be set in our path in one form or another. How will we cope? Who will comfort us? How will we be transformed? On what internal resources will we be able to call and how successfully?

STRESS AND OUR VIEW OF OUR WORLD

Returning to modern times, we find ourselves in an historical period which social commentators often depict as the Age of Anxiety or the Age of Stress (see Wilson, Galvin, & Thompson, 1983). What does this mean to be in the Age of something? In this first chapter, I hope to explore this first question. Because scientists have produced so much work on stress, we are risking losing the forest for the trees. We are not clear on the question of in which forest we wander. We must take some time to step outside the research on stress, to see its context. From outside the forest, we see its shape, its height, and its boundaries. From inside, we learn stress's rules and laws, but in a way that is decontextualized and disconnected if we do not step outside from time to time and question the very path we have taken. Perhaps by seeing both what is meant by the term *Age* and by capturing the historical Age that preceded the Age of Stress, we can begin to understand the stress paradigm better. In so doing, I hope to gain greater objectivity for this book and to lay the groundwork for a critical analysis of the subjective biases that stress researchers and theorists have made and that I will inevitably make as well.

I will argue that because stress is so central to broad social concerns outside of the behavioral sciences, stress more than other areas of inquiry has been conceptualized, shaped, and reshaped in a way that fits a certain worldview. How we see stress is not a pure outgrowth of the scientific methods of the behavioral sciences, but a combination of science and societal pressures. The concept of stress is also historically grounded, and this fairly recent history gave birth to a way of demarcating the borders of stress. Stress, as we study it, was developed out of the age of two great wars, and a long Cold War that threatened first the domination of the world and then our species' very existence on earth.

Stress also is necessarily conceptualized in a way to fit in with the current *zeitgeist* in the study of psychology, sociology, and psychiatry. Being a mainstream area of study, stress not only influences psychological thought, but also it is shaped by psychological thought. In the psychoanalytic era, if studied at all, stress would be seen through a psychoanalytic prism. Although it may have set the stage for our current conceptualizations, Freud's concept of anxiety has little overlap with how we envision the much broader and comprehensive term *stress*.

At the current turn of the wheel, and this wheel certainly continues to spin, we are in the midst of the cognitive revolution in psychology. Not surprisingly, stress is therefore mainly understood in cognitive terms. Even here, however, we see that sociology and psychiatry part with psychology. Unless psychology is wholly correct and these sister disciplines are wholly wrong, which no one in any of these fields believes, then we necessarily have only part of the picture of the stress phenomena if we do not consider these other viewpoints.

For the clinician in psychology and medicine, for the human resources professional in industry, and for educators in the classroom, stress is a foundation concept as well. By taking a step back and examining stress in its wider context, I hope to foster thoughts and questions for practice. When addressing stress in one way, we serve certain ends. By altering our vantage point, we alter the questions we ask, the way we intercede, the conclusions we make, and the meanings we impart. If stress is in the mind, we change people's thoughts. If stress is in the environment, we alter people's world, not their beliefs about the world. If stress is psychodynamic, we dig deeper and intervene earlier. If stress is endemic to life, we may even choose to leave it be and move on to more manageable pastures.

STRESS AND THE LIMITATIONS OF SCIENTIFIC PARADIGMS

If we can be humble enough to admit that the behavioral sciences are inexact, then we must follow the lead of Popper (1959) and Kuhn (1962), and pay attention to the parameters of the paradigm in which we study, analyze, and intervene on stress. Indeed, much of what and how we study in the social and behavioral sciences is largely a matter of interpretation of scant data that is always acknowledged in our scientific journals as ambiguous enough to be open to multiple interpretations. This ambiguity demands that we rely heavily on theory, and our theories are constructed within the boundaries of larger paradigms. As Kuhn and Popper write, a paradigm is not a truth. Rather, it is a way of construing scientific outcomes, as Kuhn states, we are enmeshed in a web of meaning that is the product of "the theory ladenous of facts."

When we viewed earth as the center of the universe for religious reasons, facts were scientifically interpreted to fit this paradigm. Provable mathematical theorems and logical arguments were created and quoted to support this thesis, and it is a mistake to think that this was a matter of distinguished scientists arguing empirically with superstitious clerics. There were eminent scientists on both sides of the issue. Indeed, to understand the spinning of earths and the movements of galaxies in modern scientific terms, we must resort to another unknowable—the paradigm of the infinity of the universe. Because without infinity, where does this ultimate motion transport us?

We interpret facts within the theories that are dominant. Our theories, in turn, exist within larger paradigms that often cross disciplines and define the borders of our ways of knowing. Moreover, we create facts within the ruling paradigm, and means of uncovering knowledge outside of the paradigm are deemed unscientific. Hence, it is not just that our study outcomes are interpreted in the light and shadows of a paradigm; the very methods we use are governed by the paradigm and are biased to support the paradigm.

When Anna Freud (1958) defined adolescence as a period of "storm and strife," she created a paradigm, with a small *p* according to Kuhn's model. Studies that followed were devised in a way that accepted this assumption *a priori*, and set out to define and understand the nature of this stormy period. But this existed within another, larger Paradigm (Kuhn's large *P*) that defined how the very issue of psyche was conceptualized and could be studied. The larger *P* in paradigm can be seen in Sigmund Freud's work. For S. Freud, logical positivism and its accompanying fixation on scientific measurement were irrelevant to the study of the human psyche. Hence, when sent an empirical study confirming the existence and operation of defense mechanisms, he replied on a postcard, "Gantze Americanishe, very American." The scientific method was inconsistent with the psychoanalytic method, and Freud was unconcerned that psychoanalysis was not a science of prediction. The boundaries of his paradigm served as explanation and understanding without resort to logical positivism. The paradigm Freud embraced colored the questions he asked and the data he accepted.

It is also worthwhile to point out that a paradigm may follow a set of methods as much as they might a theoretical perspective. The study of stress in psychology became nested in the questionnaire method based on the pioneering work of Janet Taylor Spence (1985) and C. D. Spielberger (1966, 1972). Spence and Spielberger developed reliable and valid questionnaires that allowed for the measurement of the internal state of anxiety. This had advantages over the psychoanalytic method, because it opened the way for the quantification of stress responses. Spielberger further aided scientific inquiry by clarifying the state versus trait distinction. He distinguished between anxiety state, being the emotional expression of anxiety during a given period of time, and anxiety trait, being the general tendency to become anxious that characterized the individual's personality. However, by developing paper-and-pencil measures of internal states, Spence and Spielberger may have also steered psychology in the direction of seeing stress as an internal rather than external aspect of the environment.

THE CONCEPT OF AGE

To better understand how the stress paradigm developed, I would like to spend some time on inquiry as to what we mean by the Age of Stress, and the cultural context which shapes and is shaped by this Age. The term *Age* comes from references to defining elements of a time of human culture. The Stone Age, Iron Age, and Age of Reason are historical periods wherein the conceptual center is that thing. It is the hub of the wheel upon which society spins. From the stone comes flint for fire, arrow, and spearheads to hunt more effectively, and the sculpting of idols to worship. Knowledge of stone becomes power. The group near the best quarries is more powerful than its neighbor, the person who can shape the stone is more powerful than those who cannot, and stone itself becomes in some way sacred. Men govern stone, and women are not permitted to shape stone. Thus it is not only that this was the period in which stone was in use, but also the period in which civilization was in large part defined by stone. Nor should we misinterpret that stone was all-defining. Tribal life, knowledge of nature, and the process of adaptation were all developing both in relation to stone and independent of it.

More abstractly, more modernly, and more connected to our own Age of Stress, we have the Age of Reason. Beginning in the 1600s and lasting until the end of the eighteenth century, Locke, Rousseau, and Descartes developed a philosophy esteeming reason as its core. The Age of Reason credited the scientific method for the advances of society and science. It saw itself as a modern, informed response to the Middle Ages, which were dominated by superstition, ignorance, and blind acceptance of authority. It was a fountainhead for scientific discovery and, at the same time, the wellspring of democracy. If humans could reason, they could advance their lot and rule themselves. Borrowing from the sciences, it saw mathematics as the basic truth and logic as the revealer of self-evident laws of nature. From the Age of Reason came not only advancement of science, but also science as power. Philosophers such as Locke and Voltaire also influenced the framework, form, and arguments that led to the American and French Revolutions. At the same time, men, especially white Northern Europeans were seen as the guardians of reason, and women and other peoples were seen as emotional and irrational (Montesquieu, 1752). These conclusions, too, were seen as empirical, logical truths.

Why, then, are we no longer considered to be in the Age of Reason? Are we not reasoning individuals, and are the sciences and society not based on the notion that reason is paramount to progress? Reason began to be criticized in the early parts of the last century for often being arbitrary. What was argued to be reason and logic was frequently tautology. Reason was also pushed aside to make room for the ideas of spontaneity, emotions, and the rise of individuality, all of which were based not on reason and its necessary call for order, but on passion. And so we have entrée to the Romantic Movement. Consistent with this change, Marx argued that the Age of Reason was not based on logic, but on the promotion of a certain class. Landed people used reason as a convenient tool to promote their class and remove them from the yoke of higher authority. He argued that mathematics did not enter into the formula of human welfare. Freud also dismissed the idea that reason governed action. By seeing unconscious processes as underpinning human behavior, Freud rejected the notion that humans were logical and that reason ruled. An ultimate romantic, for Freud, passion ruled. So total was Freud's rejection of logical order that passion not only ruled, it had us so emotionally dominated that we sexually desired our mothers and plotted to kill our fathers.

It is thus apparent that the theme of an Age, the paradigm, shapes the substance of what we believe and value. The paradigm silently demarcates how scientists inquire, how people think, how facts are interpreted, and even what we believe to be facts. We can also see that one Age gives way to another. In some ways these Ages are linked, but according to Foucault (1970), we should also pay heed to their disconnectness, and not their smooth transition.

To examine both the transition to our current age and its distinctiveness, we need then ask what preceded the Age of Stress? It is interesting that it would probably be considered the Atomic Age, if we can be allowed to call the Age of Anxiety and the Age of Stress a basic renaming of the same period. The atomic bomb ended World War II and brought a new reality to the world. Access to the bomb was access to ultimate power and possible world destruction; many said probable world destruction. Post–World War II life was consumed with the idea of the power of the bomb and how we would, or would not, save ourselves from it. People unearthed their back yards to build air-raid shelters and schools practiced air-raid drills. I cannot remember if it was weekly or monthly, but in this Atomic Age I recall a childhood of crouching under our desks or next to our lockers in order to practice the moment that we would save ourselves from the atomic blast. With the Cold War between America and Russia very much a reality, the folly was not so much our fearing The Bomb as it was expecting that we might survive it. The papers, politics, film, and art reflected our fears and thoughts. Our economy was drained to build up our atomic and strategic arsenal, and meet our need to defend ourselves against this omnipresent threat.

Another possible connection that we can surmise between the Atomic Age and the Age of Stress is the creation of a time of anxiety. The reality of the atomic bomb produced a mushroom of fear that placed a pallor over our lives. Although World War II ended with reason winning over tyranny and evil, anxiety emerged in the postatomic dust. Anxiety comes from our fear of loss, separation, and harm, and the Atomic Age found us in the midst of these fears. Socially, the Atomic Age both pressed technology forward and produced the ugly era of McCarthyism, in which the U.S. Congress investigated suspected communists and the very implication of suspicion was grounds for blacklisting, dismissal, and often imprisonment. Julius and Ethel Rosenberg were executed as spies in 1953 for giving atomic bomb secrets to the Soviet Union, against worldwide calls for clemency by such leaders as Einstein and Pope Pius XII. Anxiety was the order of the day.

The Atomic Age also saw a reemergence in the belief that science would answer our needs. Science had produced the bomb that created the nihilism and protest of the Beat Era of Ginsberg and Kerouac, with its black garb and emphasis on a return to individuality. But for most, there also existed the belief that science would bring medical advances, safety, security, leisure, and prosperity. Science would liberate us from disease and poverty and bring the 32 hour work week. Our only problem was how to spend our excess leisure time! Modern psychology was to be a part of this modern scientific revolution. And psychology clearly aligned itself with the sciences and emulated physics as its method. Moving from a realm akin to philosophy, psychology adopted the traditions of Wundt and Titchener, whose laboratories operated under the scientific method. Measurement became meaning, and statistics became the tool that replaced logical reasoning as the method of inquiry. This is not to say that statistics are inherently illogical, but where logic and statistics were in disagreement over any point, statistics determined conclusions. So, when one system of reason, psychoanalysis, was seen as either inconsistent with statistical conclusions or not given to principles of scientific measurement, it was rejected by mainstream psychology, which sought explanations of behavior that could be measured, statistically analyzed, and empirically judged.

THE AGE OF STRESS AS A PARADIGM

This brings us to analyze the distinctiveness of the Age of Stress. The cover story of *Time Magazine* of June 6, 1983 declared us in the Age of Stress. It depicted us as a society consumed by demands for our resources and threats to our well being. McGrath (1970) defined stress as a "substantial imbalance between environmental demand and the response capability of the focal organism" (p. 17). Hence, we see emerge a consensus between the lay descriptions of stress and the scientific one. The behavioral sciences defined and studied the concept, but the media went further by characterizing us as overwhelmed by stress. Howard Kaplan's (1983) definition of stress may be seen as even closer to the media's depiction of the societal phenomena of stress. For Kaplan, psychosocial stress "reflects the subject's inability to forestall or diminish perception, recall, anticipation, or imagination of disvalued circumstances, those that in reality or fantasy signify great and/or increased distance from desirable (valued) experiential states, and consequently, evoke a need to approximate the valued states" (p. 196). Of course, the *Time* article did not use these terms. Nonetheless, the essence of the article spoke to the existence of a pervasive perception that people's efforts were not forestalling the fear of losing those things they valued. Hard work and playing by the rules were not sufficient to ward off a feeling that the next threat to our well-being was just around the corner. It is probably not inconsequential that at this time, our economy was slowing from its period of unprecedented postwar expansion. Increased opportunities were no longer guaranteed, and companies were asking for greater sacrifice in exchange for lower security and a dollar that was rapidly diminishing in power. Nor is this economic trend a temporary one, as economists are well aware that the postwar economic boon was a historical period that is not sustainable.

As I have already alluded, there are different ways of conceptualizing stress. It is helpful at this stage to examine how the Age of Stress unfolded within the social and behavioral sciences. Stress in a Freudian sense is more of a battle between levels of subconscious selves than between subconscious selves and external realities. Indeed, for Freud, environmental stress, however conceived, is best seen as an unimportant factor, and even a distractor from understanding of the critical operating mechanisms in the human psyche. People's reactions to external threat were only important insomuch as they provided insight about subconscious processes developed early in life. It is interesting that Freud himself, caught in the siege of Vienna, with two sons involved in the war as soldiers, wrote about the influence of current factors on the human psyche (1917/1963). But this is an aberration by Freud of Freud, for the comprehensive picture painted by his writings depicts current affairs only as a possible passage for understanding our deeper selves, not as the cause of psychopathology. Indeed, Karen Horney was virtually disbarred by the psychoanalytic community because of her environmentally based departure from Freudian thought (Rubins, 1978). Horney, conducting research during the Depression, postulated the then heretical notion that major psychological dysfunction was often a product of such stressful life events as difficulty paying the rent, buying food, and providing for children.

Early research within psychology and physiology depicted stress in more purely biological terms. Walter Cannon (1932) began a tradition of stress study by investigation into the effects of cold, lack of oxygen, and other environmental stressors. He concluded that biological systems were resistant to low to moderate levels of environmental stressors, but that high-intensity or ongoing stress was followed by biological breakdown. This tradition was continued by Hans Selye, who many call the father of modern stress research. Selye saw stress as an orchestrated set of bodily defenses that operated in response to noxious physical stimuli (1950, 1951–1956). Using laboratory methods, he noted that organisms reacted in stages. First came the alerting response, then the resistance response, finally culminating with the exhaustion and breakdown response. As was Cannon, Selye was concerned with the physiological responsiveness to physical stressors, and he extrapolated to psychological stress based on this model.

Still closer to current conceptualizations of stress were the contributions of two Harvard colleagues, Lindemann (1944) and Caplan (1964). Their concept of crisis was an original and provocative departure from both the biological traditions of Cannon and Selye, and the psychoanalytic tradition of Freud. Both men were psychoanalysts, but my readings of their work and my personal interactions with Gerald Caplan reveal two unusual minds that were uniquely willing to question the basis of their training and the traditions of their fields.

Lindemann studied the Cocoanut Grove fire in Boston, in which hundreds were caught and many perished. What struck Lindemann and caused him to question psychoanalytic thought was a discovery of something noted earlier by Karen Horney (1937) in her work with men during the Great Depression. Like Horney, Lindemann noted marked psychopathology in survivors for whom he could find no psychopathogenic underpinnings in their early life. Here were people who should have had transient reactions to the fire, but instead remained deeply psychologically troubled. It is also notable, if we are to give realistic credence to history as influencing scientific thought, that Lindemann was a Quaker who fled Nazi Germany because of persecution. He was well aware of the influence of the Holocaust on the refugees coming to Boston in the postwar era.

Gerald Caplan was also deeply influenced by historical context. He came to Israel following the birth of the nation and was profoundly influenced by the psychological hardships of both the Holocaust and its survivors and by people's crises with the new State of Israel, ravaged by war at its birth. A psychodynamic theorist, Caplan developed the concept of *psychological crisis* that he was to take back to Harvard. According to Caplan (1964), normal individuals, when confronted with extreme challenge to their existence, their loved ones, or their well-being, could experience temporary psychological breakdown. If untreated, this temporary state could have profound, lifelong effects on their psychological well-being. In this theory, Caplan was stepping outside of the boundaries of psychoanalytic thought by concluding that major psychopathology could follow in the absence of early life trauma and experience. In so saying, he was rejecting Freud's traditional distinction between mourning and melancholy, the former, the normal reaction of grief, the latter, the pathological process that was not a reaction to current circumstances, but based on childhood experience. This man who always wore a white physician's coat and bow tie throughout his professional life was challenging the established order. He did so ahead of psychiatry and psychology, even nonpsychodynamic versions, and even went so far as to suggest that short-term crisis intervention of a few sessions was the therapy of choice for such conditions. Long before cognitive psychologists entered the scene, he suggested that crisis was critical because it undermined people's sense of mastery. He was also later, we shall see, the first to understand the importance of social support in the stress process (1974).

As we examine the development of thinking on stress, we see the influence of World War II and war in general as influencing more than Lindemann and Caplan alone. Indeed, the Age of Stress very much began as reflection on war-related stress. In accounts as early as the Civil War, we have reports of "paralysis" and "insanity" in otherwise healthy soldiers attributed to the shock of battle (Kellett, 1982). During World War I, army psychiatrists coined the term *shell shock.* Following an earlier tradition, linking victims' psychological reactions post–train crash to contraction of the spinal column (called railroad spine), army psychiatrists attributed the psychological breakdown of soldiers to the physical intensity of exploding shells. The World War I physician, T. W. Salmon (1929), saw it differently. He associated soldiers' psychological breakdown to psychosocial rather than physical causes, and recommended four basic principles: (1) Treat immediately, (2) treat near the front line, (3) share the expectation of full recovery, and (4) ensure continuity of community belonging. Salmon's thinking was so out of the *zeitgeist* as to be all but forgotten for another 40 years. Indeed, during World War II, combat stress was once again conceptualized in physical terms as a response to exhaustion, hence the term *combat fatigue.*

Two major stress theorists, who wrote directly out of their own experience during World War II, keenly influenced scientific thinking on the stress phenomena. Bruno Bettleheim (1960) and Victor Frankl (1963) both wrote of their experience as prisoners in Nazi concentration camps. Largely existential in their tone, both depicted the confrontation with stress as a search for meaning amid the challenge of meaninglessness. The concentration camp undermined human existence as it had been known for its victims. Death prevailed in place of life, a society that prided itself on culture produced the Nazi philosophy, and people were treated as subhuman and without identity—a number tattooed to their left arms. Victims were forced to live with constant threat to their lives, exposure to extreme cold and heat, physical discomfort, a total lack of privacy, lack of adequate food, sleep, or medicine, and loss of loved ones, usually to certain death. This tradition of meaning as the antithesis and healer of stress was also adopted later by Antonovsky (1979), not surprisingly, based on his work with Holocaust survivors in Israel. It has also been revisited in work by Janoff-Bulman (1992) on traumatic stress, and most recently by Meichenbaum (1994) in his work on constructionism and hermeneutics (the interpretation of people's discourse).

Two individuals who may be seen as bridge theorists between the environmental basis of stress and individual interpretation of the stress experience are C. D. Spielberger and I. G. Sarason. Both have offered a lifelong research legacy. The common thread of the fabric of their work is reflected in their separate empirical studies and in their joint pioneering series of 17 volumes on *Stress and Anxiety* (1975 to 1998). Spielberger and Sarason each advanced a view of stress as influenced in rather equal measure by environmental exigencies and personal meaning. Although they are more typically seen as personality theorists, they were each deeply involved in the community psychology movement and Spielberger was, in fact, founding editor of the *American Journal of Community Psychology*. Whether studying test anxiety, airplane controllers, emergency workers, or the process of social support, their respective research laboratories looked for the process of stress within clearly stressful conditions.

THE COGNITIVE REVOLUTION IN PSYCHOLOGY

The early 1970s saw a shift in psychology away from two formative models, behaviorism and humanism. Behaviorism, on one hand, was seen by many as too restrictive a paradigm (Lazarus & Folkman, 1984). Behaviorism denied the central role of internal processes in determining behavior. Cognitions, subconscious processes, and emotions were depicted as internal processes that could not be observed. Being unobservable, they were relegated to philosophy and outside of the realm of science (Skinner, 1938, 1953). In Seligman's (1975) original formulation of learned helplessness, the reactions of laboratory animals to inescapable punishment was thought to be the cause of helpless behavior in future challenge contexts. Stress in this model was operationalized in terms of punishment or unpredictable circumstances wherein punishment could not be avoided or pleasure achieved. There was no appeal in the original model to emotions or cognitions.

Humanism was also alive and well in psychology in the 1960s and early 1970s. The formulations of such theorists as Carl Rogers and Abraham Maslow were highly respected and the mainstay of many programs of clinical psychology. Nor can it be said that humanistic psychology was abandoned because of a lack of evidence or inability to operationalize the concepts. In both psychotherapy (Truax & Mitchell, 1971) and education (Aspy & Roebuck, 1974), it was found that empathy was a key therapeutic trait among both therapists and teachers. In other words, it was not necessarily what therapists and teachers did, as much as their acknowledgment of the client or student's positive sense of self and the communication of caring about that self that produced positive outcomes. Many of the research thrusts promulgated by humanism, such as the importance of self-disclosure, the essential nature of positive self-regard, the importance of connectedness with others, and the need for love, respect, and acceptance, were testable hypotheses that excited both clinicians and researchers. With the swing right politically in the country and the departure from the "All You Need Is Love" generation, humanism became lost somewhere in the wind.

I say that humanism became lost, because it is difficult to track its heuristic path in the research literature either on stress or in other mainstream psychology areas. This has often troubled me, because I thought that humanism deserved central stage in the study of psychology. Perhaps it was a personal inclination, but humanism felt good; it felt like something with which I wanted to be associated. In part, humanism lost its own path by splintering into some questionable practices, such as searching unscientifically for Eastern religions and "selling" them as psychology, and a tendency to employ overly optimistic jargon about the sheer wonderfulness of people. If Skinner was to be chastised for being overly deterministic, Rogers and Maslow may have been guilty of being overly optimistic about the grandeur of self-will. Not that what Rogers and Maslow theorized was wrong, but its package became increasingly inconsistent with the hard science emulation that psychology was taking. With the Love Generation beginning to fade along with the breakup of the Beatles, the inclination to follow a theory that championed love, well-being, self-awareness, and linkage to others became out of step with the social *zeitgeist.*

In part, in preparing this book, I read very carefully the theoretical work of Meichenbaum, Lazarus, and Bandura. In their writing, I have come to think that cognitive behaviorism may have grown out of a melding of these two earlier movements within psychology, behaviorism and humanism, although cognitive behaviorism sees itself as emerging more clearly out of purely behaviorist beginnings. By continuing a focus on behavior, researchers and clinicians could remain true to the push for better measurement of simpler, more basic building-block constructs, and this appealed to many. Cognitions were seen as another set of behaviors and, like overt behaviors, were accessible to the principles of reinforcement, punishment, and shaping. By focusing on the subjective interpretation of events through cognitions, cognitive behaviors were actually more closely following one of the principle contributions of humanism. Carl Rogers wrote in 1980:

> The only reality I can possibly know is the world as I perceive and experience it at this moment. The only reality you can possibly know is the world as you perceive and experience it at the moment. And the only certainty is that those perceived realities are different. There are as many "real worlds" as there are people! (p. 102)

Don Meichenbaum (1977; Meichenbaum & Cameron, 1983), a leading proponent of cognitive behaviorism and one of its founders, emphasizes that people develop problems when their cognitions interfere with their behavior. Self-statements such as "I must be perfect," "Help is only good if its spontaneous," and "Bad things happen to me because I am a bad person" are obstacles to psychological well-being because they are unachievable and inevitably interfere with positive self-regard. Trained in one of the most purist bastions of behaviorism at the University of Illinois–Urbana, Meichenbaum developed a discomfort with a system that ignored the critical role played by thought and emotions in human behavior. A direct link can be found between his thinking and early humanistic notions of Karen Horney (1937), who felt that psychological problems emerge when the healthy, real self is displaced by an unhealthy, idealized self. Likewise, we can see developmental links between Meichenbaum and Rogers (1956), who felt that the chief cause of psychopathology was the incongruency people experienced when they evaluated themselves through an introjected value system of others, because it denied them experiences that are conducive to growth.

So, for example, if I must be perfect, I cannot enjoy my experiences in research, teaching, family life, and tennis. If I must always be a parent who never becomes angry, I should never have children, because the standard is unachievable and denies me the pleasure of doing pretty well, trying very hard, accomplishing some things, and realizing that I could do better sometimes, but not at all times. Rogers and Skinner debated from their seemingly unbridgeable camps at the 1956 meetings of the American Psychological Association, but any true rapprochement of their ideas took almost 20 more years to percolate and be translated into an integrative system of thought. Meichenbaum was successful I think in identifying the strongest points in two competing viewpoints.

Lazarus (1966) and Lazarus and Folkman (1984) fostered the tradition of cognitive behaviorism in their transactional stress model. They saw appraisals and cognitions as the key to understanding the stress process. Within their model, appraisal acted in two ways. Primary appraisal was the process by which events were judged as to the degree they were threatening, challenging, or benign. Secondary appraisals were the process by which individuals judged and evaluated the extent to which they had the coping resources to respond successfully to the threat or challenge. Richard Lazarus, together with Susan Folkman, have clearly been the most influential contributors to the psychology of stress and an understanding of the stress process. Their principle contribution lies in acknowledgment of the role of cognition in interpretation of the meaning and mastery of external events that challenge individuals.

At this juncture, I wish to take a step back and evaluate the historical context of the cognitive revolution, especially as it applies to stress. By the late 1970s and the early 1980s, many years had passed since World War II and the experience of the war and the Holocaust. North American psychology was no longer so concerned with the environmental stressors that had motivated the classic study of the American GI, *Men under Stress*, by Grinker and Spiegel (1945), nor were they confronted with the stress of poverty widespread during the Great Depression that so influenced Horney. North America was relatively safe, the economy was good, and even the Cold War had settled into a stalemate with which most people were willing to live and let live. If major stressors are not omnipresent, then it makes sense that attention would turn to more garden-variety life stress. Reviewing the life event lists of Holmes and Rahe (1967), we find that although some major events were represented, many minor events were listed and more likely to be endorsed, because such events are simply more likely to occur daily.

In a major debate regarding whether cognitions were confounded with the study of stress, Dohrenwend, Dohrenwend, Dodson, and Shrout (1984) argued that much of what the cognitive model saw as stressors and coping, was actually stress outcomes. Marital difficulty was as likely to be a stress outcome as it was a cause of stress. Drinking and burying emotions in a sea of denial were listed by Lazarus and Folkman as ways of coping, but Dohrenwend et al. saw them as outcomes of failed coping. I do not wish to enter into this debate at this point, but rather want to underscore that the Dohrenwends had been studying stress in the lives of the poor, where the objective quality of the event plays a more major role in both their model and in Lazarus and Folkman's (1984). Said another way, the difference in the two models lies, in large part, in the focus of their studies, not in the ultimate truth of either theory.

But paradigms produce a slippery slope. They tend to be rapacious, devouring the intellectual territory of the range of possible discovery. Although Lazarus and Folkman (1984) emphasized the role of the objective environment as one important factor in the stress process, they clearly placed overwhelming emphasis on appraisal of those events. In so doing, objective elements, emotions, and resources play second stage as handmaidens to cognitions. Indeed, by placing all these elements in their model, they are able to deflect criticisms by virtue of being all-encompassing. Like many models, however, the case that would reject their model or any aspect of their model evaporates. To be scientific, a theory must be rejectable and the case that would reject it, in whole or part, should be possible in every study that tests the model. Measures, attention, statistics, and hermeneutics become tools of both insight and deception in virtually every scientific schema. With a microscope, we may begin to look for instruments of greater magnification to see even smaller unseen bodies, but we do not point the lens up at the stars. By making snapshots, we miss movements apparent only in natural settings and we begin to develop models that exclude, by attentional atrophy, the appendages of the model that at first only lacked emphasis.

The cognitive model fits the way stress is often studied, and as such is assumed to accurately reflect the nature of stress. Researchers typically either examine everyday events that are ambiguous as to their objective stress quality (e.g., work hassles, interpersonal interactions) or people experiencing the same major stressor (e.g., heart attack, criminal victimization). For ambiguous, low-level stressors and when all persons studied are undergoing the same severe stressor, cognitions play a defining part. Cross the boundaries in time to one of war, or the boundaries of countries to places of social conflict and upheaval, then objective elements again loom larger. What emerges is a model that may not be resilient to time, place, social class, ethnicity, or gender. Otherwise class struggle, the civil rights movement, the battle with sexism, and negotiations for peace need not occur. If they are only in the mind's eye, then we only need convince people to see things a different way. This is the strategy used by management in industry; workers are just not seeing the situation correctly, whereas labor translates stress to objective elements of the environment that require change.

In our research on women undergoing breast biopsy, we found that virtually 100 percent experienced depressed mood the day prior to the biopsy, and most were free of depression three months later if the tumor was found to be benign (Hobfoll & Walfisch, 1984). Individual differences were hardly apparent the day prior to biopsy, but were quite common three months later. Three months postbiopsy, women who faced other objective stress experiences and who were low in sense of mastery continued to be depressed. In this brief period of these women's lives, objective and subjective elements are key to understanding their reactions. Whether an environmental or a cognitive model is the best explanatory system depends, in part, on the moment in time that the psychological photograph is taken. The film of the whole process probably contains element that are best portrayed by both models.

Three months is hardly enough time to speak of history, but the translation of time into an element of the stress process serves to instruct us that models of stress have temporal elements. Most models acknowledge that time influences processes within their model, but a lack of awareness of the social–historical influences of time on paradigms precludes an awareness that a model may fit better in some circumstances than others. This said, a cognitive model or an environmental model may best describe the phenomenal space within some circumstances and not others. Paradoxically, at any one time or instance, competing models may each describe some major aspect of a phenomenon, even though they appear to obviate one another.

BEWARE WHEN BUYING A THEORY THAT FITS A LITTLE TOO WELL

Although many aspects of my own theory of stress, which I develop in the next two chapters of this volume, have a marked cognitive component, I find myself seeing cognitive influences as particularly deserving of skepticism. By this, I mean that the cognitive revolution and cognitive behaviorism are suspect in another important social–historical sense, beyond the points I have already made. When psychiatrists promote biological models of human behavior, psychiatrists are immediately suspect. Biological models place psychiatrists on the top of the intervention pyramid, as they are the only mental health professionals with full credentials to treat biologically. Psychologists, social workers, and counselors are either attendant to psychiatrists in this model or superfluous. The more purely biological the model, the more other mental health professionals are ancillary. Biological models of psychopathology also supply much greater remuneration to psychiatrists than psychosocial models. Chemical treatment of depression, anxiety, and obsessive–compulsive disorders pays two to three times the income to a psychiatrist that psychotherapy pays. A psychiatrist can bill four to six patients an hour, in which she might only see one patient in psychotherapy. In a similar manner, many are suspect of psychoanalytic models, because in challenging them, we were told that if only we understood them, we would necessarily believe them. Hence, only a psychoanalyst could judge the validity of psychodynamic theory. In both cases, the principle proponent of the model is also its chief benefactor. This does not *de facto* dismiss their perspective but gives us reason for pause.

When psychologists promulgate a cognitive model of behavior, we must be equally suspicious. Cognitive research is not only more straightforward than psychodynamic research, but also it is easier and probably less expensive than studying biological, sociocultural, and emotional bases of behavior. Cognitive models are most easily given to questionnaire study. They can apply equally well to community residents as to college sophomores, and they are readily given to quantification. If you wish to know what people think, ask them. The fact that in real life psychologists seldom just believe what clients say seldom comes into discussion. Cognitive therapy, because it is most easily studied, becomes the therapy of choice. Is this because we respect science or simplicity? Are we sacrificing insight in the name of parsimony, before we have looked hard enough and deep enough? Psychologists would tend to answer "yes" in the case of biological models versus psychosocial models but become less aggressive in promoting the need not to sacrifice complexity for expediency when competing psychosocial models are considered. In this Age of Stress, we must be more self-aware as we don the robes of what Perry London (1964) so insightfully called the secular priesthood in which psychologists become the shamans of society.

With pressure to conduct therapy in no more than 8–10 sessions, cognitive models may have the best fit with economic demands, but this does not make them better models in any theoretical sense. Indeed, managed health care organizations, by confusing efficiency with effect, are increasingly demanding chemical treatment of psychopathology. Fast food is not *haute cuisine*, and should not be confused with it because its efficient. In better economic times, more long-term therapy may allow easier fit for other intervention models. On another level, psychosocial change might even be more efficient because it is potentially cost effective to affect thousands. Community organizing, fighting crime, training people for better jobs, and combating racism may be both effective and efficient. However, psychologists have not been on the forefront of such study or intervention. If they were, they would probably be more environmentally oriented. But they are not, and social action has always had the problem of lack of a third-party payer. How convenient that cognitive models emphasize personal interpretation; otherwise, they would have to leave their offices and promote social change—it does not pay well, it is not prestigious, and it is somewhere either off in social work, or in Community Psychology, a movement within psychology which, not surprisingly, was center stage during the late 1960s and early 1970s, the heyday of social change, before social change was *démodé*.

Indeed, cognitive psychology has attempted to dislodge itself from other domains of psychology by renaming itself cognitive science. This is an old strategy, but it does no more than calling a hall a foyer. It is an attempt to make more scientific a realm of psychology by association with the harder sciences on campus. It is a paradigm change by force *majeure*, rather than by actually being more scientific. Astrology is astrology and physics is physics;

any tampering with labels is marketing. But it is marketing that is interpretable, and it speaks to the pressures within psychology to be associated more closely with physics than with anthropology or sociology. It is an attempt to place psychology with different bedfellows by denying our history and the nature of our intellectual family tree. It is all too convenient when cognitive behaviorism becomes the model of choice. Indeed, the attempt is already breaking down with the rising acknowledgment of the place of emotion (Lazarus, 1991; Spielberger, Jacobs, Russell, & Crane, 1983), implicit cognitions (Schacter, 1987; which look astoundingly like subconscious processes), early life attachment (Hazan & Shaver, 1987), and existentialism, now explored through cognitive interpretation of the meanings implied by personal narratives (Meichenbaum, 1994).

Like the case of "biologicalization" of behavior in psychiatry, we must at least suspect cognitive psychology, because it makes psychology king. Cognitive models are most consistent with psychological theory and have been, for the most part, championed by psychologists such as Lazarus, Bandura, Meichenbaum, and Seligman. They place psychology at the head of the intellectual pyramid and the intervention food chain. If they do not dismiss psychiatry and social work, they ensure psychologists to be major players. The paradigm fits in place all too neatly. We have ended up a little too near a place that puts us on Park Place and Boardwalk to believe that the scientific role of the dice was entirely free of tampering. Psychology has too much stock in things working out just this way not to be more cautious and scientifically introspective.

DOES A SOCIOHISTORICAL APPROACH MISLEAD US?

This chapter has critiqued stress theory from a sociohistorical perspective, but I do not imagine that I can now set the stage for an alternate paradigm that is free of sociohistorical impact. Rather, it has been my thesis that we continue to be rooted in history. When we study the influence of religious belief on stress, we are examining this psychological phenomenon at a certain time with a certain cohort. Social scientists originally believed that people become more religious as they became older, that the elderly turned to religion. This is partially true; however, it also represents a cohort effect that is historical (Payne, 1988). People who are older at this point in time grew up more religious, and when they became older, they did not so much return to church inasmuch as younger people began to attend in fewer numbers. When we saw church pews filled with the elderly, we assumed that older people were attending in greater numbers. Instead, people who always attended church were getting older. Likewise, how people react to stress and what they find stressful is shaped by sociohistorical processes that shape their lives. Again, from inside the forest, it is hard to tell the trees.

A sociohistorical approach is more humbling than a purely scientific one that relies religiously on logical positivism. Heralding science as the process that will lead to understanding is dangerous. It is not only dangerous because science can create an atomic bomb as well as it can a vaccine for polio, but also it is dangerous because it assumes that science always moves forward. Indeed, this view is unscientific. Science is a process for studying our world. Whether science progresses is itself an empirical question. Not only do avenues of science sometimes lead to dead ends, but also there are many diversions along the scientific route. As such, the current state of the art, as it is called, may have failed to incorporate earlier advances. I have tried to illustrate that because the state of the art is usually consistent with wider research and social trends, it may actually act to censure earlier, contemporary, and future knowledge that is inconsistent with the current paradigm.

Minimally, because research trends tend to be narrow in order to be precise, science tends to shave off ways of viewing phenomena that are inconsistent with those trends. Said another way, we find rooms only behind doors we open. When we enter a room looking for our missing keys, we are unlikely to notice things as dominant as the color of the wallpaper or the Picasso on the wall. We then are in danger of extrapolating to the conclusion that our focus is the inherent, central organizing principle and adopting the false premise that other factors are tangential.

We also have to be careful of considering sociohistorical context because "knowledge is power." I mean this more in the sense of Nietzsche, who questioned Bacon's original idea. Certainly, knowledge creates power, and those who have knowledge are powerful, as Bacon would have it. But, as Foucault (1980) writes, knowledge and power are one. The institutions that create knowledge have power and create further knowledge in ways that foster their power. When knowledge is produced by a certain class (e.g., scientists who are themselves upper middle class and looking to government for research grants), they will not produce knowledge that undermines their power or their attachment to powerful sources of funding. Hence, historical context is critical to understand the nature of power and the knowledge that power produces. Study of Darwinian evolution is linked to capitalism; Lamarckian evolution was historically linked to communism. Capitalism promoted survival of the fittest. Communism wished to see a world in which acquired traits could be passed on to the genetic code of future generations. Arthur Koestler (1971), in his important book *The Case of the Midwife Toad*, observed that evidence of Lamarckian evolution was witnessed in Western laboratories until specimens pointing to its existence on the footpads of midwife toads were destroyed by agents provocateur in the laboratory that produced it. Such evidence could not be tolerated.

Communism similarly disdained the study of behaviorism and placed obstacles to its advancement. Although such active censorship was not practiced in the West, the funding for behaviorism was strongly supported with research dollars, thus promoting its prominence in psychological thought. More recently, funding for research on the biological basis of behavior in the United States has increased proportional to the decrease in funding of psychosocial research. These trends are linked to a period of conservative government that wished to unlink poverty, crime, and success to the environment, and wished to make these problems a matter of personal responsibility. This is the meaning of knowledge is power, or, as some philosophers state, *powerknowledge* (Foucault, 1980).

If we live in the Age of Stress, we must realize the potency of these broader historical trends within society, scientific trends within psychology, and ulterior motives for explaining stress one way or another. This is not to be confused with conspiracy, as most scientists I know are only armchair politicians and, as a group, prize their scientific integrity above any possible political motivations or personal gain. Nevertheless, psychology would not find that talk therapy is especially effective for depression, while psychiatrists herald the biological basis of depression and its treatment if not for the financial, social, and political constraints and reinforcers that divide these two close professions (Pearlman, 1992). Looking at the same data, surgeons suggest radical mastectomy (complete breast removal) for breast cancer, whereas oncologists suggest lumpectomy (i.e., removal of the tumor and immediately surrounding tissue). The problem cannot therefore lie in the integrity of the evidence. It is easiest sometimes to see these influences, however, when we are looking as an outsider, and not a member of the scientific community in question.

In the chapters that follow, I argue against a strictly cognitive view of stress. I suggest from the outset that the cognitive revolution has misled us in our understanding of the stress process. But this should not be construed to mean that elements of the stress phenomenon are not cognitive, or that cognitive psychology does not provide valuable insights into our understanding of stress. Rather, I will argue that cognitive notions have colonized too much of the territory of inquiry into stress, have misinterpreted elements of the stress process that are environmental as being a matter of appraisal (as opposed to objective reality that is perceived), and have served a Western view of the world that emphasizes control, freedom, and individualized determinism. I suggest instead that resources, not cognitions, are the *primum mobile* on which stress is hinged. Indeed, I argue that many resources are cognitive. However, I would reason that people's economic and social resources primarily shape cognitions, not vice versa (see also Allen & Britt, 1983). Cognition is a player, not the play.

I must clearly acknowledge at the outset that I am subject to the same influences, biases, and blinders as others. To say otherwise would make me guilty of what Mandelbaum (1979) calls the *self-excepting fallacy*, whereby I see paradigms as ladening others' facts with theory, but not my own. Both cannot be true. One of the most influential lectures I recently attended was by Don Meichenbaum, who spoke of how his view of psychology was influenced not in the hallowed halls of academia insomuch as it was a reflection of his mother's kitchen table. He spoke about how her view of the world and the nature of the insights gleaned in their conversations became the essence of his mode of intervention and his model of psychology. I thought this was a major insight and instructive on Meichenbaum's part. In thinking about what he said, I find myself seeing the environment as critical because I struggled with rough city life in childhood, and because of the years I spent in Israel, where what is occurring around you is a matter of life and death, and where crowded buses are silent on the half-hour to hear the news broadcast. My own cognitive leanings depend, at least in part, on my early exposure to a Jewish way of arguing at the table over points of religion, politics, and social issues, endless conversations in which persuasive argument, tinged with spirituality and a large dose of emotionality won the day, and the respect of elders.

In this vein, drinking alcohol was disdained in my upbringing, not because it was bad for you, but because it clouded thought, and thought (read cognition) was what separated us from other nations (*goyim* in Yiddish). Clouded thought was disdained like the plague. In so saying, this model that I was raised with, and which is imbued in the culture that defined the perimeters of my upbringing, also prized emotionality. You were to feel emotion, express emotion, and cherish emotion. Thought, free of emotion, was as foreign as not thinking. Finally, discussion at our kitchen table placed social action on the forefront, as it was critical to an historical period when Jews were moving from the shadows of anti-Semitic America to vocal expression of Jewish causes, be they fighting anti-Semitism and anti-Jewish quotas, promoting Israel, or liberating Soviet Jewry. Treating the environment as the status quo was entirely inconsistent with this cultural context, even as I rebelled against it in the mandatory "What does religion offer me?" period of late adolescence. When others preached that blacks needed to appreciate their place, or that "Things aren't really that bad" (i.e., change your mind, not the problem), my family, my rabbi, and my teachers answered that Jews must align with African Americans because prejudice is real, exists in both overt and covert behavior, and must be fought by social change. To imagine that I am not biased in my perspective by the sociocultural world created in my parents' and grandparents' kitchen would be as naive as thinking that the way I raise my children, interact with my wife, or the food I enjoy are independent of the long historical caravan upon which I have been traveling. In the coming chapters, I hope to continue this discussion of sociohistorical influences; respect for the contributions of the philosophy of science makes no other route possible, logical, or, in the end, scientific.

> This is something I owe to the historians of science. I adopt the methodolgical precaution and the radical but unaggressive scepticism which makes it a principle not to regard the point in time where we are now standing as the outcome of a teleological progression which it would be one's business to reconstruct historically: that scepticism regarding ourselves and what we are, our here and now, which prevents one from assuming that what we have is better than—or more than in the past. (Foucault, 1980, p. 49)

Finally, although this sociohistorical viewpoint may be less well traveled in psychology, I can take little credit for having a unique perspective, as there is a rising tide of voices adopting a more socioculturally rooted viewpoint. American psychology's devotion to Cartesian logic attempts to isolate the nature of knowledge, and its method attempts to ensure that "representations correspond to reality—so a fixed reality means a fixed method" (Rorty, 1986). Skinner spent as much time arguing for the philosophical correctness of his determinist position, as he did in the laboratory producing data (1948, 1953, 1978). The Hegelian tradition, more popular in a European view of science than an American one, assumes that what we depict as rationality is to be viewed relatively, and in the framework of social and historical trends. We see cracks and fissures opening in the Cartesian tradition in recent contributions, and sometimes in direct attacks from the quarters of feminist, ethnic minority, and qualitative scholars in psychology and sociology. By adopting a more relativist tradition, I hope that we can both explore the phenomenon of stress and understand the influences of greater social forces on our methods, models, and interpretations.

2

The Evolutionary and Cultural Basis of the Stress Experience

What we now call stress is obviously not new to the world. What we have done is psychologize the concept. This process has taken two forms, as I discussed in Chapter 1. First, we have made the concept consistent with Western world-view in what we have called the Age of Stress. Second, it has been couched in a time when psychology is overwhelmingly cognitive in its approach. These paradigms have resulted in a stress concept that is decidedly mentalistic, individualistic, and internal. It has detached stress from the external world and from the problems that people confront. It is almost devoid of culture and context. Both the Age of Stress and the cognitive revolution in psychology will fade with time, but we will be left with an age-old problem of our having to combat difficulties in both a physical and psychological sense. It is therefore a worthwhile exercise to depsychologize the stress process and examine what people find stressful.

In this chapter, I explore how widening the study of stress to broader social, cultural, and contextual considerations might change the way we view the stress process. My goal is to move from a psychology of stress based on individual appraisal to one that incorporates the self-nested-in family, nested-in social organization. I first consider the evolutionary basis of stress as it evolved as an integral aspect of the basic properties of culture that are constructed to ensure survival. This will take my arguments to the development of the market village as a primary social structure that defines the stress experience through our own times. From this account, I argue that resources are the primary unit of interest in the stress process. By considering perspectives of East, West, and Africa, I also illuminate not only the stress experience in those cultures, but also how insights from other cultures help us understand the blinders we have used in constraining our Western, psychological view of stress. I argue for a new stress viewpoint that bridges individualist and collectivist cultures.

EARLY EVOLUTIONARY AND CULTURAL ASPECTS OF STRESS

People's first goal is survival, just as it is in all species. Because without survival, there is obviously no continuation of the self, family, or species, it is of primary concern. Survival is biologically not an individualistic concept. Sacrifice of the self for the family or tribe is as much a part of survival as survival of the individual, and perhaps more integral to what Darwin meant by survival of the fittest. The joint survival of the individual-in-group is the fundamental motivation of our species. Indeed, the twisting of Darwinian concepts to promote the idea that survival in any way relates to the fittest *individual* is a strictly political reinterpretation of Darwin's species-specific theory (Koestler, 1971). No individual has the genetic variation fundamental to change the transfer of the genetic payload to future generations. Rather, a large set of individuals must share a variation for the promotion of that type of individual in the genetic competition. The perishing of an individual has no influence on the species' domination of a niche, and individual survival does not ensure the transfer of its genes unless those genes are shared by enough members of the group to allow creation of a new genetic template for the species.

> I saw, also, that the preservation in a state of nature of any occasional deviation of structure ... would be a rare event; and that, if at first preserved, it would generally be lost by subsequent intercrossing with ordinary individuals.... I did not appreciate how rarely single variations, whether slight or strongly marked could be perpetuated ... if a single individual were born, which varied in some manner, giving it twice as good a chance of life as that of other animals, yet the chances would be strongly against its survival. Supposing it to survive and to breed, and that half its young inherited the favourable variation; still,... the young would have only a slightly better chance of surviving and breeding; and this chance would go on decreasing in the succeeding generations. (Darwin, 1859, pp. 97–98)

In contrast, supporting the collective nature of variation Darwin writes:

> Natural selection will modify the structure of the young in relation to the parent, and of the parent in relation to the young. In social animals it will adapt the structure of each individual for the benefit of the whole community; if the community profits by the selected change. (p. 93)

Focusing on this level of analysis, stress becomes those events or circumstances that stand in the way of survival. Tempests, floods, attacks by neighbors or wild beasts, failure to find food, and an inability to mate are stressful. Some of these threats can be met by coping resources. For example, diligence in hunting can be seen as a coping resource; as long as this resource is not overtaxed by winter's thinning of the herds, stress can be seen as offset. However, wherever circumstances potentially threaten survival of the individual or group, they are experienced by the species as stressful. Even if it does not overtax resources on a dozen occasions, the individual, group, and tribe will be vigilant because the stakes of miscalculation or the inappropriate response are so high.

With cultural advances, humans create social conditions that make survival more easily obtainable and at the same time infinitely more complicated. From tribal hunting emerges trade for objects of survival that a second group produces in more plenty, such as grain. With time, some valued commodity such as gold or silver becomes a substitute for goods and acts as an intermediary to trade of the goods for survival; eventually, money takes the place of gold and silver. By this process, these new resources inherit the properties of more fundamental survival resources, and threats to them become, by this same process, sources of stress.

On another level, the seeking of status within the group is transformed from hunter status to the status of those who can produce the most goods for their family in the more complicated contexts of our current society. The search for status and concomitant self-esteem, however, is a common thread across time and societies. Survival, which includes mating, association with others, and accomplishment of life tasks, changes in the course of cultural development, but the fundamentals are more or less constant. The associated social conditions and structures pertaining to social status are therefore to be diligently protected, just as are the more basic elements of survival. Social status acquires importance along with food for the table and finding a desirable mate, precisely because the three are interconnected.

As culture evolves further, survival becomes increasingly taken for granted, especially if we consider survival from this tribal level of existence; that is, the tribe will survive, if not certain members of the tribe. As survival becomes less questionable, humans are unique in creating a symbolic layer of goals, with a desire to possess goods, status, and success. Some of these are indirectly related to survival. For example, the seeking of wealth may be related to a more primitive need to ensure that no instance will bring financial ruin. Accumulation and valuing of other fetish objects—for example, *objets d'art*—may be related to the need for status in the group. Still, culture creates a system in which these resources are distant from survival. Nonetheless, they are diligently sought. At this stage, conditions that threaten these tertiary social structures and goals, some linked to survival, some more peripheral, induce stress.

This argument takes us to an appreciation that with the advance of culture to its modern expression, survival becomes a matter of obtaining money, position, job security, and status. These resources ensure mate selection, creation of progeny, and their protection—properties that link them across culture and history. In terms of stress, what is stressful are circumstances that either overcome people's ability to ensure the attainment and maintenance of these goals or that diminish these goals directly without regard to people's capabilities. Hence, losing one's job is stressful if a reasonable alternative position is not readily available or if the loss of the job is accompanied by a loss of status or self-esteem. Individuals strive to maintain the elements necessary for survival and the goals that culture creates as structures related to survival, advancement, and protection of valued ends.

Indeed, culture itself can be said to be created to ensure the establishment and maintenance of survival of the tribe or nation. DeVries (1995) theorizes that culture provides a system in which social structures and relationships are constructed to maintain adequate distribution of physical and social resources that allow sustained distribution of goods, assurance of the capacity to organize each of the stages of the human life cycle, and the securing of human reproduction. Within culturally patterned social structures, roles, and anticipated life-span transitions, cultures create a context in which stress and coping responses are defined and delineated. The individual experience of physical and mental functioning to a great degree is outlined by this cultural frame of reference.

What is stressful then? Stress is the state in which valued goals are threatened or lost, or where individuals are unable to create the necessary conditions for obtaining or sustaining these goals. On a primary level, these goals are related to survival of the group (see also Kaplan, 1983). This means that individuals will value the conditions that ensure survival of themselves and the family and tribe. On a secondary level, they will value the cultural structures that are created to ensure survival on a more primary level, hence the valuing of employment, knowledge, and church. On a tertiary level, status itself becomes a goal, possibly because it is related to power on a more primary level. Hence, we see a structure such that the goals of survival of the individual and group, and the resources that may ensure these ends, are valued. This then includes the direct objects of survival and the social attachments made possible by sustaining the family and tribe. It includes the knowledge, tools, social structures, and fetish objects that either are valued in their own right, or that may be exchanged or utilized to obtain valued objects or states.

This treatise may seem obvious, but it stands in stark opposition to current thinking about stress. Let us examine some prominent stress definitions:

Psychological stress is a particular relationship between the person and the environment that is appraised by the person as taxing or exceeding his or her resources and endangering his or her well-being. (Lazarus & Folkman, 1984, p. 19)

Stress refers to that quality of experience, produced through a person–environment transaction, that, through either overarousal or underarousal, results in psychological or physiological distress. (Aldwin, 1994, p. 22)

Most definitions of stress emphasize the relationship between the individual and the environment. Stress is the consequence of a person's appraisal processes: the assessment of whether personal resources are sufficient to meet demands of the environment. (Taylor, 1995, p. 219)

What is common to these stress definitions is a reliance on the individual's perception of his or her environment. This suggests that we have to ask individuals what is stressful to them to know what is stressful. There is no inherently stressful condition. Kasl (1978) cogently discusses the circularity of these definitions, as by basing the existence of stress on perception, we cannot disentangle whether we are receiving report of the stressor, the emotional response, the perceived difficulty of coping, or the amalgam of all of these. Beyond the circularity, which might be methodologically overcome, the individualistic, mentalistic conceptualization suggests an infinite array of stressful circumstances, equal to the number of individuals in the world, multiplied by the infinite number of circumstances they might have.

By tying stress theory, instead, to more anthropological roots, we can obtain a more finite set of circumstances, although still quite large, in which individuals are likely to experience stress. These circumstances are those that remove them or threaten obtainment and maintenance of survival of the self, family, or tribe, or the knowledge, tools, social structures, and fetish objects (including money, diamonds) that either are valued in their own right, or that may be exchanged or utilized to obtain valued objects or states.

THE CULTURAL BASIS OF APPRAISAL

This more anthropological formulation does not disqualify the importance of appraisal either. The difference lies in its suggesting that most appraisals will be primarily a product of the evaluation of objective, observable physical and social circumstances. That they were perceived is a methodological artifact, as we may obtain cultural information by other means. If we know what is valued for people in general and in a given culture in particular, we can predict what will be stressful in most circumstances. Individual differences beyond these jointly shared appraisals will be important in a number of circumstances and these can be immediately delineated. Individual differences will assume greater importance:

1. When circumstances are ambiguous (e.g., minor events or events that have a large unknown factor as in the case of rumors of layoffs).
2. When circumstances are constant for the group (i.e., comparing individuals with similar resources that have undergone a similar threat (e.g., married, insured, employed middle-class men who have experienced heart attack that is similar in impact and who are free of other health problems).
3. When individuals are so deeply psychologically disturbed that fantasy has been substituted in large part or wholly for reality.

Beyond these conditions, common perceptions of commonly valued conditions will be the key factors. As Haan (1993) proposes,

> Despite our seemingly contradictory recognition that stress is in the eye of the beholder, we well understand the commonsense meaning of stress in our everyday lives. We know when we and others are stressed. Of course, we may have special, deeper understandings of another person's plight if we have experienced the same stress. Acknowledgment that stress has common, shared human meanings is the underlying justification for the methodology used in life events research.... Its meanings are commonly understood even though some people's histories may be especially vulnerable to certain kinds of stressors. (p. 258)

I have often presented my argument about the commonality, as opposed to the individuality, of the stress experience to groups of researchers, business people, and lay groups. Typically, their first reaction is one of disagreement. Then I ask them what I will ask you next. What are the things that have been most stressful to you in the last few years? Unless you have been rarely blessed with a period of few major life stressors, you will think of such things as severe health problems, loss of a cherished loved one, job loss, financial difficulties, divorce, or serious interpersonal difficulties. Would these events not be stressful to others? Were these matters not objectively stressful? Would altering your appraisal alter the essential stressfulness of the events? Of course, how you or another individual eventually cope is a matter, in part, of individual differences, but let us leave coping to a later discussion. The perception of stress must be appraised by the individual, but it is our Western, individualistic cultural bent that has us imagine that it is a matter of personal, individualized perception. Our perceptions are joint, and they are tied to our cultural heritage and our species.

The exaggeration of individualism is a post–World War II phenomenon. It is evidenced in society as what is often referred to as the chief trait of the baby-boom generation, specifically the "I, me, mine" culture (Light, 1988). American families, in particular, enjoyed unprecedented wealth and economic prosperity at the same time that most families had fewer children allowing them to indulge children's individual needs. The war, too, had produced a great appreciation for children, the antithesis of war and death. Because many had to postpone having children due to the war, children were all the more cherished, and individualized. It is apparent in the watchwords of the generation: *"Do you own thing!"*

In psychology, we also see a revolution against the pluralistic theories of both Skinner's behaviorism and Freud's psychodynamics. In these theoretical approaches, both Skinner and Freud were joined by a common thrust; the phenomena of which they spoke held for all people. Individual differences were minimized. From humanistic psychology, in contrast, was born individualism. Maslow's (1954/1987) theory is the best example of this trend, with the pinnacle of his theory being self-actualization. It is interesting to examine this appealing concept, a goal toward which much of psychology hoped humanity would aspire, for what lies underneath it.

Maslow's theory in actuality not only distanced him from notions of communalism, but he also relegated close attachments to the status of weakness. For Maslow, self-actualizers have a tendency toward detachment and a deeply felt need for privacy. They are autonomous beings and therefore tend to be independent of their social environment and culture. Their attachments are deep, but they make these attachments with few others and act in an inner-directed way, more or less independent of social norms. "Some of them recover so quickly from the death of people close to them as to seem heartless" (Maslow, 1954/1987, p. 146). They are strong enough, says Maslow, to be independent not only of the opinions of others, but also of their love and affection. To the heart of the matter, they are unlike "deficiency motivated" people who must rely on others for love, safety, respect, prestige, and belongingness.

My argument here also reveals a bias of the perspective that I offer as an alternative when I speak of the species- and culturally based nature of the stress phenomenon. An emphasis on culture and communality emanates in part from current movements that may be called tribalism. Positive ramifications of this trend are people finding stronger identification and pride with their group and culture. It is a time of return to families, increase in religious attendance, and emphasis on mother tongue. Its beauty lies in its generating open arms of belongingness of people searching for roots. Its ugly underbelly is also apparent, as we have an unprecedented level of ethnic hostility in Eastern Europe and the former Soviet Union, and in promulgation of intergroup conflict generated by White Supremacists and Farrakan's Nation of Islam in North America. Just as Francophones find greater shared esteem in the preservation of their language and culture, the separatist movement they create is felt as discrimination by Quebec's Anglophone community who, indeed, are fleeing the Canadian province in large numbers. Just as communalism generates a place of attachment for young black males, so badly needed in the face of racism, it seems to come at th⸍ price of xenophobic beliefs in the existence of a Jewish Cabal that seeks from its secret chambers to undermine black ownership and advancement, an age-old anti-Semitic myth.

By questioning individualism, we fall into the potential trap of idealizing culture and communalism. Temperance and evenhandedness tempt us to split the difference and compromise at some middle ground. However, this too is a dangerous scientific course, as it prejudges the evidence. It is probably best that we examine how these philosophies impinge on the subject of the appraisal of stress in a more open fashion, not moving to side too quickly with one philosophy or the other, or with an amalgam. If I am correct in my thesis that we have been most guilty of imagining that the study of psychology and stress in particular is value-free, then the most prudent scientific course is to design, analyze, and interpret studies from multiple viewpoints and note the differences that emerge in our conclusions. I would suggest further, however, that because individualism has been so dominant in the stress literature, we must actively promote more communal theories of the stress process, investigating shared perceptions, common threats, and cultural underpinnings of what appears on the surface to be individual perceptions.

Perception as an Iceberg

The appraisal of stress can be seen metaphorically as an iceberg, meaning that we are only seeing the tip above the surface when we ask people for their appraisal of stressful circumstances. The misinterpretation of the meaning of data based on people's self-report, I believe, resulted from a belief, not directly examined, that what people reported was inaccurate, biased, subjective, and personalized (see Figure 2.1). The jump was made that if individual appraisals, which are assumed to be inaccurate, are good predictors of outcomes, then a personalized (biased) account must be the main ingredient in stress. I believe and hope to illustrate that this is a misrepresentation of the data and is the sole product of a methodological bias in psychology, whereby, when we want to know something, we typically administer self-report questionnaires and in a few cases interview people. Because the appraisals came from individuals, we make the connection that they are individual perceptions. Stemming from the fact that we do not ask for cultural, group, or family-based reports, we do not interpret our data beyond individual interpretation. Hence, what we have are appraisals of individuals, not individual appraisal.

By an iceberg, I mean that above the surface lies individual perceptions. Below the surface are (1) objective factors that the individual is reporting

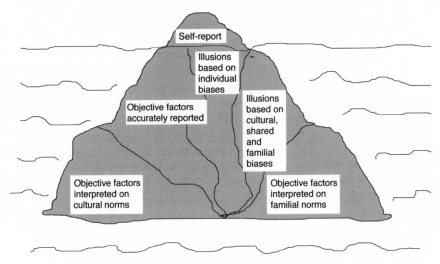

Figure 2.1. Perception as an iceberg.

with fair accuracy (Brown & Harris, 1989), (2) objective factors that the individual is interpreting based on culturally based biases shared by members of his or her culture (deVries, 1995), (3) objective factors that the individual is interpreting based on familial norms and rules (Brown & Harris, 1989), (4) illusions that the individual has created based on individual, familial, and cultural biases (deVries, 1995), as well as (5) illusions based on individual biases. Seen this way, it can be seen that most individual self-reports could be obtained through objective accounting, accounts of others who are members of shared groups (i.e., family, culture), and normative data taken from observation of members of those groups (i.e., reported by no one referring to themselves). Idiographic (i.e., individual-specific) perceptions are only one aspect of what lies beneath the methodological artifact of our way of acquiring information about people's stress experience.[1]

A fact that has been totally lost in this debate is that the very concept of stress appraisal was based on research concerning the ability of individuals to make accurate estimations of physical properties of their environment. Writes the originator of the famous and most widely used Social Readjustment Scale, known to many as the stressful life event list:

> In 1962 the answer to our problem found us, arriving in the form of Dr. Eugene Gallanter. Gallanter gave a lecture to our faculty at the University of Washington in which he spoke on the new field of psychophysics—the study of the psychological perception of the quality, quantity, magnitude, and intensity of physical phenomena.

Gallanter explained how he and S. S. Stevens had demonstrated the ability of subjects
to make reliable subjective magnitude estimations of physical dimensions such as length
of object, intensity of sound, brightness of light, number of objects, and so on. Dr.
Richard Rahe and I saw the relevance to our problem immediately. Applied to the field
of psychosocial phenomena, the subjective magnitude estimation technique could give
us a method for quantifying life events. (Holmes, 1989, pp. 29–30)

Hence, Holmes and Rahe created a method based on subjective appraisals,
because of the *general accuracy* of these *reliable* judgments and because
people are good catalogers of their surrounding. In subsequent research,
Harmon, Masuda, and Holmes (1970) and Woon, Masuda, Wagner, and
Holmes (1971) illustrated the cross-cultural stability of estimates of the
weight given different life events across cultures. Across cultures, there were
important differences, but the striking finding of these studies was the
similarity of ratings of stressful life events and the amount of readjustment
they required in their wake. Holmes and Rahe also saw the importance of
the individualization of responses, but their technique and perspective
emphasized the entire iceberg and the essential element of people's percep-
tual accuracy and commonality.

Aldwin (1994) counters that only for overwhelming environmental
phenomena are objective aspects of the iceberg predominant in the stress
process. She states that "most environments are more ambiguous and more
subject to individual interpretation." (p. 39). She goes on to provide examples of complex social stressors and minor hassles as examples. I would
agree that as ambiguity increases, people drift from objective characteristics
of the phenomena to more symbolic ones. However, even when the situation
is ambiguous, people know when an argument with their spouse has crossed
the line of being serious within their culture, even if an Italian or Jewish
family may have higher baseline volume than a WASP family. Even given
some ambiguity, it is not this individual perception that may be pivotal as
much as culturally general interpretations that would be common across
broad classes of people. Because we have ignored studying the sociocultural
level of the stress experience, we have been able to deny its potentially
central role.

Socially Based Norms and Standards

A major argument in favor of the primary role of individual appraisal
has been that people's self-report (and therefore their appraisal) of
stressors is a better predictor of their well-being than is an observational
(and therefore objective) report. The argument follows that if this is the
case, individual perception must be more central to the stress process than
are socially available standards (Lazarus, 1991).

However, what we call perceptions are often not personalized appraisals, but more objective accounts than the external viewer can provide. Kowalik and Gotlib (1987) insightfully explain why observers are often poor judges of what is actually objectively occurring. In viewing couples' interactions, Kowalik and Gotlib point out that the observer only has a few frames of the film version of the couple's life together. When he says to her, "You did a great job cleaning the house" the observer sees this as a compliment. However, if she knows that he is against her working outside the home, she may accurately translate his comment as a criticism that she does not do this more often. Psychology has interpreted this as meaning her appraisals are more important than objective facts, but the comparison and logic of this conclusion is specious. What has been compared is her fuller cataloging of objective facts against the observer's cursory recording. She saw the whole film; he saw the film clips of one brief sequence. The superiority of her viewpoint is a methodological artifact, ironically related to her ability to have more objective information. Now, does she also add an idiographic interpretation that is specially hers? Yes, certainly, but this is not what has been tested here, and the conclusions of such comparisons cannot be taken in any way as confirmation of the appraisal model. Instead, as Coyne (1976) and Gotlib and Hooley (1988) theorize, people in large part create their social reality, which they then perceive. Rather than a distortion, however, they see more or less what they have created and what has been created around them.

The appraisal model emphasizes individual differences, not as an important factor, but as the central factor. A socioenvironmental viewpoint, in contrast, does not rely on cold objectivity, which is what lies on the opposite end of the spectrum from appraisal. Instead, a socioenvironmental assessment relies on socially based norms and standards. Thus in Moos's (1984, Moos & Schaefer, 1993) groundbreaking socioenvironmental work, he did not rely on calculating objective aspects of social environments. Instead, he sought to create a metric of group impressions by people who shared social settings.

By recognizing the importance of cultural, environmental, and individual perspectives, we may be finding a common meeting ground between the environmentalists and the cognitive theorists. As Aldwin (1994) states, "A similar problem may be appraised ... very differently depending upon indigenous belief systems." (p. 202), thus recognizing the dual interplay of the social basis of individual perceptions. However, to date, cognitive theorists in the stress field (Aldwin, 1994; Lazarus, 1994; Lazarus & Folkman, 1984) minimize cultural and social-structural patterns as distal and less relevant, stating that personal experience is primary. Hence, although there exists a continuum here, the distance on that continuum between theorists such as Moos and Lazarus is considerable. More telling, the research that has followed heuristically from the individualist perspective has only recently, and quite superficially, even considered cultural or social-structural components.

Interestingly, although many mental health clinicians subscribe to the cognitive model, they do not so often make this transformation from individual report to the importance of appraisal alone. For example, leading cognitive therapists emphasize a need to balance individual perceptions with objective and social standards. Ellis (Ellis & Greiger, 1977) virtually fights with clients to get them to see the folly of their false views of the self. Meichenbaum (1994; Meichenbaum & Fitzpatrick, 1993) has clients create a narrative (their own story) but helps them shape their perceptions to fit with a balanced reality, recognizing that self-illusion is often the pattern that created the anxiety, depression, or other psychological dysfunction. Bandura's (1982, 1997) approach demands that we shape people's perceptions through small wins, but these small wins need to be actual, real, tangible wins that create a concrete foundation for mastery. From these small mastery experiences, efficacy will emerge when larger wins are sustained. Taylor (1983) (Taylor & Brown, 1994) has suggested that mental health may come from slanting facts to more favorable interpretations. But in all her writing, Taylor is clearly speaking of slight variations of reality, tantamount to shading a bit of a different hue of a photograph. Never does she suggest colorizing a black-and-white photograph, let alone painting a blank canvas with a preferred reality.

On an individual level, I think that clinicians compare each case to the normative base that they have read about and experienced through their contact with other clients. Although they accept clients' accounts of their own experience as important, they compare them to other cases and develop expectations based on a model that they and their field have developed for similar people who have undergone similar circumstances (the basis of diagnosis and all nosological systems). Indeed, although we can understand someone's past through them, we can only predict the future by placing individuals in a model that pertains to them and others like them. Radical existential therapists (Binswanger, 1963) are perhaps the only school that theorized an entirely individualized system of explanation of behavior, and such as approach has few adherents. Logically, we could not otherwise predict a future course, because each case would be entirely, not partially, different from others.

The tendency to argue from the perspective of individual appraisal in the extreme form that psychology often follows reflects a cultural ethic. This ethic teaches that "each person is an individual, there is no other like him or her." Stress theorists have often taken this adage quite literally, but its current iteration stems from a philosophy, promoted in its contemporary form beginning in the 1960s, as much as it follows from any psychological evidence. It is no more, or less, true than the adages "Each person is like every other person," "No man is an island," or "the family of man." From the earliest Biblical writings, both messages are strongly emphasized because they speak to our duality. The very expression that we are each created in the image of God contains both messages according to Biblical scholars because God is conceived as endowing us individuality and shared humanity. These philosophies percolate through society, and at different times, the individuality message has greater fidelity and at other times the "people as part of a global village" concept gains fidelity.

Stress theory has been so individualized at this point in time that even models of shared familial appraisals have seldom been explored (Hobfoll & Spielberger, 1992). In family systems theory, the therapist translates the report of family members jointly in order to interpret the family dynamic, that is a dynamic that cuts across individuals. In Olson's (1989) circumplex model, adaptability to stress emphasizes the relative need of families to retain the status quo, some being more flexible than others. Families interpret challenges to the family according to a family-common pattern. This pattern is influenced, in turn, by the nature of other structures of the family—family leadership style, level of parental control, methods of discipline, and degree of family attachment. Likewise, according to Minuchin (1974), the structure of the family controls perceptions of events, not vice versa. These family systems theories hold at their root the assumption that individuals' appraisals are products of familial templates. They are not independent, idiographic appraisals.

Family-based perceptions are seen differently when we consider Asian philosophies. Understanding these Eastern cultural interpretations provides insights into the Western family, because they both aid our appreciation of Asian cultures and highlight aspects of Western families that the Western way of viewing families camouflage. In Chinese culture, Confucian ideals produce a certain configuration of the extended family (*jia*) and shape one's thoughts on the family. This includes unmitigated respect for elders, subordination of women marrying into the family to the mother-in-law, and subordination of women to men. What one did and thought about such relations was sanctified and beyond question (Lee, 1953; Hsu, 1971). The tie between family structure, behavior, and perception is so strong that Chinese familism may be the one social practice to survive communism (Jenner, 1992). Westerners may be more "individualized" in their thinking, but not so much as psychology's Western orientation has led us to believe. Western families have many of these same attributes, and we must incorporate these insights to broaden the asocial, individual *zeitgeist*.

Some, mainly ethnic, minority psychologists are considering what a culturally sensitive model of psychology would look like in North America, and it is interesting that they frequently look to Africa and the East for insight. This expands further on some of the themes raised by family systems theorists and highlights the more contextualized overview made possible when shared appraisals and objective evaluations of environmental contingencies are incorporated. In work on integrating Afrocentric worldview with cognitive models of treatment, Parham (1989; Parham & McDavis, 1987) discusses the need to focus simultaneously on individual perceptions of difficulties and joint perceptions of the world as experienced generally by African Americans. These African American perceptions are seen as related to traditional African ways of experiencing the world that have been reshaped by the shared experience of African Americans through slavery and subsequent oppression.

Because the dominant culture chooses the governing models within academic disciplines, they choose models that support the cultural conditions that favors the majority group. Watts (1992), a theorist concerned with the development of the African American male, expands on this point, arguing that a focus on individual perceptions belies a mentalistic process that places thought and individualism as the progenitor of important human behavior. He reasons that if psychology had been created by African Americans, the communal–environmental nexus would have been the central organizing feature, and individualism would have been in the blurred background. According to Watts, a racist culture creates a multitude of obstacles and impediments to healthy development of ethnic minority men. Psychology, by focusing on microsocial interactions, avoids illumination of the macrosocial conditions that underlie oppression, racism, and sexism. In psychology, this leads to an emphasis on individualism and the self as a sufficient entity for study. Solidarity and awareness of shared social conditions are neither foreground nor background; they are ignored in the equation.

The Allowable Margin of Misjudgment

A major debate in the stress literature concerns the accuracy of people's perceptions of real-world phenomena. This debate is critical to our understanding of the stress process and development of a cultural view of stress as something that is general to humans and that is further specified by culture (Baumeister, 1989).

One line of research examined the accuracy of self-report of stressful life events. In general, investigators have found that people's report of midlevel and major life events are fairly accurate (Brown & Harris, 1989;

Dohrenwend, Raphael, Schwartz, Stueve, & Skodol, 1993). Over time, there is a tendency toward telescoping, a process whereby some events are exaggerated and some minimized, as if we were looking through one or the other end of a telescope. However, these distortions may also be attributable to ways that original events were shaped. For example, recall of a divorce may focus accurately, but on two different aspects of the divorce, or on two different time periods in the evolving conflict and resolution. So one might recall the storm-and-strife period more than the period of separation and finding peace when being asked about stress but remember both periods accurately. Even in the case of hassles, where ambiguity makes individual interpretation greatest, Brandt (1993) notes in the study of police that they report common elements of their job that they find to be irritants, such as paperwork and supervisor scrutiny. Again, how different officers respond to this stress may or may not be a more individualized process, but I wish to separate coping with stress from identification of stress for the time being.

A second, and intriguing, line of inquiry questions whether depressed individuals are in fact more accurate than individuals who tend not to be depressed. Taylor (1983) theorized and provided considerable supportive evidence that depressed individuals accurately perceive life's potential and actual tragedies. Nondepressed individuals view the world with more rose-colored glasses. Others have suggested from studies in more naturalistic settings that accurate appraisals are prerequisite for mental health and that depressed individuals are more likely to distort reality (Colvin & Block, 1994; Colvin, Block, & Funder, 1995). However, neither side of this debate is speaking of major distortions of reality. The debate is instructive, nevertheless, because if we turn the debate inside out, as it were, we see a very different point being made.

As illustrated in Figure 2.2, the "accuracy of perception" debate is arguing over spaces to the right and left of reality. They have focused on the margins, holding the centerpiece where both sides agree most perceptions exist, as not relevant to either side's position. My argument instead highlights the point that they deemphasize—the centerpiece of shared reality is the broadest region of perception in both models. Baumeister (1989) suggests that by making only slight distortions, people can benefit from reality-based judgments and still profit from some relief from the brute force of reality. Moving outside of this slight margin of inaccuracy is adaptively dangerous and potentially disastrous.

Where neurotic processes may come into play is in the extent not that individuals distort, but the amount of time they spend thinking about the negative aspects of life and life's circumstances. Seen this way, some individuals do not need to have any distortion of reality to become depressed and

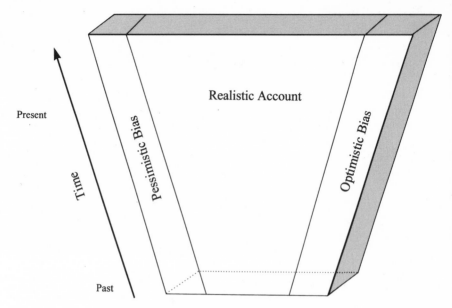

Figure 2.2.   Allowable margin of misjudgment.

others need no optimistic distortion to avoid depression. Rather, life offers a cornucopia of troubles, and although these fall more to some than others, we all receive a share. If our direction of attention is on the troubles, and if we do this across life's various domains, then there is no need to add the construct of distortion into the picture. Or, perhaps, distortion must be viewed differently, in terms of the direction of the concentration of our thoughts and efforts.

Still, I fall back here on the insights offered by Coyne (1976), who theorized that chronically depressed individuals create a certain reality that permeates the important domains of their life. Their depressive style results in a rejection of others, likely work failure, and an active sabotaging of potential domains of success. Hence, although we must at this state of research remain open to the question of distortions, there is ample evidence that their actual life circumstances offer adequate fuel for depression, anxiety, and anger. Moreover, where they add their own measure of interpretation, those interpretations are largely dictated by culture and shared experience. Their perceptions are of a world that they themselves sculpted by their own behavior. Hence, although perceived, it remains anchored by objective circumstances.

Distinguishing between Stressful Circumstances and Distressed Individuals

A major impediment to understanding the nature of stress has been a clouding of the distinction between the very concept of the self and the environment. Following the philosophical lead of existentialism, and more recently, social constructionism, psychology has come to equate the self's experience of the world as the world. If this philosophical stance is an accepted assumption, then there is no need for empirical inquiry as to the extent real events influence individuals independent of their perceptions. There are no real worlds.

Following this viewpoint, stress researchers and theorists have often equated the retrospective reporting of experiences by depressed and other psychologically distressed individuals to be stressful, environmental circumstances. So whatever the person reported as stressful was stress. If more depressed people reported greater difficulty with certain circumstances, then those kinds of situations were seen as stressful. Indeed, Lazarus and Folkman (1984) went as far as to call inner torments, which have no environmental basis, stress. Seen this way, stress is the reaction of the individual and demands no environmental anchor whatsoever. Let us explore this notion.

Are the imaginary demons that a paranoid schizophrenic battles stress experiences? Are the imagined insults that an individual with borderline personality perceives from his or her environment stressful experiences? Are the hassles in every nook and cranny of life that many anxiety neurotics see stressful experiences? If we equate backwards from psychopathology to the environment, we see the world as in a Bosch painting. Bosch, the fifteenth-century artist, depicted a world infested by demons seeking to enter at every crack of reality. Like the medieval practice of Bosch's time, however, we may be better to send these madmen off in ships than harbor them as part of the stress experience. If the definitions of stress are allowed to cross this border, then stress becomes everything and there is little hope of conceptual clarity.

This is not to say that hassles are not stressful or that paranoid schizophrenics cannot also be impacted by stressful experiences. However, if we lose the distinction between the inner self and the outer world, then we truly need never again look at the environment. However, I would further argue that stress research has little to offer for an understanding of the nature of the workings of the inner self of deeply disturbed individuals. Indeed, the richness of the stress area was in its introducing the notion that current events may influence individuals and produce forms of psychopathology that *resemble* those evidenced among individuals whose psychopathology is more deep-seated and emanating from early life experience or biological underpinnings. This major insight allowed psychology to distinguish stress-induced responses from long-term, psychopathology-based processes. In turn, this led to crisis modes of intervention that prevent transient psychological distress from becoming more fixed due to inattention that would allow them to become more firmly entrenched in personality (Caplan, 1964).

Costa and McCrae (1990) and Depue and Monroe (1986) examined the question of distinguishing stress responses from psychopathology. They suspected that much of the relationship between stressful appraisals and psychological distress was a product not of response to the outer world, but the inner world; that is, they argued that it was not so much that stress produced depression, but that depressed individuals reported events as stressful. They found evidence that the relationship between environmental events and the appraisal of those events as stressful was deeply colored by underlying psychopathology and that the supposed relationship between stress appraisals and psychopathology was confounded by the underlying tendency for more neurotic individuals both to perceive stress in their world and torment within themselves.

Nor is perception the only potential confounding factor here, or necessarily the principal one. In this regard, more neurotic individuals will encounter more stressful events, make decision errors that will exacerbate potentially threatening events, and behave in ways that will result in further problems. They are more likely to create interpersonal problems and less capable of ameliorating interpersonal problems that arise (Coyne, 1976). Through these behaviors, they would appear to be more distressed owing to environmental stress, but their underlying psychopathology might actually be the culprit in this complex relationship.

This confusion between psychopathologically based perceptions and the negative psychological sequelae of stressful life events continues to be an area of confusion. Its disentanglement will be paramount to separating environmental from individual influences in the stress process.

STRESS BASED ON A MODEL
OF SOCIAL DEVELOPMENT AND INTERDEPENDENCE

Although I may wish to depsychologize the stress process to some degree, at the same time I do not want to lose psychological insights into the stress process. A model of social development may act as an effective bridge or vantage point connecting sociological, anthropological, social-psychological, and clinical-psychological views of stress. By social development, I mean that the midpoint of my argument sees individuals nested in social context and culture—both individual and context are vital. Relationships with macrosocial structures, such as nations, are loose and ephemeral, making them less relevant to a psychosocial understanding of stress. Midlevel social structures, those that fall between the level of family on one end, and village on the other end, may be a more profitable contextual background for our purposes. They allow us to peer beyond the individual, but avoid risking the loss of the self in macrosocial structures. These midlevel, mesosocial structures include our attachments to families, religious institutions, employment organizations, charitable institutions, neighborhoods, and ethnic groups.

From the Emergence of Market Economies to the Right to Self-Esteem

Exploring how mesosocial institutions and associations evolved and how they led to principles evidenced today in psychology may be instructive in developing an understanding of the social context of the stress experience. In the mid- to late Middle Ages in Europe, there were few towns, and what towns there were had simple market structures for the buying and selling of local goods. People were attached to the land and under the protection of liege lords. This meant that there was an absence of social structures between the family and the local governance structure. Interestingly, accompanying such minimalist structures was a lack of rights afforded to other than the few landed individuals. Serfs were the property of their lord of the manor. He could bed their wives, demand their labor, or literally take their lives.

Knights who had no property emerged in associations with peddlers who had wares to sell but were unable to do so without the knights' protection, because travel away from the local castle was treacherous. Joining the now mobile band of knights and peddlers came skilled workers who could not be supported by a single region with its dispersed population, but could offer services for a time for profit and then move on. These associations naturally found market day to be a desirable time to arrive in an area and would join with local farmers to create a more varied marketplace. As the power and size of these groups grew, they were able to traffic in material from farther regions and to allow trade across a greater network of persons. From small bands, they became like fairs, arriving with goods, entertainment, and social–judicial services, for now a troubadour, prostitute, traveling clergy, scribe, money changer, and judge could travel under protection. This protective demand also grew as the group became a more desirable target for organized assault of larger bands, brigands, and disenfranchised soldiers from recent wars.

From this association grew a more complicated and socially evolved system of interdependence. The knight offering protection, but without owning expanses of land, required the payment of others and their goodwill. He needed to protect them to ensure his profit and could no longer act with immunity toward them. The judge had to be paid by the general group in some form of tax, because the group required justice to ensure their social and economic endeavors in turn. Not inconsequentially, the landed lord lost much of his power, because sources of sustenance other than serfdom developed. Eventually, these traveling bands became so large and cumbersome that it became easier for them to settle in one place and become a town, joining forces with the nonmigratory population of some small village. A select spot near a riverway allowed them access to trade elsewhere. But unlike the earlier towns, the emergence of a middle class of artisans, traders, and professionals was now seeded (Beresford, 1967; Konvitz, 1985).[2]

Soon after, tradesmen associated and organized among themselves—silversmiths with silversmiths, bakers with bakers—to further increase their power. From this also grew other midlevel social institutions in the form of schools, colleges, local press, hospitals, cultural organizations, and charitable institutions. This brings me to a key point. The independent market economy made possible an array of new organizational structures—schools, local press, hospitals. These structures, in turn, led an emergence of a different view of individual rights and the valuing of men as free. True, this expanded expectation of rights and freedom was at first limited to men of a certain religion and social class, but the liberal foundations of the emergence of an independent middle class would eventually lead to others' shared privileges, although not with ease! I would highlight that these institutions have at their core the goals of increasing the resources of the middle class through group resource investment in hopes of larger gain. Now, not only those at court could hear the work of Haydn. Silversmiths and bakers could send their children to schools and universities, where they could secure a higher social position or further economic opportunity. In France, Japan, and China, these institutions made possible entrée to the esteemed bureaucracies or leadership of state-owned business that came to a man of letters (Fukuyama, 1995).

Similarly, the free press was the voice of the middle class and the guardian of its resources, for whom there was formerly no pulpit to combat the edicts of the titled wealthy. Indeed, the systems of democracy and communism are social institutions whose purpose is to increase and ensure the resources of the many. They represent in their pure forms an expansion from societies in which resources and power over resources are held by the few, into those in which they are communally fostered and shared. It is also notable how often these systems revert back to political orders that attempt to reconstitute resources and power to an inner circle.

Defining Resources and Stress

By stopping history at this point of village life, a number of insights are revealed. As Fukuyama (1992) argues, social interdependence, such as that expressed in the market village, is a level of society that crosses all cultures and to which all people aspire. At this level of social organization, people come to see themselves as deserving of esteem, status, and the rights to earn a livelihood, which, it is not inconsequential to mention, are also the underpinnings of the notions of democracy. I call these things that individuals value, to this level of social construction, *resources*:

Resources include the objects, conditions, personal characteristics, and energies that are either themselves valued for survival, directly or indirectly, or that serve as a means of achieving these resources.

So just as food is a resource, money for food or employment to purchase food, are resources. Because personal esteem and freedom are valued as elements of this system, they too are resources and what contributes to them are resources. At earlier levels of society, there may be a need for self-esteem that is expressed by each member of the tribe, but not necessarily the concept of deserving such. This latter viewpoint of deserving esteem is only accorded to the privileged members of the tribe, not those that are lower in status, and certainly not to those that are chattel. It is only accorded as a "right" to those at the lower levels of the social hierarchy in the more advanced cultural orders of the market economy.

The social basis of people nested in larger social structures allows a further defining of resources, which although broad, prevents an overextension of the concept.

It is therefore necessary to delimit the range of resources to be resources that are valued by a broad class of individuals and that are seen as highly salient for people in general as well as the self.

At this level of social history, we can culturally define stress, remaining true to the personal psychological and sociocultural foundations of the concept. As I have defined elsewhere (Hobfoll, 1988, 1989) but elaborate more culturally here, and which I will be developing through much of this book, according to Conservation of Resources theory,

Stress is predicted to occur as a result of circumstances that represent (1) a threat of resource loss, or (2) actual loss of the resources required to sustain the individual-

nested-in, family-nested-in social organization. In addition, because people will
invest what they value to gain further, stress is predicted to occur (3) when
individuals do not receive reasonable gain for themselves or social group following
resource investment, this itself being an instance of loss.

Resources can be subcategorized into object resources, condition resources, personal resources, and energy resources. Their common thread is being intimately related to survival of the individual within this level of social organization. The interweaving of these resources can be seen in how closely tied the most personalized resource of self-esteem is with having shelter and food (object resources), family membership and employment (condition resources), job and social skills (personal resources), and money, credit, and knowledge (energy resources) (see also Maslow, 1962). Moreover, the social basis of these relations depends on sharing a common culture that rules norms of behavior, values, and practices that define the individual's world and shape his or her perceptions and judgments.

According Baltes (1987, 1991), psychology has been able to minimize the central role of resources by relying on stress research with young adults to those of middle age, and not children or the aged. In so doing, psychology is observing phenomena at the age of maximum independence. Adding to this equation that most research participants are middle class, we can see how psychology created an understanding of stress that is relatively independent of resource loss and the need to adjust in response.

As soon as we study the aged, however, we see how resources play a primary role not only in their stress, but also in the interface of all age groups with the greater cultural forces that exist for them. As Baltes (1987, 1991) has cogently argued, the chronologically oldest members of society exist within the youngest culture, because we are only recently confronting the needs of such a substantial element of older individuals. By "young culture," he means that the institutions, practices, supports, and rituals that are associated with being this old in our society are immature and have had little time to develop. Paradoxically, because of potential health and economic problems of aging, the old are likely to, like the youngest members of society, have greatest need for culture (see Figure 2.3 here). Loss of resources inevitably occurs for the elderly, and the cultural structures that should be available to compensate for these losses are marginal and early in development.

Margret and Paul Baltes (1982, 1990) emphasize in their theory of compensation with optimization that stress is a sociocultural phenomenon and that individuals' stress experience is a derivative of social and cultural processes involving their resources and the resource demands of the culture that follow a developmental course. Although this process is magnified for

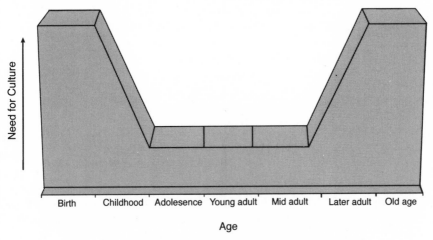

Figure 2.3.   Differential need for culture of different age groups.

the elderly, it holds true for any age group and becomes spotlighted whenever there is a clash between cultural demands and individuals' resources.

Conclusion: Maintaining Sociocultural Context

The redefining of the stress concept developed in this chapter spans individualism and communalism. As Etzioni (1994, 1997) has described, in all cultures, we depend on each other and are interdependent with one another. Insomuch as resources exist across important life domains that are inherently social in a cooperative (e.g., work, family) or competitive (e.g., who obtains more resources) sense, the threat to resources and efforts to garner and protect them will embody the stress experience across cultures that vary in their degree of individual versus collective orientation.

Cultures will nevertheless foster certain resources in preference to others. Resource priorities emerge that reflect the sociocultural fabric as it exists and this is a key point of my thesis. Max Weber's *The Protestant Ethic and the Spirit of Capitalism* (1904–1905/1930) argued that the culture of Protestantism allows ultimate reinforcement of individualism by offering individual salvation detached from a Church, and through worldly endeavors. More communal cultures, whether embodied in Chinese Confucianism or Italy's close-knit family hierarchies, tend to emphasize and sanctify familism. Instead of prizing the personal initiative or self-confidence of Western Protestantism, familism seeks family connections and the sustained social position of the family (Fukuyama, 1995). Advancement occurs through group initiative and shared goals. Hence, based on the framework of the social fabric in Western, North American culture, psychology has not depicted self-sacrifice as a resource, whereas it is central to Asian and Italian culture. Indeed, it is difficult in Western terms to conceptualize self-sacrifice as a personal trait. But self-efficacy seen as a trait may be just as foreign in some cultures at the same time that it is paramount in Western research on coping resources (Bandura, 1982).

Paradoxically, Fukuyama argues in his groundbreaking work *Trust* (1995) that individualism may foster extrafamilial trust, whereas familism inhibits trust outside the family. Weber (1951) called these "sib fetters" in describing the Chinese family—restrictive family bonds that breed suspicion. Maoist China's revolution purged these family structures because they created a shackled peasantry with few rights or prospects. Familism also produces hierarchal structures, and men are uniformly heads of household. Although women are more communal than men across cultures (Kashima et al., 1995), the rights of women, the belief that women deserve equal status, and even the expectation of physical safety from kin have seen more advances in individualist cultures. In Japan, women must still speak to men using a subservient level of discourse, and Latin American countries similarly assert men's superiority and power over women.

It is interesting that in Judaism, which is an amalgam of strong individualism and communalism, women received greater economic rights and status than in either individual or communal cultures. Although, arguably, still of second-class status, Jewish women received contractual guarantees in marriage that afforded them definite rights and privileges. Indeed, the rights of women to hold property is the only Old Testament instance in which God personally intervened in an earthly judgment of the law that he had essentially entrusted to male judges, this judgment predating women's property rights by some 3,500 years in most societies.

"Why should the name of our father be done away from among his family, because he had no son? Give unto us a possession among the brethren of our father." And Moses brought their case before the LORD. And the LORD spoke unto Moses, saying: "The daughters of Zelophehad speak right: thou shalt surely give them a possession of an inheritance among their father's brethren; and thou shalt cause the inheritance of their father to pass to them. And thou shalt speak unto the children of Israel, saying: If a man die, and have no son, then ye shall cause his inheritance to pass unto his daughter.... And it shall be unto the children of Israel a statute of judgment, as the LORD commanded Moses." (Numbers 27:4–11)

These cultural considerations and nuances serve to illustrate that social context creates and preserves the particular combination of resources that will serve individuals and groups' goal attainment. These social structures also delineate which circumstances act as stressors, because they create the conditions within which acquisition, protection, and maintenance of socially linked resources operate. This point is well made by Fukuyama (1995), who describes why familism was an essential value and resource (i.e., being attached to family) in China.

> In this [Confucian] sort of environment, a strong family system can be seen as an essentially defensive mechanism against a hostile and capricious environment. A peasant could trust only members of his own family, because those on the outside—officials, bureaucrats, local authorities, and gentry alike—felt no reciprocal sense of obligation to him and felt no constraints about treating him rapaciously. With most peasant families living perpetually at the edge of starvation, there was little surplus with which one could be generous to friends or neighbors. Sons—as many as one could afford while one's wife was of childbearing age—were an absolute necessity, for without them there was no way one could hope to support oneself in old age. Under such harsh conditions, the self-sufficient family was the only rational source of shelter and cooperation available. (p. 88)

In Japan, unlike China, extrafamilial bonds grew parallel to familism, creating a society in which family-relevant and broader socially relevant resources were prized and sustained. These are found historically in the evolving of nonfamilial groups called *iemoto*, which center around master–disciple relationships and practice of traditional arts such as Kabuki theater and flower arranging. These types of relationships have been extended to alumni of the same school or colleagues at work. Not surprisingly, the Japanese culture places honor and obligation as key resources that evolve from these sociocultural roots. Individuals in Japan prize honor and perceive the most subtle undermining of it. These appraisals are individual, but, for example, when an honorific code is transgressed, others in the room are aware but look away from the victim of the effrontery so as not to compound his or her disgrace. An act by one individual to save another's "face" can be seen as repayable only by extreme obligation in gratitude because of the public awareness of personal appraisals of acceptable codes of interpersonal behavior (Shelley, 1993).

We may have esteemed individualism to such an extent that we have lost sight in stress research and theory of the social context of the stress experience. Although our culture is less communal than many, it is more communal than others, and differences exist within the multicultural mix in our midst. On a recent trip to North Dakota, I consulted with the Red Cross regarding the chronic flooding disaster of Devil's Lake. They were surprised at the insights about the nature of the stress experience that we were able to jointly derive when I suggested we consider the cultural roots of the Norwegian and German settlers. Their initial response that these were "Americans from North Dakota; they have no culture." What unfolded from their thinking in terms of culture was an understanding that flood victims would disproportionately value the concept of homestead over its financial equivalent, and this explained why many had refused buyouts. They would also be reticent to accept help because of their principles of independence. At the same time, they had little trust for government and the possibility that government could help them solve their dilemma. Help had to grow endogenously because of their further distrust of outsiders. For them, the "self" in self-esteem and self-efficacy is magnified, and the "social" in social support and social cooperation is minimized. Again, this is perceived by individuals but holds for the group, because these resources were necessary to create, maintain, and protect the more basic resources we all value related to survival and the family and tribe that emerged from their culture and heritage.

By depicting stress and resources within a biological context that is situated in a socially derived culture, we avoid seeing stress as either biologically determined or as purely socially derived. We retain the importance of people's perceptions but can retain them within the context of our species and the divergent cultures that our species has evolved. We can appreciate the individual component of perception but not lose sight of its being nested in a certain biology, culture, and context. We may feel uncomfortable because such a working definition of stress can only be understood multidisciplinarily, but we may be less feted with the biases of any one discipline as well. Moreover, we may be less fixed to a particular paradigm that is embedded in a particular psychology at a particular time, and that may have little elasticity to applications across cultures and time periods.

NOTES

1. The reader will also note with some irony that Freud used this same metaphor to make a somewhat opposite point, that being that the subconscious is the iceberg below the waterline. Still, I think that the metaphor is useful here.
2. This is only one of a number of paths by which towns and cities came about. Some were new cities, created by decree. Others developed from ancient Roman towns that had dwindled in importance. Each of the paths by which towns developed, however, could be used to illustrate the themes of social independence, advancing of human rights, and codependence of individuals with groups larger than the family (Beresford, 1967; Konvitz, 1985).

3

Conservation of Resources Theory
Principles and Corollaries

I have developed the thesis in the first two chapters that stress has biological, social, and cultural bases in terms of the demands on people to acquire and protect the circumstances that ensure survival, and distance themselves from threats to survival. Although stress's foundations are biological and related to biological requirements, it is further, and significantly, shaped by cultural experience. Stress emerges from the difficulty achieving the common goals that members of a culture pursue, beginning at a shared biological level and extending to complex social relations and rituals reflected in that society. As deVries (1995) theorized, culture itself is formed to ensure the successful coping of the tribe or people. Behavior that leads to survival becomes codified within the culture and even ritualized such that much behavior becomes automatic within social roles. Moreover, stress is largely culturally determined because many of the major demands placed on people have a social context, and culture is largely a social phenomenon. Family discord, work-related problems, health concerns, and threats to liberty all have a central social component. They may be caused by social forces and their solutions often lie in the utilization and management of social contexts.

Whenever social patterns repeatedly reoccur and have importance to survival or maintenance of society, they become incorporated into norms and cultural standards. The connection between individual needs and social needs is most clear in Confucian societies such as China and Korea, where family and social harmony are the *sine qua non* of well-being. In

Northern European and American cultures, the self has a more central role, but even this self is usually seen as being defined by social comparison, social roles, and social standards (Cantor, 1990; Markus & Nurius, 1986). When appraisals are made regarding threats to the self, they are contextualized within social standards and markers, and people look to their social environment for feedback about the threat, preferred responses, and solace.

People are biologically primed and further learn to acquire and protect things that are valued. Many of these things are related to mastery of the environment. Mastery, however, is not the same as control, and perhaps a more accurate description of my meaning is *mastery of the ability to negotiate the environment in order to meet reasonable needs.* This negotiation is imperfect, works through trial and error and modeling, and accepts compromise as a natural course. Antonovsky (1979) came away from his studies of Holocaust survivors suggesting that acceptance of a reasonable level of control and predictability is the underpinning of what he called a sense of coherence— the sense that people can reasonably predict their future, that there is meaning in what they do, and that internal and external forces tend to serve their benefit. Hence, we have mastery of success and acceptance of at least occasional failure interwoven, and we have personal control and giving up control to other, we hope, benevolent powers balanced. By this process, individuals and groups set goals, work toward their acquisition or achievement, evaluate progress, and reassess goals in a cyclic manner.

Rosenbaum (in press) has theorized that the control of acceptance of things as they are is a key paradoxical aspect of mastery, underscoring the point that mastery does not imply complete control. Rather, to retain mastery of what in effect are negotiated, partial successes, people must learn both to control and to relinquish control. This process can be seen on an individual level, as when young children attempt new skills such as skipping. They attempt to copy a model, evaluate their progress, and often accept a rather awkward version, which although unrhythmic, gets them where they are going. More complete success awaits another day. Adults follow a similar course in making career or relationship goals, working toward them, and adjusting goals to match their partial progress.

The family and tribe are social structures that allow for a decrease in individual effort for goal attainment. The society creates institutions and traditions around work, marriage, education, health care, and other important life domains that facilitate individual and societal advancement in concert. A market economy acts further to diversify effort and ease individual demands and the need for any given individual to have a complete array of resources (i.e., all possible resources). One might immediately ask why, then, do we work so hard in advanced cultures? The answer is that because group effort is so much more efficient, we increase the expectation for output disproportionately. An assembly line produces thousands more cars than could individuals were they working singly on assembling automobiles. If an individual had to hunt his or her own food, prepare that food, plant, harvest, process grain, make cloth, and stand guard, he or she would never sleep, or would have to make do with a meager, subsistence existence. Thus, as culture advances, individual resources and social resources become more closely enmeshed.

I speak of individual, familial, tribal, and greater social goals together, as they are inextricably linked in life. Disciplinary study has balkanized the investigation of these different levels, but when we examine personal, familial, group, and broader social goals, we immediately see the connections. Psychology's individualistic bent has detached the individual from these ties, but there is a clear resurgence of interest in reconnecting the individual with family, tribe, and culture that probably has come as a response to the pendulum of individuality swinging too far, even for psychology. This emphasis to rejoin individual psychology with broader social structures is evidenced in the writing of leading cognitive psychologists, exploring one of the most individualistic areas of study, the self-concept.

> The pool of possible selves derives from the categories made salient by the individual's particular sociocultural and historical context and from the models, images, and symbols provided by the media and by the individual's immediate social experiences. Possible selves thus have the potential to reveal the inventive and constructive nature of the self but they also reflect the extent to which the self is socially determined and constrained. (Markus & Nurius, 1986, p. 954)

> Individuals set tasks for themselves, distilling from the many culturally prescribed and biologically based demands of social life and survival a set of personal life task goals for which to strive. (Cantor, 1990, p. 736)

Linking these self-schemas to stress, Markus and Nurius suggest that a central role of self-schemas is the creation of goals and a contextualizing of fears and threats that might inhibit these goals. Of interest here as well, Markus has been concerned with how these self-schemas guide the individual through major stressors such as death of a family member or loss of a long-standing relationship (Markus & Nurius, 1986). How the individual behaves in reaction to stress and the emotions that are matched to situations is largely derived from social norms and constraints.

RESOURCES AND PREDICTION OF STRESS

Through personal experience, modeling, and other forms of learning, people come to recognize what is important. As a matter of course, they also acquire a knowledge of what they need in order to assure the acquisition and possession of what is important directly, indirectly, and symbolically for success within their culture and sheer survival. They come therefore to value these things. As delineated in Chapter 2,

> *I will call these things that individuals value* RESOURCES. *Resources include the objects, conditions, personal characteristics, and energies that are either themselves valued for survival, directly or indirectly, or that serve as a means of achieving these ends. I delimit the range of resources to be resources that are valued by a broad class of individuals and that are seen as highly salient for people in general as well as the self.*

These include primary resources such as food and shelter, which are directly required for survival. Next, we have what might be called secondary resources, such as sense of mastery, health insurance, and transportation, which are "tools" that increase the likelihood of obtaining or protecting primary resources. In this way, as cultures advance, other major life goals substitute for biological survival. More distally but still important are tertiary resources, such as social status (e.g., title, luxury home), which are only symbolically tied to survival and may be linked to more primitive social hierarchies (e.g., dominant male in the tribe), as well as the desire to distance oneself from possible critical resource loss by producing a thick, protective barrier between the self and challenges to survival. For example, although a luxury home is unnecessary for survival, it serves a similar symbolic value as plumpness and white skin of the upper classes in medieval Europe, these being outward signs of the distance of the wealthy from the plight of the poor, which included a struggle for food and exposure to the elements that aged the skin.

Recent work by Diener and Fujita (1995) defined resources similarly and applied their work to the study of subjective well-being and life satisfaction. Resources were defined as the "material, social, or personal characteristics that a person possesses that he or she can use to make progress toward his or her personal goals. Resources can be external possessions (e.g., money), social roles (e.g., being a chairperson), and personal characteristics (e.g., intelligence)" (p. 926). Consistent also with conservation of resources (COR) theory (Hobfoll, 1988), Diener and Fujita outlined the role of resources as means of achieving sense of competence and mastery and of fulfilling psychological and physical needs. They found the sum of resources possessed to be one of the strongest predictors of both life satisfaction and subjective well-being noted in the literature. Furthermore, they found that these relationships were almost unaffected by extroversion, a personality trait that might underlie both assessment of resources and well-being. Although based on a student sample, this would actually make this study a conservative test of resources' importance, because college students tend not to differ widely on health, financial, and role resources.

Diener and Fujita also noted individual differences, such that those who valued a resource more were more influenced by that resource. However, the individual differences, while significant, tended to be much smaller than the general influence of resources on subjective well-being and life satisfaction. This study is also consistent with Diener, Diener, and Diener's (1994) cross-cultural finding that a nation's ability to provide the basic biological resources of clean water, food, and health care was related to national subjective well-being and argues in favor of a theory that bridges from individual to macrosocial phenomena.

Central Tenet of COR Theory

This discussion brings us to the central tenet of COR theory, that:

> *People strive to obtain, retain, and protect that which they value (Hobfoll, 1988, 1989). I would add to this now that people also endeavor to foster that which they value.*

Hence, people work to obtain resources they do not have, retain those resources they possess, protect resources when threatened, and foster resources by positioning themselves so that their resources can be put to best use. Major life stressors are likely to have significant impact on resource acquisition and protection, but even minor hassles may collectively act to diminish people's capacity to cultivate and guard their resources. Also from this tenet, I highlight that people are directed to cultivate resources, even when there is no current stress. Such anticipatory coping has been generally left unstudied but is key to people's stress-response strategies (Aspinwall & Taylor, 1997).

From this tenet, COR theory, as I have defined elsewhere (Hobfoll, 1988, 1989) but elaborate more culturally in this volume, develops a definitional structure for stress:

> *Stress occurs in circumstances that represent a threat of loss or actual loss of the resources required to sustain the individual-nested-in family-nested-in social organization. Furthermore, because people will invest what they value to gain further, stress is predicted to occur when individuals do not receive reasonable gain following resource investment, this itself being an instance of loss.*
>
> *Hence, stress occurs when (1) resources are threatened with loss, (2) resources are actually lost, or (3) there is a failure to adequately gain resources following significant resource investment.*

By individual-nested-in family-nested-in social organization, I imply that although we can separate these levels for study, they are enmeshed. There is no organization or family without individuals, and individuals must rely on social attachments for well-being, self-esteem, and survival.

Resources are further subcategorized into object resources, condition resources, personal resources, and energy resources. Their common thread is their being intimately related to survival for the individual, existing within a social network of family, friends, and organizations. Because of the common basis of human survival, most of these resources are valued across cultures. Because cultures seek to protect individuals who are in particular ecological niches (e.g., agrarian, hunting, or industrial society), and because cultures themselves develop and adopt chaotic paths that are only partially linked to their origins, the order of importance of resources will differ along with differing values (Schwartz & Bilsky, 1990), and some resources may even be evidenced in some cultures and not others.

For example, American culture is founded largely on individualism, as noted in the early part of the nineteenth century by Alexis de Tocqueville. Tocqueville (1945) did not fail simultaneously to recognize that Americans were aware of the need to cooperate with others, but did so to preserve their self-interest. This tradition stems from Anglo-Saxon liberalism that sees humans as isolated, self-sufficient individuals. They engage in social relationships, according to the seventeenth-century philosopher John Locke (1952), to achieve what they cannot on their own, but otherwise prefer isolation as a natural state.

One might therefore surmise that American individualism would have made only individual resources of importance. However, the tendency to such extreme individualism was tempered both by realistic needs as early as the original Puritan communities, and by the merger of more familial non-Anglo-Saxon, non-Germanic cultures in America. Italian immigrants, largely from the highly familial culture of southern Italy and Sicily, for example, carried with them a strong family-based tradition in which the needs of the family outweighed the rights of the individual. Jewish immigrants from Eastern Europe were similarly ensconced in a culture of family and community, which even dictated that a minimum of 10 men settled together so that they could organize prayer. Jews could and did also unite, as most shared a common language of Yiddish, independent of their country of European origin. Irish immigrants not only aggregated in linked communities, but also made concerted effort to gain control of important community organizations such as the political machines of Boston, Chicago, and other major northern U.S. cities and their respective police and fire departments. Today, the impetus of the more communal Hispanic and African American cultures is also making its mark on society.

Thus, whereas America is seen as an individualistic culture, the self is not so isolated as some of the theoretical roots of American ideology would suggest (Sowell, 1981). Nonetheless, America can be seen as a culture in which people value the self more highly than does Confucian culture or

Afrocentric culture. This translates to self-oriented resources being primary, but not sufficient without the connective tissue afforded by more collectivist resources. Nor is the self necessarily devaluated in Eastern societies. Individual achievement is highly sought in Japan, China, and Korea, and senior positions are coveted. Nevertheless, the cultural differences reflect niches that required different resources and thus created different hierarchies of resources.

CATEGORIES OF RESOURCES

There are a number of ways to demarcate taxonomies of resources. I have found three methods of categorization to be especially helpful in understanding the stress process, although only one, the simplest and probably least valuable, is typically employed.

Internal versus External Resources

This first and simplest level of abstraction is to categorize resources into internal and external types. A number of researchers have relied on this distinction (Hobfoll & Walfisch, 1984; Holahan & Moos, 1987; Sarason, Sarason, & Shearin, 1986). Internal resources include those that are possessed by the self or are within the domain of the self. They include self-esteem, job skills, optimism, and sense of mastery. External resources are those resources that are not possessed by the self, but are external to it. Principal among these are social support, employment, and economic status. The value of this distinction is that it is simple and organized around a central psychological concept—the self. The weakness of the distinction is that it is too broad to be helpful in understanding important differences within categories, and it has no theoretical basis. Sarason et al., (1986) have also questioned whether external resources such as social support are not internal resources when they are measured as perceptions made by the self (i.e., perceived support).

Notwithstanding the simplicity of the internal–external resource dichotomy, there is certainly some value in this distinction. Kobasa and Puccetti (1983), Holohan and Moos (1987, 1991), and Hobfoll (1988) and Hobfoll and Lerman (1989) have relied on it to examine how internal resources may be seen as managing systems for external resources. For example, mastery may operate as a management system for decisions on how to use social support in different stress situations (Kobasa & Puccetti, 1983). Hobfoll (1985a, 1985b) has also made the point that internal resources may be more immediately accessible, whereas external resources demand greater mobilization time and possible inheritance of obligations that may be burdensome. Perhaps it is best to call the internal versus external distinction a building block for the more complex study of types of resources.

A Structural Resource Classification

In my earlier work on COR theory, I used a four-part classification, dividing resources into (1) object resources, (2) personal resources, (3) condition resources, and (4) energy resources. An advantage of this structurally based system is that it divides internal and external resources into further types that have meaningful differences. Object resources include resources that have a physical presence, such as a home, transportation, and fetish objects (e.g., diamonds, valuable household items). Many objects' worth is related to their direct survival value, whereas others have acquired value because they are linked to status or self-esteem. Although there is little study in psychology of materialism, either for survival or for status, people invest enormous efforts in order to obtain, retain, protect, and foster object resources, in part to sustain life, and in part to gain social dominance and sense of self-worth.

Personal resources include both skills and personal traits. Personal skills resources include occupational skills, social aplomb, and leadership ability. Personal trait resources include self-esteem, optimism, self-efficacy, and hope. Personal resources tend to be learned and are products of modeling, education, nurturance, and role adaptation. Underlying these traits in some instances may also be biologically based temperaments (Strelau, 1995) that may make some individuals more likely to develop, for example, sociability, a positive outlook, mechanical ability, and high activity level. Key to many of these traits are early and ongoing developmental experiences having to do with secure, loving attachments (Ainsworth, 1979, 1989; Bowlby, 1980). Much developmental literature speaks to how self-esteem, hope, self-efficacy, and sense of trust emerge from a nurturant parental bond that encourages developmentally appropriate exploration of the environment and eventual launching from the nest. This may be why so many of the major personal trait resources are strongly linked to one another (Ainsworth, 1989; Bowlby, 1980).

Condition resources are important because they lay a foundation for access to other resources. Conditions are resources when they are structures or states that allow access to or possession of other resources. Because of their broad acquisitional and protective role, they become valued in their own right. They tend to be studied more by sociologists than psychologists because they are in the realm of social roles that until recently have not been of major interest to psychology. Condition resources include being healthy, employment, tenure, seniority, marriage, and, in some societies, being first-born males. Some conditions are earned, such as tenure and a good marriage. Others are proffered by nature of inheritance or social rank, and some are partially biologically based (e.g., stamina, health). Condition resources tend to be slow to acquire. Tenure, seniority, and a strong marriage require great resource investment. Interestingly, they may be lost rapidly, such as when a job layoff or marital indiscretion ends a resource's longevity. Because they create access to pools of other resources, condition resources are often greatly coveted and valued.

Energy resources derive their value from their ability to be exchanged for resources in the other three categories. Energy resources include money, credit, and knowledge. These resources can be invested or retained in order to enhance resource acquisition, protect against resource loss, or combat loss cycles once they begin, Money, for example, has no value in and of itself, and if its exchangeability weakens, it loses value, as in the case of hyperinflation. Knowledge may be seen as valued in and of itself, but again, as with money, if knowledge cannot be used for other purposes, it is not esteemed. Another characteristic of energy resources is that they are more valuable prior to exchange than after their exchange. For example, a new car is immediately worth less than the money that purchased it, because the flexibility to use the money in other ways has been lost. This occurs before the car is even driven from the showroom floor. Likewise, knowledge loses value when it is released. Many inventors left major technological corporations because they had knowledge that if released to the company would be worth less than if developed under their personal copyright or patent. Energy resources may, however, gain fetish value and be stockpiled, as in the case of the wealthy who live without enjoying their wealth.

This four-part nomenclature's principal weakness is that it is a categorization made by type, rather than by some theoretical formulation. As in other classification systems, not all resources are easily categorized, and this also presents a problem. For example, whether health is a condition resource or personal resource is ambiguous. Likewise, social support is in some ways a condition resource and in some ways an energy resource that lies in wait to be mobilized. We may need to settle for the compromise that it has attributes of both resource types. The possible strength of this taxonomy lies in the fact that there are some general properties that do distinguish resources in the different categories, and that do operate differentially in the stress process.

Centrality of Resources to Survival

A third type of resource classification that I had not considered earlier in work on COR theory (1988, 1989), nor seen others utilize may be especially heuristic because it is most theoretically based. This system is based on the proximity of the resource to survival, as I previously mentioned. Primary resources are those that directly relate to survival. They include adequate food, clothing, shelter, mastery to negotiate the environment (e.g., occupational skills, knowledge of how to grow food), and those resources that ensure safety. Secondary resources are those that contribute indirectly to primary resources. They include social support and attachment to the group or tribe, marital or romantic ties, hope, and optimism. Tertiary resources include those things that are symbolically related to primary or secondary resources. These include money, resources that signify social status (e.g., a luxury home or automobile, jewelry), and workplace and social conditions that allow great availability or access to secondary resources (e.g., friendships, organizational memberships).

One might discredit social status resources as superficial, but an enormous percentage of Western economy is geared toward their acquisition and maintenance. Although people may be aware on some level that status objects are superficial, it is hardly unusual for parents to lose site of their children in the race for acquiring the trappings of luxury. Also, many status resources are important because they are intimately tied with stability of other resources, such as employment, salary, and social recognition (Siegrist, 1996). Siegrist (1986) also underscores the fact that when status is threatened, it undermines people's basic sense of identity and their view of themselves and place in the world.

A classification made on the basis of proximity to survival might be helpful because it is hierarchical and may indicate how impactful a loss or gain would be at different levels of the hierarchy. It may also provide insight into research on how resources come to be valued. Work by Baltes (1987, 1991) would similarly suggest that culture plays the role of supplementing resources that are meaningful for survival. According to Baltes, young children and older adults especially must rely on culture for this reason, because their ability to live independently is more limited than during the middle years. By studying which resources are needed as people age, information about the relative value of resources could be placed in a more developmental framework. No single categorical system will answer all research or theoretical requirements, but these three classification methods may prove helpful used separately or in combination.

THE ROLE OF SOCIAL CONFLICT IN RESOURCE ACQUISITION AND PROTECTION FROM RESOURCE LOSS

Until this juncture, I emphasized the value of social linkages in the process of resource acquisition and prevention of resource loss. To understand resources and their interplay in the stress process, I wish to develop another point that I have not found covered in theories of stress in the past, nor previously considered. I speak of the role of social conflict and its contribution to the process by which resources are sought, obtained, protected, and fostered. Because resources are commonly valued, and because they are often finite, social conflict often results. Consequently, social conflict and competition for resources become major underpinnings of the stress process. Furthermore, because societies cannot sustain outright violence and constant social upheaval, this competition for resources becomes routinized within individual and social endeavors. For hunters in a subsistence economy, this translates into territoriality. In liberal democracies with free market economies, competition occurs for money, power, position, and social status. We might imagine that this competition for resources is not relevant to personal resources such as self-esteem. However, although self-esteem is potentially an unlimited resource, even here, because of status seeking and social comparison processes (Rosenberg, 1965), some individuals gain more self-esteem and others are afforded less.

I do not know if social conflict is endemic to the human endeavor, but it is most certainly widespread across cultures. It can be seen in the caste system of India, the highly delineated social status system of traditional Japan (which had its own untouchables), as well as the aristocrat-based cultures of England and France. In southern Italy, families could hardly see fit to contribute to common social organizations, less they offer undue gain and advantage to other families (Banfield, 1958). In American inner cities, where resources are scarce in the face of an affluent society, social conflict can be seen in terms of warring gangs of Los Angeles' Bloods and Crips, and Chicago's Blackstone Rangers, who vie for territory and market share of the lucrative cocaine business. In each of these cases, people are in conflict with others over the acquisition, possession, retention, and growth of available resources. This, in turn, places people themselves in conflict as beating adversaries or diminishing their chances of success become major preoccupations and their results key factors in the stress process. Ideally, communistic society sought to end this very competition as the central thesis of communism by proposing that individuals be required by law and social forces to act toward the common good. However, outside of the Israeli kibbutz, which is communistic on a much smaller, community scale, communism's downfall came in part because of internal competition for scarce resources and the inability to match competition-based economies.

Thus, social conflict is another important communal mechanism by which societal ties are orchestrated in a push for resources. Because individuals often see themselves as outmaneuvered by powerful social forces in this conflict, they also are motivated to further organize to obtain, retain, protect, and foster resources; that is, survival does not only mean survival against the natural elements, it also means competing for resources that are sought by others and naturally (e.g., food that is scarce due to drought) or artificially (food that is destroyed to increase prices) limited. This includes family structures, unions, corporations, and governments (for the services they render to protect and organize resources). At times, such social groups can be altruistic and have as their goal the sharing of resources with those less fortunate, as in the case of public charities. At other times, they are formed out of hatred for another group's real or imagined advantage, as in the case of White Supremist and neo-Nazi organizations. In Confucian society, these associations are a matter of obligation, such that one's ties to the Emperor and one's parents are derived from a common set of social values. In contrast, in Anglo-Saxon culture, they are necessities promulgated to secure individual rights. But in all societies there is a common understanding that these associations will secure the individual-nested-in-family's well-being.

Most importantly for COR theory, and the point I hope to make here, social competition ties the individual to the social group such that individual resources such as self-esteem, sense of hope, and occupational skills become intertwined with group membership, religion, and guild or union association. So self-esteem comes to a large extent from being part of the right group. Hope is institutionalized and inspired by the teachings of the Church or Koran. Unions label workers according to strict job classifications to maximize salaries and prevent companies from using less highly skilled (and paid) workers for higher status jobs. The personal scripts that individuals develop are to a sizable extent the outgrowth of these broader social role conflicts. The importance of resource scarcity becomes especially salient in the latter part of the twentieth century and for the foreseeable future because global competition has meant a competition for more limited resources and a demand for greater research investment with the risk of less payoff (Siegrist, 1996).

RESOURCE LOSS'S SALIENCE: PRINCIPLE 1

Two major principles and several secondary corollaries follow from the basic tenet of COR theory. The first principle, and perhaps the most important, is:

Resource loss is disproportionately more salient than is resource gain.

In other words, given an equal amount of loss and gain, loss will have much greater impact. This principle is critical because it distinguishes COR theory from both change or homeostatic theories of stress, and from more straightforward reinforcement theory. Gains and losses could otherwise be depicted as rewards and punishments, as reinforcement theory would have it, but this would fail to distinguish a differential amplitude or effect for reinforcers versus punishers. According to COR theory, it is loss and the threat of loss of resources that principally defines stress ontologically, ontogenologically, and culturally. Although it is difficult to calculate how much more powerful loss and the motivation to avoid loss is from gain and the motivation to obtain gain, COR theory posits that the distinction is significant. The degree of difference, favoring loss, probably depends on the resource being considered. Loss versus gain of $500 might favor avoidance of loss as the more powerful motivator, but only slightly. Loss versus gain of a lover might have a much larger differential.

Historical Notions of Loss

The importance of loss in psychology has a long tradition. Robert Burton in his *Anatomy of Melancholy* (1624) wrote of the importance of loss of loved ones in the formation of melancholy.

> Montanus makes mention of a country woman that parting with her friends and native place, became grievously melancholy.... If parting of friends, absence alone can work such violent effects, what shall death do, when they must eternally be separated, never in this world to meet again? This is so grievous a torment for the time, that it takes away their appetite, desire of life, extinguisheth all delights, it causeth deep sighs and groans, tears, exclamations, howling, roaring, many bitter pants, and by frequent meditation extends so far sometimes, that they see their dead friends continually in their eyes. (p. 234)

Nor did Burton limit this to loss of a loved one.

> There is another sorrow, which arises from the loss of temporal goods and fortunes, which equally afflicts, and may go hand in hand with the preceding [i.e., loss of loved ones]; loss of time, loss of honour, office, of good name, of labour, frustrate hopes, will much torment, but in my judgment, there is no torture like unto it, or that sooner procureth this malady and mischief: ... "Loss of friends, and loss of goods make many men melancholy, as I have often seen by continual meditation of such things." (p. 236)

And generalized the effects, saying they could occur by

> accidents ... shipwreck, fire, spoil and pillage of soldiers, or that loss soever, it boots not, it will work the like effect, the same desolation in provinces and cities, as well as private persons (p. 237).

In 1812, Benjamin Rush, the father of American psychiatry, wrote that intellectual derangement was more commonly from "mental" than "corporeal" causes. Rush was influenced by Pinel, the eighteenth-century French pioneer of "moral treatment" of the mentally ill. Rush quotes Pinel, who surmised that of 113 cases in the Bicêtre Hospital, 34 were from domestic losses, 24 from loss of love, and 30 from distressing events of the French Revolution, possibly threat of loss of life or witnessing of traumatic events. At the Pennsylvania Hospital, Rush reported that of 50 "maniacs," 7 were from loss of love, 7 from loss related to grief, and 7 from loss of property. Other causes of mental illness were certainly mentioned as well, including 2 cases of winning the lottery leading to mania and death, but the loss theme was conspicuous.

This thinking by prominent early psychiatrists is not so far from current notions. Loss of primary attachments in early life has been associated with major psychological disorder and functional difficulties (Ainsworth, 1979; Bowlby, 1980). Freud (1917/1963) saw loss as critical to psychological development, associating it with (the unfortunate) fulfillment of oedipal fears (i.e., the fulfilled wish to kill the parent). Loss has been particularly associated with depression (A. Lazarus, 1968, 1972). The link between interpersonal loss and depression followed psychodynamical theory that argued that the loss was internalized as guilt (i.e., "Its my fault") or because the loss meant that early childhood needs that contribute to a positive sense of optimism were undermined. Paykel (1985) found that loss or exit events were associated with depression, whereas entrance events (e.g., birth of a newborn, entering a challenging new job) were not. However, reviewing the literature, he also noted that the previously asserted link between loss events and depression was unjustified and that the association was more generalized to a number of psychological disorders.

Cognitive Bias and Loss

That loss has a more salient impact than gain has also been developed in work by Tversky and Kahneman (1974) and Kahneman and Tversky (1979) in their prospect theory. Prospect theory postulates that the gradient of loss is steeper than the gradient for gain, resulting in a bias in favor of loss. In laboratory experiments, for example, they found that people will expend more resources to prevent the loss of a cup that they received upon entering the laboratory than they will to gain the same cup; that is, once they possess the cup, its loss is more valued than would be the gain of the cup were they not to possess it. In other experiments, they show that when problems are understood in terms of loss (e.g., loss of life), greater risk will be taken than if the same situation is framed in terms of potential gain.

Loss and the Life-Events Tradition

Investigating people's grief reactions, Lindemann (1944) and Parkes (1972) were among the first to link loss events during adulthood to psychological distress. Earlier work had suggested that if losses did not occur in childhood, they might lead to mourning but not melancholy (Freud, 1917/1963), that is, sadness but not depression. This theme is easily forgotten so great is the influence of the stress paradigm, because we forget that only a few decades ago, a link between crises originating in adulthood and psychopathology was thought to be theoretically untenable (Caplan, 1964). The pioneering work of Holmes and Rahe (1967) on life events during adulthood transformed the entire fields of psychology and psychiatry and called attention to the fact that life events during adulthood could have major psychological consequences.

Holmes and Rahe (1967) theorized that it was the *readjustment* that followed life transitions that was stressful. Indeed, the concept of stress as change so permeated the literature that it remains a dominant principle held by clinicians. Holmes and Rahe calculated life change units, or the amount of change that was required to adjust to a particular event. Unfortunately, they were misled by an artifact of their method. Specifically, they had mixed clear loss events (e.g., death of a spouse, imprisonment) with ambiguous events (e.g., change in financial status, change in living conditions). The loss events were more clearly related to psychological distress, but the ambiguous events were somewhat positively related to distress and illness as well. By asking people to merely indicate change, respondents endorsed an event that had either positive or negative change indistinguishably. In subsequent analyses of studies that separated loss versus gain events, loss events were found to have a more profound effect on psychological distress and illness than gain (Taylor, 1991; Thoits, 1983). In fact, Cohen and Hoberman (1983) found that positive events were related to a decrease of psychological distress, and even buffered the potential negative impact of loss events; that is, not only are positive changes not stressful, they act to inoculate people from some of the deleterious impact of negative events.

Unpacking Loss Events

The "event" is increasingly being seen as the wrong unit of analysis. This insight was first and most passionately made by Brown and Harris (1979, 1989). They argued that the event list method aggregated many subevents that were the actual operating mechanisms in the stress–distress association. They instead developed a careful interview method in order to tease apart the nature of the stressful event and its meaning. Their use of the term *meaning* was not the meaning ascribed by the individual, but the meaning that could be taken from the actual circumstances that the person experienced, that is, the meaning that could be generally socially ascribed to such events by trained observers. Similarly, the unpacking of events into constituent subevents has also been advanced by Dohrenwend et al. (1993), who use a semistructured interview to dissect events. Dohrenwend et al. make the point that the way life events are typically used (e.g., divorce, illness as events) is too inclusive, and that the impact is better revealed when the sequence of the event is delineated.

A resource perspective takes a somewhat different course. The resources lost and gained are the unit of analysis that is critical. We would not speak of negative life events or positive life events, but the extent to which resources were lost and gained in the process. Hence, a divorce as an event is only a starting point. Outcomes will be a product of the resource losses and gains that come of the event. If a woman loses finances, insurance, self-esteem, and trust, but gains freedom and hope, it is the balance of these that will influence her. If loss is more salient than gain, then the losses will also loom larger than will the consummate gains.

In examining stressful event lists (see Table 3.1), we can see that all of the major life events are clearly loss-concentrated and that where more minor events are stressful, they are likely to cue a loss progression. Of the most stressful events, there are loss of a loved one, economic difficulty, imprisonment, loss of employment, and divorce. These usually are accompanied by an array of losses, albeit with some possible attendant gains. More mundane events such as minor violations of the law, family discord, or work hassles are not likely to be as devastating, but nor are the resources lost likely to be as large. The literature has continued to chart these as "negative life events" and leave the rest up to individual perception, but again, these perceptions are likely to be related to whether actual loss or gain of resources emerges. If we do not delineate the constituent resource changes that occur, of course, perception will be a more powerful predictor than events, because individuals will by and large be fair arbiters of what occurred to their resources (Baumeister, 1989).

The origins of people's bias in exaggerating the importance of loss may be both biological and cultural. Biologically, people were on the edge of survival for millions of years of evolutionary development. Loss of a tooth, food source, or the tribe's toolmaker spelled disaster. Resource gains also had survival value, but gains could seldom be accumulated prior to the advance of market-oriented culture, and then for some classes of people more than others. Hence, tribes would fatten and store food for the winter, but by spring, many would still have died and all would be at survival's edge with severe vitamin and nutritional deficiencies. This would result in a biological priming for being loss attentive. The biological and cultural underpinnings of loss are noted in a recent study by Diener et al. (1995), who found that lack of resources was the principle determinant of low life satisfaction across many disparate cultures that encompassed comparisons

Table 3.1 Social Readjustment Scale

Rank	Life event	Mean value
1	Death of spouse	100
2	Divorce	73
3	Marital separation	65
4	Jail term	63
5	Death of close family member	63
6	Personal injury or illness	53
7	Marriage	50
8	Fired at work	47
9	Marital reconciliation	45
10	Retirement	45
11	Change in health of family member	44
12	Pregnancy	40
13	Sex difficulties	39
14	Gain of new family member	39
15	Business readjustment	39
16	Change in financial state	38
17	Death of close friend	37
18	Change to different line of work	36
19	Change in number of arguments with spouse	35
20	Mortgage over $10,000	31
21	Foreclosure of mortgage or loan	30
22	Change in responsibilities at work	29
23	Son or daughter leaving home	29
24	Trouble with in-laws	29
25	Outstanding personal achievement	28
26	Wife begin or stop work	26
27	Begin or end school	26
28	Change in living conditions	25
29	Revision of personal habits	24
30	Trouble with boss	23
31	Change in work hours or conditions	20
32	Change in residence	20
33	Change in schools	20
34	Change in recreation	19
35	Change in church activities	19
36	Change in social activities	18
37	Mortgage or loan less than $10,000	17

Source: Holmes and Rahe (1967). Reprinted with permission of Pergamon Press, Ltd.

of wealthy and poor countries worldwide. This included both material and more abstract resources such as freedom.

As culture advanced, most individuals were still left in a state of appreciable poverty. The rise of a relatively comfortable middle class is a very recent historical development. Safe banking is even more recent, having long made even middle-class life tenuous indeed. People naturally learned to guard against the insidious effects of loss and there was little hope for gain. For farmers or industrial workers, wages and earnings were almost universally only enough to subsist. Drought or recession spelled disaster, as there was little ability to create reserves. Thus, culture taught traditions of loss saliency. The peasant families of China and the American farmer had to produce as many sons as possible to work the fields. Working-class families of southern Italy and Welsh coal miners had to retain tight family associations to produce a sufficient economy for survival of the members of the family. Even though the middle class has broadened substantially in this century, the cultural traditions of loss laid the threads of bias favoring loss vigilance. For the poor today, current realities are enough of a reminder.

THE VALUE OF GAINS

With all the attention to loss, it would be easy to ignore the importance of resource gain altogether. However, COR theory sees resource gain as an important facet of stress, even if secondary to loss.

Resource gain is less salient than resource loss, but its importance is defined in terms of loss's critical nature; that is, resource gain is important because it is intertwined with loss. First of all, although loss is more impactful, it may be prevented, offset, or forestalled through resource gain. Money can be invested to prevent financial loss outright, and time and energy can be invested to prevent loss of love by contributing to one's family. If initial losses occur, previously stockpiled resources can be utilized to minimize loss's impact. A love rejection may still be painful, but by turning to friends and family who were given support in the past, an individual can see him- or herself as nevertheless loved and cherished. In line with this supposition, Kessler, Turner, Blake, and House (1988) examined workers who were laid off from their positions. Those with financial reserves did not experience the same deleterious effects of job and economic loss as those who lacked savings. However, prior to the experience of the job loss, the savings had little positive impact.

The entire insurance industry is predicated on people making sizable investments of their resources into insurance in order to forestall the losses that would otherwise transpire from financial setbacks that could come from death, fire, flood, or lawsuit. These investments are obviously inequivalent to the ultimate gain that one will likely receive, and the margin of difference between the value of such investments and their worth is the profitability margin of the insurance industry. This is to say, people invest disproportionately in order to offset possible resource loss. If otherwise, there would be no profit in selling insurance. Much of the investment of resources (i.e., establishing gains) in times of low stress is done in order to build resource reserves for future hard times.

Resource gain or possession of resources is also made important at times of loss or where loss is threatened; that is, gain increases in meaning in the face of loss (Frankl, 1963). This, in part, occurs because people take stock of their resources when loss occurs. In deciding how to act, people must consider their repertoire of coping behaviors and the resources from which they can profitably draw. The fact of loss also focuses gain's greater clarity, as we are aware of things around us by contrast. Even in the face of great personal tragedy such as loss of a loved one, people come to tell of and remember their blessings.

Therefore having and not having arise together.... The ten thousand things rise and fall without cease (LAO TSU, 6th Century B.C.E.).

People enact gain cycles in the wake of loss, in part to offset current resource loss, but also because they become more aware of future losses and look to prevent them. Again, gain here becomes more important because resource loss has served to draw attention to the severe consequences that may follow if loss cycles continue or some future, more pervasive loss occurs. Having experienced loss, gain strategies that might shelter the individual or social group on future occasions are learned and people seek to implement them.

EMPIRICAL EXAMINATION OF LOSS'S SALIENCE: PRINCIPLE 1

If loss is more salient than gain, resource loss should have greater impact on psychological distress than gain. In order to create a resource list to begin to test this principle, we first had groups of students, community residents, and psychologists nominate things they valued. We sought input from university students, church groups, hospital patients, and community residents in the process. After initial groups created a preliminary list of nominated resources, we had additional groups add resources that they felt were important, but that did not already appear on the list, and delete resources that they felt were not widely valued. Groups were also allowed to condense or split apart resources if they felt there was an overarching resource that was descriptive, or where a resource was too overarching. So, apartment and house were combined, but hope and optimism were seen as distinguishable and not covered by "having a positive outlook." This process continued with some 50 small groups, until no new resources were added that had not been deleted by more than one prior group, and until no new deletions were deemed necessary that had not been reinstated previously.

The final list of 74 resources is presented in Table 3.2. In a daylong workshop with a group of Dutch psychologists sponsored by the Dutch Heart Foundation, a similar exercise was conducted without knowledge of the original list. Participants were split into small groups and the nomination and deletion process was repeated. In 3 hours, 56 resources were nominated, all being listed on the original form. The smaller number of resources was probably due to the shorter time element, but whether cultural differences would emerge given more time is open to empirical examination. Nevertheless, the cross-cultural relevance of the list is apparent for at least these two cultures. Although probably not a complete list, it can be seen as comprehensive.

Having the resource list in hand, we had 255 students and 74 community residents indicate whether they had lost or gained each of the resources "recently" and then during the past year (Hobfoll & Lilly, 1993). They did this on two occasions, separated by 3 weeks. Respondents also completed the state and trait versions of Spielberger, Gorsuch, and Lushene's (1970) State–Trait Anxiety Inventory and the Beck Depression Scale (Beck, Ward, Mendelson, Mock, & Erbaugh, 1961). The influence of loss versus gain on psychological distress was then analyzed,[1] relying on both measurement periods to increase the stability of the associations.

The results for the community and student sample were virtually identical. Neither recent resource gain nor resource gain during the past year had appreciable positive (or negative) impact on psychological distress. The effect of gain was essentially zero. Recent resource loss and resource loss during the past year, in contrast, had major negative repercussions for psychological distress. The (absolute) influence of resource loss was 34 times larger on psychological distress than the (absolute) influence of gain in the least distinguishable case.[2] It is also instructive that the effects of resource loss were sizably larger than typically found for life events (Rabkin & Streuning, 1976), suggesting further that the resource method may depict the more central element that is stressful in events. People were deeply and negatively affected when they lost resources but hardly impacted whatsoever when they experienced gain of the selfsame resources.

We also had respondents rank the importance of 74 resources from 1 to 7 (*Very important* to *Not at all important*) (Hobfoll, Lilly, & Jackson, 1992).

Table 3.2. COR Resources

Personal transportation (car, truck, etc.)	Sense of humor	Adequate financial credit
Feeling that I am successful	Stable employment	Feeling independent
Time for adequate sleep	Intimacy with spouse or partner	Companionship
Good marriage	Adequate home furnishings	Financial assets (stocks, property, etc.)
Adequate clothing	Feeling that I have control over my life	Knowing where I am going with my life
Feeling valuable to others	Role as a leader	Affection from others
Family stability	Ability to communicate well	Financial stability
Free time	Providing children's essentials	Feeling that my life has meaning/purpose
More clothing than I need*	Feeling that my life is peaceful	Positive feeling about myself
Sense of pride in myself	Acknowledgment of my accomplishments	People I can learn from
Intimacy with one or more family members	Ability to organize tasks	Money for transportation
Time for work	Extras for children	Help with tasks at work
Feelings that I am accomplishing my goals	Sense of commitment	Medical insurance
Good relationship with my children	Intimacy with at least one friend	Involvement with church, synagogue, etc.
Time with loved ones	Money for extras	Retirement security (financial)
Necessary tools for work	Self-discipline	Help with tasks at home
Hope	Understanding from my employer/boss	Loyalty of friends
Children's health	Savings or emergency money	Money for advancement or self-improvement (education, starting a business)
Stamina/endurance	Motivation to get things done	
Necessary home appliances	Spouse/partner's health	Help with child care
Feeling that my future success depends on me	Support from co-workers	Involvement in organizations with others who have similar interests
Positively challenging routine	Adequate income	Financial help if needed
Personal health	Feeling that I know who I am	Health of family/close friends
Housing that suits my needs	Advancement in education or job training	
Sense of optimism		
Status/seniority at work		
Adequate food		
Larger home than I need*		

*Although luxury resources, groups repeatedly admitted investing more in these two luxury resources than other resources they deemed more important.

There was large overlap among the student and community sample, but consistent with developmental notions already discussed, the younger sample was more concerned with achievement and material resources necessary for this stage of life. The community sample was more concerned with health and family-related resources. Nevertheless, for each sample, resource loss was the critical factor.

Gain's Secondary Function

We examined the influence of resource gain using a second analytic strategy, again following COR theory. COR theory, as I outlined earlier, predicts that gain will become important in the context of loss. This was noted in two ways. First, those who experienced more loss of resources also reported more resource gain. In a number of studies, we have noted this pattern, which is typically of low order but stable across samples. Also, if resource gain is important in the context of loss, those who have experienced loss should find gain more important. This is precisely what we found. Resource gain acted to decrease psychological distress, but its impact was felt in the context of people having experienced losses. So, for example, the gain of time with one's family, of money, and even of love in itself is not heralded by people as terribly salient, at least in terms of their mental health. However, when people experience a period of resource loss, then the gain of these same resources becomes important to their psychological well-being.

The value of resource gain may also have a strong appraisal component. What I mean here by *appraisal* is not appraisal as bias, but appraisal as focus of attention. During times of high stress in particular, a number of researchers have found that people pay more attention to what resources they have during such periods. Antonovsky (1979), Bettelheim (1960) and Frankl (1963) all made special note of this in their studies of Holocaust survivors. Their common finding was that meaning was for many found in its most significant sense amid the ultimate resource losses of the death camp experience. This also may explain, in part, why the participants in our study of loss versus gain report greater gains as losses increase. The fact of their losses turns their attention to their resources, and they are motivated to look for positive aspects of their lives that may aid their stress response in the face of losses. They do so in order to cope emotionally, which would be adaptive in itself. This process may also be the product of a resource search strategy as people are keyed to respond to the destructive sequelae of major losses and the secondary losses that are likely to follow in their wake. By focusing attention to resource gains and resources that are possessed, they can better array and align their resources to respond, survive, and emerge to a more hopeful future.

A number of personality theorists have argued that negative events may be keyed to negative affect and positive events to positive affect in a kind of dual channel of emotionality (Watson & Pennebaker, 1989; Zautra & Reach, 1983). This might suggest that our findings concerning the salience of loss compared to gain is an artifact of our studying negative emotions. According to this argument, were we to examine positive emotions, we would find that gain is more impactful. Furthermore, others have questioned whether the reporting of positive and negative events is little more than a matter of personality style (Costa & McCrae, 1990; DePue & Monroe, 1986). More negative, or neurotic, individuals thus might be reporting both negative events and negative emotions, and not necessarily experiencing negative events. These questions were addressed by Suh, Diener, and Fujita (1996) in a study of college students. They found that negative events, where resources were likely to be lost, were related not only to greater negative affect, but also to less positive affect. Positive events, which were likely to result in resource gains, were unrelated to negative or positive affect. Indeed, negative events had 254 times greater impact on positive affect than did positive events! Interestingly, negative and positive events had equivalent impact on life satisfaction, suggesting that resource gain may influence this particular aspect of well-being.

Suh et al. also investigated whether the influences of negative and positive events were sustained after neurotic, or negativistic, style was controlled. They found here that neither extroversion nor neuroticism appreciably reduced the significant impact of negative events on either positive or negative affect. This evidence both supports COR theory and defends it against some important alternative interpretations.

RESOURCE INVESTMENT: PRINCIPLE 2

Principle 2 of COR theory states:

People must invest resources in order to protect against resource loss, recover from losses, and gain resources.

A number of stress theories have underscored the role of resources in the stress process. Lazarus and Folkman (1984) suggest that resources set the stage for what people appraise as stressful and the type of coping they employ. Holahan and Moos (1991) have studied how personal and social resources act in tandem to buffer the negative impact of stress. Antonovsky (1979) saw a sense of coherence as orchestrating other resources in defense of the self when stress was encountered. Each of these models, when referring to psychological resources such as self-esteem or sense of control, tie into the earlier psychodynamic tradition that depicted ego resiliency as a central dimension of mental health and especially of the work of the ego psychologists such as Karen Horney (1937, 1950) and later Eric Erikson (1958), with his focus on the formation of a strong personal identity. When more concrete resources such as employment, marriage, and finances are referred to, they link to more sociological traditions that have long considered material resources to underpin mental and physical health (see Allen & Britt, 1983).

COR theory builds on these traditions, but also departs from them in meaningful ways. Other theories place resources as a progenitor of coping, but COR theory suggests that resources are the central organizing feature of the stress experience. Stress occurs when resources are lost or threatened, and people use resources to prevent or offset loss and to make other resource gains. This investment of resources occurs by a number of mechanisms. Although I couch this discussion in economic language as denoted by the very word *investment*, I illustrate that it is not a cold or detached economy and is commonly used as much in the language of love as of finance.

The first mechanism of resource investment is the outright expenditure of a resource. This may occur, for example, where money or time is invested in order to prevent other resource loss, protect against multiple losses, or invest in hopes of further resource gain. Once invested through the process of outright expenditure of the resource, the resource is lost (Schönpflug, 1985) and this price must be mapped in the equation of the value of such coping efforts. We hear this in the expression, "Is that time well spent?" Knowledge is a resource that similarly loses value when invested. If someone has knowledge, it is valuable to the extent it is not "common knowledge." A secretary who knows the file system is indispensable, unless the system is known by others. A professor who knows only what others know has no special advantage. Knowledge is often artificially guarded through patents and copyrights exactly for the purposes of preserving its value when it is invested. This artificial mechanism allows those with special knowledge to use it for some common good without having its value diminished. Indeed, this is currently one of the major trade disagreements between two of the largest world economies, China and the United States, as China has not developed a system, or perhaps an inclination, to guard proprietary knowledge that the United States might import to her.

A second kind of resource investment involves risking the resource, without outright expenditure. On a concrete level, money or property can be placed as collateral. One can continue to live in the collateralized home, but it is lost if the expected gain by which the investment was made does not transpire. Trust in others is a much more abstract resource but can be seen in similar terms. We invest our trust in relationships. If the relationships succeed, trust grows. However, if we are deceived, our trust may be damaged, especially if it is a significant relationship. Likewise, we can see how self-esteem can be risked. A surgeon states in a case conference how she views a complicated case, perhaps disagreeing with a senior colleague. Making her views public, she has taken a risk-investment approach, putting her self-esteem on the line. If in subsequent weeks the case develops as she argued, her self-esteem will be enhanced. However, if she is wrong, the senior colleague might well make it known in a later case conference, and her self-esteem will be publicly effaced.

Resource investment may also occur directly or through substitution. Following a loss of love, an individual may look for a new loved one. Losing money, another might try to develop a secondary strategy for financial gain. These would be examples of direct investment—resource for resource. Often, however, individuals substitute resources. A failure at love might motivate someone to seek self-esteem by investing further in his career. A financial failure might lead a second individual to seek a sense of personal accomplishment by investing in spiritual endeavors. Because many basic resources such as self-esteem, sense of mastery, shelter, and food may be achieved through multiple paths, either direct or substitute investment can often act well enough, if not equally well, to obtain, protect, and foster key resources.

Resource investment may act to offset the loss, protect against threat, or contribute toward gain of the same resource or another resource. Social support may be employed to bolster self-esteem (Cohen & Wills, 1985), such as when individuals call on social support to preserve their self-esteem in the midst of a divorce. But social support may also be used to garner further social support. For example, in order to gain support on a job search, someone may call on close friends and family to help him or her make important business connections.

In each of these instances, the investment of resources comes at a price, or at least a potential price. Favors require implied or declared obligations, money invested in one direction is unavailable for other use, and time spent cannot be revisited. Schönpflug's (1985) work in this area is important because he outlines both theoretically and in carefully conducted laboratory analogs how individuals consider and evaluate resource investment. Again, this is as true in love as in the stock exchange, as it is not just financially that we consider the cost of our investments. Indeed, many people are more comfortable taking financial than interpersonal risks, and the arena of love is perhaps the most carefully guarded.

How people determine which investments to make and in which instances to make them is on one level a matter of individual decision making. People consider their options and their goals and make choices accordingly. According to Pearlin (1993), however, many of these choices are actually elements of people's social roles, and so not so much choices as following of established role patterns. Retribution for an insult in eighteenth-century British upper-class society required "satisfaction," which meant a public apology or a duel. Duels were so common that the officer corps of the

British Navy and Army had to outlaw them so as to not see their best officers (or perhaps second-best) decimated. Such a course would be more common today for members of rival street gangs. In societies guided by strong community norms, such as Japan, the social role requirements that dictate stress response are rather strict. Similarly, in close communitarian societies such as among Mormons or Hasidic Jews, there is an expectation to rely on the wisdom of ritualized laws and elders to determine stress response. Within the Catholic Church, guilt and anxiety are assuaged through penance meted out by a priest. Stress-related decisions, such as whether a Hasidic Jew should have another child if a child is lost, or if a woman has had difficult pregnancies, is made by the Rebbe (the spiritual leader of the community). How to grieve, how long to grieve, and when to return to partial and then full functioning following death are all prescribed. Individual responses are limited within demarcated boundaries of behavior.

In the United States, where these norms are looser, we see the rise of more legalistic, contractual relationships to guide retribution (Fukuyama, 1995). However, even within the United States, Nisbett (1993) has discussed the historic herding roots of the culture of many white, Southerners which, in turn, are a product of Celtic culture from the borderlands of Scotland and Ireland. Those descendants of this culture, being more bound by honor, are more likely to find insult or threat stressful, and therefore more likely to respond violently. Seen this way, one of the most ruggedly individualistic responses—the shoot from the hip response—is depicted as a culturally ingrained cognition with a prescribed stress response for alleviation of the attendant distressing emotions.

The terms of stress reactions, which resources were to be invested and how, were in many instances carefully dictated by the Bible. Quite opposite its common usage, the adage "an eye for an eye" comes from Biblical text that ritualized terms of resource allotment in order to avoid violent overreactions commonly following a stressful loss. The meaning of the text is that you were *not allowed to take more than the worth of an eye* if an eye was lost. Hence, if a laborer lost an arm at work, the employer was bound to repay the family the worth of that arm and not more (Hertz, 1958). Thus, when a stressful experience required revenge to expiate the emotional upheaval of the wronged family, the family could without resort of violence have their grievance redressed and find personal peace at having righted the wrong done their loved one. Criminal courts today have only recently allowed victims of crime to know of the sentencing and parole of the wrongdoer, for similar reasons of limiting their stress response.

And if a man smite the eye of his bondman [indentured servant], or the eye of his bondwoman, and destroy it, he shall let him go free for his eye's sake. And if he smite out his bondman's tooth, or his bondwoman's tooth, he shall let him go free for his tooth's sake ... and if one man's ox hurt another's, so that it dieth; then they shall sell the live ox, and divide the price of it; and the dead also they shall divide. (Exodus 21: 26–35)

Thus, a code was laid down not only to decide grievances but also to limit the emotional distress derived from that grievance in a manner that allowed people to live in a community. Still, especially in a society where cultural traditions are weakened, there are many individual choices to be made in how resources are invested in the service of stress responding. In part, these choice follow logical paths, because people attempt to optimize their resource investment based on past experience (Baltes, 1987). However, individual appraisal (Lazarus & Folkman, 1984) and false self views (Markus & Nurius, 1986) are likely to bias personal reactions and create greater individual differences. As noted by Shore (1996), "Not all experience is culturally modeled to the same degree. And cultures differ in the extent to which certain classes of experiences are modeled for individuals" (p. 46).

Examination of Principle 2

Schönpflug (1985) conducted innovative and elegant experiments to test the principle of resource investment and its costs. He developed computer simulations wherein participants were allowed to invest resources to solve stressful problems. Although a laboratory analog, he illustrated how decision making under stress allowed for consideration of the costs of the resource investment. Prior work on stress had concentrated on the benefits and outcomes of coping but ignored the costs. The amount of action to take and, indeed, the decision to not act are all possible stress responses.

Interestingly, only when we consider the cost of action can we fully understand the choice not to act. Given the overwhelming bias in favor of control-taking strategies, nonaction has been depicted as a poor coping response. Schönpflug's work illuminates how, under low resource conditions, nonaction can be a favored strategy, as people employ nonaction to conserve resources for everyday challenges or future stress circumstances that might not allow a choice as to the need to act. His research also reveals the class bias of stress research, in that by assuming action or active problem solving as the best course, theorists were not accounting for the depleted or impoverished resource reservoir of the poor. Not that the poor cannot have high self-esteem and sense of mastery, but the likelihood of sustaining such high resource levels and the number of circumstances demanding the investment of these resources places the poor at a considerable disadvantage. Bold action is a strategy consistent with a richly endowed resource reservoir.

In general, the strategy for employing the military is this: If your strength is ten times theirs, surround them; if five, then attack them; if double, then divide your forces. If you are equal in strength to the enemy, you can engage him. If fewer, you can circumvent him. If outmatched, you can avoid him. Thus a small enemy that acts inflexibly will become the captives of a large enemy.... One who knows neither the enemy nor himself will invariably be defeated in every engagement (Sun Tzu, 6th Century B.C.E., p. 178–179)

In order to further examine the costs of resource investment, we investigated the influence of loss and gain of resources on a sample of 92 middle-class, mostly European-American pregnant women who were either primarily homemakers versus those who also worked outside of the home (Wells, Hobfoll, & Lavin, 1997). We hypothesized that according to COR theory, resource loss would have a greater impact on women's anger and depression than resource gain, as predicted by Principle 1. We further hypothesized that women who had multiple roles would be making additional resource investments and that, according to Principle 2, this would make them more vulnerable to resource loss. Because they have invested greater resources, they had greater expectations for gain and were less resilient to resource loss because so many resources were already fully taxed. In this regard, repeated research has found that women who work outside of the home and have families expend much greater effort, have less free time, sleep less, and work a much greater total number of hours than homemakers (Hochschild, 1989). However, they are generally sustained by the greater rewards attendant to these multiple roles. COR theory predicts that when these gains are not made, their distress will be greater because they have made greater resource investment, and hence experience greater net loss.

These hypotheses do not necessarily follow from other stress theories. Baruch and Barnett (1986) have predicted that overall role quality is what influences both employed and unemployed women. COR theory suggests instead that negative role qualities in the form of resource loss are predominant, whereas positive role qualities in terms of resource gains will have less influence. Furthermore, resource investment hypotheses have suggested that women with multiple roles have a general stress advantage due to their greater access to privileges and rewards (Marks, 1977; Waldron & Jacobs, 1989). COR theory does not diverge from this point, but specifies a special case, such that if under conditions of high resource investment resource losses do occur, women with dual work and family roles will be especially vulnerable.

Our results provided support for our hypotheses. Resource loss was strongly related to both greater depression and anger. Resource gain, in contrast, was related marginally to lower depression, but unrelated to anger. The magnitude of the influence of loss compared to gain is remarkable,

9.5 times greater in the case of depression and 33 times greater in the case of anger.[3] This further supports the notion that positive change is not stressful, and that it in fact limits stress, albeit more moderately than negative change induces stress. Finally, although resource loss was related to greater depression for both groups, the influence of loss was significantly greater for the employed women. We followed up women postpartum and again found similar influences for resource loss and gain, suggesting that these are causal processes. The longitudinal data give credence to the argument that it is not the case that depressed people accentuate their losses and minimize their gains, but rather that resource loss and gain have prospective influences over time, as COR theory posits.

The work of the German sociologist, Johannes Siegrist has been particularly instructive on the issue of resource investment. Siegrist presents a model consistent with the COR thesis that investment of resources without adequate compensation is a highly stress-generating condition. His studies are both insightful and methodologically sophisticated, because he crosses from the individual level to the level of social structures in a manner that is unusual for either a psychologist or sociologist. By using medical and physiological outcome data, he also avoids the potential confounding of self-report that dominates in this field of research. Siegrist (1996) postulates that conditions of high effort and low reward will produce high stress levels and translate to heart disease and related disorders. In keeping with the general thesis of this volume, he also emphasizes that what is particularly threatened in these circumstances is the stability of attachment to social structures that ensure and preserve identity and economic viability. When effort is expended at work without adequate reward, the fabric of the social contract between people and society is itself threatened.

In a series of elegant studies, Siegrist and his colleagues find solid support for their theorizing and by extension for this prediction of COR theory (Siegrist, 1996; Siegrist, Peper, Junge, Cremer, & Seidel, 1990). For example, in a large sample of blue-collar workers, he illustrates substantially increased odds of coronary heart disease, sudden cardiac death, and acute myocardial infarction of between 6 and 8 times under conditions of high effort–reward imbalance; that is, when workers have to contribute a high degree of effort (resource investment) with little reward (resource payoff), their risk of serious heart-related ailments increases substantially. In a separate examination of middle-class managers, Siegrist shows increased risk by a factor of 3 to almost 7 for dangerous levels of LDL cholesterol and hypertension, respectively, under the combination of high effort–reward imbalance. As Siegrist cogently emphasizes, such conditions are often unavoidable due to the need to remain employed and the risk to resources if one attempts to exit from these stressful circumstances. Hence, there may be added stressfulness because as high investment–low reward conditions continue, individuals become increasingly aware of not only the difficulty of their situation, but also the decreased control they have over their destiny.

RESOURCE SPIRALS AND THE LINKAGES OF RESOURCES

Until now, I have been discussing resources as an aggregate notion. Four corollaries of COR theory outline a set of rules that allows for specific predictions as to how resources operate over time. Evidence supporting these corollaries will await later chapters, but it is instructive to outline them along with the basic tenet and two central principles of COR theory presented in this chapter in order to complete the theoretical basis of COR theory.

> COROLLARY 1: *The first corollary of COR theory posits that those with greater resources are less vulnerable to resource loss and more capable of orchestrating resource gain. Conversely, those with fewer resources are more vulnerable to resource loss and less capable of achieving resource gain.*

This corollary further suggests that for those who are low in resources, gain spirals will be fragile. Moreover,

> *those who lack resources are more likely to experience extreme consequences, as without adequate resource reserves they are less likely to have resources to invest in the wake of initial losses.*

Corollary 1 follows from the fact that resources may be used either individually or in combination and that stress often makes multiple demands that call for different combinations of resources. Those with greater resources may parlay resources off one another. Social favors can be used to bolster self-esteem or be exchanged for financial credit in the form of a cosigner on a loan. Because offsetting resource loss demands so many resources and may fit only specialized resources, those with impoverished resource pools are less likely to have the resources that best fit the particular stress demands and may not have any resources available in reserve to meet the specific situational challenges presented. This same corollary follows for families, organizations, and communities, as when individuals join in social groups their combined resources act as a common defense and lack of resources makes them jointly vulnerable, be it economically, socially, or psychologically.

Following job loss, a woman who has a broad resource pool, including education, social support, savings, insurance, and a sense of mastery, has a combination of resources that she can rally in her defense. As her sense of mastery ebbs, she may call on social support to lift her spirits and confidence (Pearlin, Leiberman, Menaghan, & Mullan, 1981). Without salary, she can call on savings and favors to make her passage through a job-search period (Kessler, Turner, & House, 1988; Wellman, 1985). Her counterpart who lacks these resources will be more greatly affected because he not only experiences the initial loss but also lacks a resource armamentarium that can be called on to address the initial and subsequent losses entailed in job loss. With little education, he has poorer fit to possible new job opportunities. He lacks social support or receives the kind of support that encourages his poor sense of mastery (Hobfoll, Shoham, & Ritter, 1991; Kobasa & Pucetti, 1983) and feels more greatly threatened because, lacking insurance, he is aware of his further vulnerability.

COROLLARY 2: The second corollary of COR theory is that those who lack resources are not only more vulnerable to resource loss, but that initial loss begets future loss.

Because individuals, groups, and organizations rely on resources to address losses, and because stress results from resource loss, at each iteration of the cycle, there are fewer resources to rally in defense or to invest in gain cycles that might counteract the influence of stress. With a depleted resource pool, future challenges are increasingly less likely to be met and a downward spiral increases in momentum. This further suggests that loss cycles will have initially higher velocity for less resource-endowed individuals, as they are from the beginning in a resource-challenged state and likely to have their resources already organized in protection of the self, family, or social system. Thus, this corollary predicts that loss cycles will have advancing momentum and strength (i.e., speed and impact). This point was made cogently in the last century by John Stuart Mill (1848), who stated that wage inequality and other rewards tend to be disproportional to equitable principles of compensation, such that those low in resources are neither adequately rewarded nor adequately protected from ongoing resource loss.

Returning to our prior example, the initial job loss may well have reduced the woman's sense of mastery. The process of a job search places further challenges on this same sense of mastery in its now weakened state. What might be a normal family challenge to finances, such as a major household repair, taxes the financial reserves that were set aside for groceries, rent, and heat. At each spin of the cycle, fewer resources are available and greater impact is felt. Like the retreat of an army, if the retreat is organized and supplies are plentiful, it can be made with little loss of life. However, a disorganized retreat with broken supply lines quickly becomes a rout. Still, she is much better off than her male counterpart, who began the loss cycle already in some jeopardy. For him, even the original losses may prove devastating, and his ability to respond will quickly deteriorate.

On the systems level, a community that confronts a major layoff at a local factory will likewise have greater resilience in weathering the storm if other businesses can offset the overall economic strain and sense of malaise that invades the community with large numbers unemployed. Other businesses can absorb workers, provide social welfare, and invest in job diversification if the community is well endowed with resources. If they are not, initially, losses will be quickly followed by collateral loss that can envelope the community, because each loss meets a less resilient system with weakened and committed economic, social, and psychological resources (Giel, 1990; deJong, 1995).

> COROLLARY 3: *Corollary 3 mirrors Corollary 2, but pertains to resource gains and gain cycles. Because loss and gain are inequivalent, however, they are not exact opposites and differ in meaningful ways. Corollary 3 states that those who possess resources are more capable of gain, and that initial resource gain begets further gain.*

Different processes underlie gain investment than loss defense. Gain typically involves risking resources in order to meet goals and aspirations. As such, the motivation for gain either is a product of desiring to better one's self or the social system (e.g., family, organization) or may be intended to offset future potential loss (Aspinwall & Taylor, 1997). In either case, the need for gain is not as imminent as the need for acting to offset loss. If initial gains are made, still greater resources become available for investment, as with resource surpluses individuals and social systems are less vulnerable and so do not necessarily need to rely on these resource surpluses for reserves. Because resource loss is more potent than resource gain, gain cycles are also predicted to have less momentum (e.g., speed) and less impact than loss cycles.

A rural farm family with enough children, shared confidence in their ability to succeed, and credit may look to acquire new land and perhaps send a child to the university for advanced training in agriculture. Initial gains might increase knowledge of how best to bring crops to market and allow for further investment in machinery, and may change family beliefs about their educational abilities. A rural farm family with few children, little money, and no shared sense of competence or credit is more likely to refrain from attempts to acquire new land and may need to send older children off the farm to find local employment in order to provide cash for groceries. This further weakens the ability of the family to plant and harvest crops. Because loss is a more powerful motivator than gain, however, even the resource-rich family will likely be cautious with investments because it must plan for a potential poor harvest that would hit harder were it to have its resources already committed elsewhere.

COROLLARY 4: Corollary 4 posits that those who lack resources are likely to adopt a defensive posture to guard their resources.

This strategy is often denigrated by resource-endowed individuals and social organizations, because it is seen as shortsighted. However, it is actually a logical and sound strategy. With few resources, Schönpflug (1985) has clearly shown that costs of resource investment may outstrip demands and make the individual or organization dangerously vulnerable. A defensive posture holds a maximum of resources in reserve for the possibility of having to forestall the impact of some future, major loss sequence. The poor farm family is correct in refraining from resource investment, because there are enough likely threats that before its investment can pay off, it will have its position compromised. Again, this may sound overly financial and pertain to more material investments. However, research also suggests that those who have experienced attachment losses may be less willing to commit trust to new relationships (Hazan & Shaver, 1994). Similarly, many economically advantaged dual-career families have decided to have few children, not because they cannot financially afford them or might not want them, but because they recognize that nurturance requires time and energy and these are resources in which they are impoverished (Hobfoll & Hobfoll, 1994).

Corollary 4 also explains why those who lack resources may utilize denial, even though this is ostensibly an inefficient defense mechanism (Breznitz, 1983). By using denial, they allow for a blunting of the emotional impact of loss and can still keep resources in reserve. Those with greater resources are less needy of the use of this defensive posture, but for those with few resources, it is a fair choice.

INDIVIDUAL PERCEPTIONS, SHARED PERCEPTIONS, AND SOCIAL REALITY

The cognitive revolution in psychology initially may have encouraged a construal of the reality of stress as nothing more than that which is in the mind of the beholder (Aldwin, 1994; Lazarus & Folkman, 1984). This idiographic approach may be criticized as overly mentalistic and denying the reality that people face, but in actuality, it also allows for an anchoring of perception in real-world phenomena. Placing it on a continuum with other stress-related theories, it is the most individualistic, the least culturally based, and the least social. However, it is a viewpoint with social value, because ultimately perceptions of resources are individualized. In cases where the target group is homogeneous on key resources (e.g., shares a common social class, education, and setting), differences in individual impressions of those resources will be paramount. Also, appraisal theories are not acultural. Rather, they allow the individual to be the final arbiter of all phenomena that are perceived historically, culturally, familially, and phenomenologically. It is also fair to say that the appraisal advocates criticize COR theory as failing to do more than replace appraisal with other terms, such as *valued resource*, which themselves are products of appraisal (Aldwin, 1994; Lazarus, 1991).

However, even within the individually based cognitive revolution there is increasing acknowledgment that construals of reality are based on social roles, societal norms, cultural boundaries, and patterns that are implanted developmentally in accordance with social class and status (Cantor, 1990; Markus & Nurius, 1984). Moreover, minority and feminist scholars have strongly argued that resources and differential access to and possession of resources is the primary mechanism by which such stressful social phenomena as racism and sexism operate (Allen & Britt, 1983; Blumberg, 1991; Watts, 1992). Loss of objective resources is also thought to be the primary mechanism challenging the elderly according to Baltes's (1987) groundbreaking work on aging and culture. These theorists also acknowledge the role of individual perception, but emphasize the objective qualities of resources and the shared evaluation or appraisal that is generally common to individuals of a given culture, class, or family.

It is, of course, possible, as Diener and Fujita (1995) and we (Hobfoll et al., 1992) have attempted to assess individuals' appraisals of resources that are commonly held to be valuable. Such an approach allows for a joint understanding of personal appraisal, taken in the context of a pool of resources that is culturally valued. By knowing individuals' culture and setting, we are made aware of their likely set of values. Once we know this, there is certain utility in then knowing their personal appraisals.

This debate has enormous political ramifications that psychology and psychiatry have judiciously avoided. For example, many psychotherapists subscribe to an individualist appraisal model and believe that stress is best conceptualized via the self-report of their clients. Others have challenged this approach as encouraging racist, sexist, and classist patterns, because it leads directly to the supposition that change is also in the mind's eye and not in meaningful social or personal action (Adleman & Enguidanos, 1995; Aponte, Rivers, & Wohl, 1995). A battered woman who is without financial resources may justify her partner's violence, because as Laing (1969) has argued, she is mystified by a system that encourages her to play a victim's role. Change must be behavioral, and resource limitations are likely to be the stumbling blocks upon which intervention falters. For this reason, Rappaport (1981), arguing for empowerment, does speak of perceived empowerment but bases it on the real needs versus rights conflicts that are omnipresent in our society. Individual perception of empowerment, in the absence of actual empowerment, may be the most disadvantageous position.

COR theory and other resource-based perspectives do not deny the value of appraisal, but as outlined in Chapter 2, they suggest that appraisal has a substantive cultural and objective component. Appraisal theorists' tendencies toward individualization and mentalization are phenomena that are the product of rugged individualist culture and have never been broadly accepted outside of psychology. In this regard, sociologists have typically relied on social structure and social roles (Merton, 1968; Parsons, 1951), and anthropologists have focused on culturally based patterns that hold across individuals (Shore, 1996). Although clinical psychologists and psychiatrists are most likely to do their work in isolated offices with isolated individuals, this is not the only, or even necessarily the optimal, mode of intervention. Rather, it is a culturally derived norm that London (1964) aptly called the work of the secular priesthood. So saying, it is also critical to acknowledge that if individualism is a product of a given culture, that those who are members of that culture may be the best served by the corresponding rituals, To the extent that people are isolated, cognitively oriented, and live lives in which they become decreasingly involved in organized religious or cultural groups, their personal perceptions will have greater play (Shore, 1996).

Nevertheless, culture is actively transferred today through the media, which often define how we think, what we value, how we dress, who we admire, and how we behave. This tendency is so pervasive and insidious that not only countries that overtly detest American culture, such as Iran, limit their population's exposure to American movies and the American "way of thinking;" France also has limited export of American films, and the development of a French Disneyworld was fought on the basis of its Americanizing French culture, which many felt was already changing its values to a more individualistic and less social model than French cultural advocates would like. Hence, although we may not immediately recognize the power of our own culture on individuals' cognitions within an individualistic society, these processes are nonetheless at work.

> Human thought is both social and public—that its natural habitat is the house yard, the marketplace, and the town square. Thinking consists not of "happenings in the head" (though, happenings there and elsewhere are necessary for it to occur) but on a traffic in ... significant symbols. (Geertz, 1973, p. 45)

CONCLUSIONS

As I have sought to illustrate in this chapter, COR theory makes specific predictions that can be placed in either a larger cultural context or more personally defined individual space. The hypotheses that derive from the theory are comprehensive, but testable, and as such serve the scientific requirement of being available to rejection (Popper, 1972). Initial research suggests that a resource-based perspective has considerable heuristic value and that predictions tend to be supported with greater strength than has typically been noted in the stress literature. The magnitude of this difference is significant.

Questions will continue to arise as to where on the continuum from objective reality, to socially shared reality, to individual perception, to outright fanciful appraisal the stress process is best represented. COR theory allows for an approach that may apply to various points on this continuum, but that may be best represented by the midrange on the spectrum. As Guisinger and Blatt (1994) have proposed, evolutionary and cultural pressures result in two developmental lines that are simultaneously represented, interpersonal relatedness and self-definition, and any theory that adequately addresses and provides insights about the stress process must answer to this inherent dialectic between an objectively delineated environment, which is in large part social, and an inwardly defined self.

Perhaps most important, COR theory signals a change from reinforcement-based, end-goal-oriented approaches that have dominated in psychology since the time of Skinner. Specificially, people are not motivated so much to receive reinforcers and avoid punishment as they are motivated to construct and preserve the conditions that will allow them to do so. This differerence is fundamental, because it emphasizes process, not outcome. It means that people seek to obtain, retain, protect, and foster resources not only to ensure a single outcome, but also to preserve and enhance their "average" outcome over time. This translates to their constructing pathways within their own lives, their family traditions, and their broader social network that will ensure the preservation of means to these ends. Moreover, it suggests that rather than the achievement of reinforcers, people will make conservation-based efforts first toward preservering what resources they have. Once these resources are solidified, they will direct themselves toward enhancing further resource gains, but always with an eye on guarding against resource loss and diminishment.

NOTES

1. Analyses were conducted using structural equation modeling. For a complete description of analyses, see Hobfoll and Lilly (1993).
2. "Absolute" here refers to the size of the relationship, ignoring its sign or direction. So, a correlation of $-.50$ is larger than a correlation of $+.25$, because we ignore the minus and plus signs. The effect size of the underlying relationship is greater.

3. This is the second instance in which I compare the effect size of loss versus gain as an indication of the enormous influence of loss compared to the rather marginal influence of gain. I should point out, however, that effect-size calculations are misleading in the case where one relationship (that between resource gain and outcomes) approaches zero. I include the effect sizes simply to state the point that resource loss has an appreciably greater direct impact than gain.

4

Majesty, Mastery, and Malignment

Stress theory has proceeded under the most naive of assumptions that all persons are subject to the same set of rules governing stress resistance. What I mean by this is not that people are confronted with different stressors based on gender, ethnicity, and class, for this is well accepted. Nor that people have different resources, perceptions, or way of dealing with stress, because this is the essence of most stress research today. Rather, there is the assumption that given the right resources, appropriate appraisals, and the equal amount of stressful demands, there is an equivalence across persons. In this chapter, I develop a new model that extends Conservation of Resources (COR) theory based on the premise that environments and people interact differently based on individuals' social status, gender, ethnicity, and personal attributes. Said simply, for different classes of people the rules change. Rather than seeing the environment as static, this model emphasizes that what we view as individual traits and resources are given differential worth, flexibility, and potency dependent on social structures evidenced in the society. Rather than soft, background characteristics, I argue that this influence is a defining process in stress and coping.

I term this addition to COR theory, the FALL model, which is an acronym for **F**itting, **A**ccommodation, **L**imitation, and **L**eniency. These four principles are expanded using COR theory as a backdrop and further developing the theme that stress is a phenomenon concerning *individuals-nested-in families-nested-in social organizations*. A basic premise of the FALL model is that modern social structures[1] allow and ensure that people will operate under different sets of rules, while at the same time strongly asserting that they are being treated the same. This paradox crosses boundaries of games, work, family life, and other challenging settings. Indeed, we assert the principle of fairness in order to justify the actual inequality and to perpetuate it. I begin with a few examples.

Majesty is a concept that may be drawn on to understand how the *differential rules paradox* operates. Privileged people or those who are of a privileged class are allowed greater leeway in their behavior. It is generally acknowledged in professional basketball that those with greater talent, the superstars, are treated differently by referees whose absolute and unequivocal job is not to treat anyone by anything other than the rules. As superstar Michael Jordan glides toward the basket, suspended in air, defying gravity and the rule that you are only allowed one and one-half steps after stopping to dribble the ball, no referee's whistle is blown. In the very next play, the move is copied by some upstart rookie and the shrill blast of the whistle fills the building. The league and its commissioner are unequivocal in asserting that that this does not occur, at the same time knowing that all know that it does and will continue. It is part of the game, and all but the purist can forgive it because basketball is, after all, only a game. However, a similar paradox applies to those with greater social status, defined by being attached to the group that is the rule-keeper, those in power. This means that the principle of majesty operates in classrooms, workplaces, and even the home.

Mastery and self-efficacy have been taken to mean a personal attribute, the sense that one believes or that one actually can successfully negotiate through environmental demands (Bandura, 1996; Pearlin & Schooler, 1978; Pearlin et al., 1981). However, what is mastery or self-efficacy if the rules are molded to fit the person-nested-in setting? It is no longer a personal attribute alone, but now becomes a more dynamic concept that includes prejudicial rule keeping within settings. This means that those with mastery may be better able to adjust to their changing position, as status is relative and people change their status based on surroundings. The junior, assistant professor is the senior to her graduate assistants, who are senior to their undergraduate supervisees in a college laboratory setting. Status changes depending on who is present. This also means, however, that those with high status vis-à-vis the society in general are proffered mastery nearly independently of their behavior. Contrariwise, those with very low status, the untouchables, are *persona non grata* across most settings, even within their own homes, they are reminded of their place. Hence, the scope of his mastery is narrowed and limited. General MacArthur could wear non-regulation, personally tailored clothing in an army that demands uniformity of dress and behave belligerently in an army that is intolerant of belligerence, because he was the commanding general. Except, to his commander, President Truman, who was the only individual who could, and did, sanction him.

Malignment occurs for those who are lacking in status, almost independent of their behavior. In law, the rights of a criminal in the United States are greatly reduced (i.e., officially maligned) and the statutes of the 14th Amendment, which guarantees no abridgement of the "privileges or immunities of citizens of the United States," nor any deprivation of "life, liberty, or property," become legally curtailed. In a family setting, a child who becomes the family scapegoat has the sins and transgressions of the family cast upon him, whatever his behavior. In many Native American cultures, the shaman could alternatively punish or cure an individual by maligning a symbol of the person or a symbol of the person's demon. Raised status through attachment to a soul could heal, just as lost status through absence of a soul could end in death (Rogers, 1982). In each of these examples, those who are low in status (i.e., maligned) are not allowed to utilize their resources or must have a greater amount of those resources to receive the same value exchange.

I illustrate in this chapter how these ideas add to and in some ways challenge the assumptions of stress theory and lead to a different way of approaching the stress phenomenon and understanding the stress process. I argue that most of those whom we have asserted are successful copers and the attributes that we have associated with them are in large part illusions of a process by which cultures and social organizations offer a differential set of rules *a priori* and independent of actual coping efforts. Real attributes of persons certainly exist, and those with greater personal resources, such as self-esteem, self efficacy, and mastery, are better equipped to negotiate challenges, threats, and losses that occur. However, the extent to which these resources are actualized, utilized, and realized is in large part a product of differential stigmatization and enobilization.

FITTING RESOURCES, NOT RESOURCE "FIT"

How resources are utilized given environmental demands was highlighted by the work of French and his colleagues (French, Caplan, & Van Harrison, 1982; French, Rogers, & Cobb, 1974), who saw the crux of stress as the fit of resources with environmental demands. Their model significantly advanced stress research at the time of its introduction. Indeed, they were ahead of their time, as their insights have still not been fully incorporated in stress research.

French et al. suggested that it was not the amount of threat or challenge that faced individuals, nor their coping capabilities, that created either stress or its solution. Rather, they argued that it was the fit, or lack of fit, between demands and coping abilities that determined whether stress would occur, and whether individuals would be positioned to overcome challenges. Their major innovation was the concept that the environment and people's resources interacted, and that stress was to be found in their interplay. Furthermore, their model suggested that one could determine the nature of the fit if one knew the character of the stressful demand and the repertoire of resources people had in their resource pool. This model makes a number of assumptions:

1. Individuals have a finite amount of resources.
2. Environmental demands can be answered by specific resources.
3. If individuals have the requisite resources, they will be able to withstand or overcome stress, or even prevent it from occurring.

The resource fit model advanced thinking about stress resistance, because it helped explain why not all individuals were equally influenced by stress and why some resources worked well in particular settings or circumstances, but not others.

Although it is relevant and valuable in its application to any setting, the model has typically been applied to the workplace. Because work tends to be viewed as rule-based (e.g., you have a designated task), this may have also led to the principle limitation in the fit model. Specifically, the fit model is typically depicted in static and mechanistic terms, and its best metaphor as it is studied is the model of the lock and key, wherein both lock and key have fixed properties.

The fit model may have most commonly been applied to work because of both the reality of work and certain myths about work success. It is a reality of work that the stressors are often ones that can be answered by specific skills, as opposed to the more amorphous skills that, say, family stress requires. Thus, only a qualified engineer can design a bridge, and only a creative and qualified engineer can design a product that answers problems that are new or present some advance. Likewise, sales require certain social skills and earning a commission, and keeping one's position often depends on the use of these skills, all the more so in the stress of a shrinking market or greater competition.

The myth of fit, on the other hand, occurs in that businesses have traditionally operated as Old Boys networks and that they wish to believe that those who are coping with the high demands of business are surviving because they are the fittest. This premise is roundly challenged in the work of Korman (1988), who illustrated the differential advancement of white, male Episcopalians in major corporations, many times their *per capita* representation, and at greater rates than Jews, Catholics, and Baptists, even if also white. Powell (1969) similarly found that Episcopalians and Presbyterians have a positive promotability bias working in their favor of five times the level of comparably qualified Jews. Rather than superior adaptation in the face of stress, this illustrates the work of prejudice and the frequent promotion of more inferior employees, the point being that the French fit model promotes the myth that the system is fair and that there is survival of the fittest, embodied as those who have the best resources. This premise, although true to a degree, is also largely false.

French et al.'s model is actually stronger than its presenters allowed, as the theory itself offers a potentially ecologically "thick" model for analysis. The concept of fit, if it is allowed to be a flexible, changing fit that operates within social forces, has exciting ecological promise. It potentially leads to exploration of environmental pressures, demands, and challenges, and the subsequent response and reshaping of environments by those who occupy these settings. Unfortunately, the theory quickly lost its ecological advantage, because French et al. emphasized "perceived fit" rather than dimensions of the ecological space. Moreover, perceived fit was typically conceptualized as a single summary score of the type "How do you judge the perceived fit of your resources with the demands of your job?" The actual demands of the environment or the resources that people bring to bear to combat these demands are seldom measured.

Hence, whereas the fit concept has a richness that allows for a more contextualized understanding of persons-nested-in settings, French et al., and others who adopted their model, removed the settings by highlighting perceptions of fit despite giving objective and subjective factors equal weight in their original theoretical treatise. Perception of resource fit to environmental demands is one dimension of the phenomenon, but we must study both objective and subjective factors in order to distinguish the two. With the switch to perceived fit, we now can no longer know, for example, if women are reporting poor perceived fit in executive positions because they lack certain resources, are being subjected to greater demands, or have a poorer sense of their own worth in a more general sense. Since perceived fit is strongly correlated to self-efficacy, those with a strong sense of self-efficacy perceive the ability to be successful across settings (Bandura, 1997). This relationship suggests that self-efficacy may be the resource that "fits" the challenge, yet it is possible instead that other resources (e.g., social support, status) are answering their demands, but they have been taught to ascribe their success to self-efficacy. It is even possible that they are actually failing, but are laboring under a myth of their own success. A most serious kind of confounding emerges here in terms of backward attributions, such that individuals who feel that they are coping well also may make the backward attribution that it is because their resources matched their demands.

In businesses that objectively measure performance and make personnel decisions based on clear performance criteria, this mythmaking would have to face objective feedback, but this is more typically not the case. More often, work creates workplace cultures that are self-perpetuating. Not just civil service jobs are rife with this problem. Once advanced, many less than competent individuals can enjoy a high degree of perceived fit because others are doing their jobs. Work tasks are often vague, and the actual fit of resources with demands may be avoided, obfuscated, or mythologized. Once a reputation for success or a certain level of stature is obtained, organizations are subject to whim and fancy in making evaluations. Indeed, a trend of the 1980s and early 1990s has been to flatten organizational structures because much of middle management was seen as obsolete, having no contribution to make that warranted their continued employment (Skagen, 1992). Many executives who had perceived fit had their illusions shattered rather abruptly.

Fit and Social Support

Cutrona (1990) and Cutrona and Russell (1990) adopted the resource fit model and creatively applied it to the investigation of fit of different kinds of social support to varied stress circumstances. They also took a methodological step that most workplace investigators avoided, in that they attempted to define the nature of different kinds of stress demands and why certain types of social support would fit those specific demands. This was an adventuresome step, as it avoided vagaries that are often present in stress research that usually adopts a simpler model that allows respondents to jointly assess their resources and the environmental demands in some summary impression of their fit to the setting. Rather, based in part on COR theory, they theorized that emotional support would be more likely to help those who were under emotionally challenging circumstances, especially where there were uncontrollable losses. This followed, they argued, because, given the uncontrollable event, it is emotions that can be modified. Instrumental aid, in turn, would be more likely to fit those who confronted a challenging task where it was possible to control outcomes.

Their results are instructive. Specified types of social support did fit the particular demands of the different kinds of situations they examined. However, the most robust finding suggests that emotional support and esteem support had generalized positive influence across different stressful circumstances; that is, rather than emotional or esteem support having good fit with specific demands, those who possessed these similar kinds of support could fit it to circumstances. This makes a critical point. Fit, as introduced by French et al., indicates a static state, whereas Cutrona and

Russell identified a dynamic molding process whereby a robust kind of support could be shaped to fit the needs of various circumstances. Rather than a lock-and-key approach, this work suggests that people shape the key, and maybe even the circumstances, so that there is a process of fitting. Because Cutrona and Russell (1990) ventured to define the particular characteristics of the resource and demand separately, they were capable of making a breakthrough in disentangling the role of social support in the stress resistance process. In general, this supports the earlier thesis of Cohen and Wills (1985) that emotional and esteem support have broad stress-limiting influences across types of stressors, as they can be translated to fit a variety of needs.

Moving from Static Fit to Dynamic FITTING

The idea of fitting rather than static fit of resources can also be inferred by theoretical work of Thoits (1994). Thoits proffered that certain higher level resources could be seen as what might be construed as management resources. Those who possessed, for example, high levels of mastery might be more capable of selecting, altering, and orchestrating their other resources to match stressful demands. Those lower in these central management resources, in contrast, would not be as facile in managing the symphony of resources that might be at their disposal. Add to this the COR principle that resources contribute to the gain of other resources and it is also apparent that those who possess these higher order resources will likely have more enriched resource armamentaria from which to select, modify, and manage. By suggesting that resources are managed, Thoits avoids the pitfall of depicting stress in the static lock-and-key framework and hints at a more strategic, active, and proactive method of stress responding.

Hence, the first step of the FALL model is the recognition that people actively and reactively act by FITTING resources to demands.

They do so by shaping resources, building an array of resources that have high potential to fit demands, and orchestrating environmental demands to select aspects that they can adjust to given the resources they have at hand or can acquire. We can construct a number of steps in the strategic act of fitting of resources that is implied in this first step of the FALL model.

1. *Shaping one's resources to increase invulnerability, irrespective of circumstances.* By shaping resources proactively, individuals adopt resources that insulate themselves against the potential influence of stress. For example, by accumulation of power in work settings, or of love in more relational

settings, individuals forestall the possibility of resource loss or threat, albeit never in its entirety by any means.

2. *Positioning oneself such that one cannot be easily threatened with resource loss or lose resources.* This is different than building and shaping resources and more in line with what might be called stage setting. By this, I mean that it is often possible to shape the setting so as to limit the potential for loss. For example, by nurturing others who may as a consequence wish to return the obligation or love, or protect their own position, depending on the kind of setting and circumstances (e.g., workplace, family, etc.), one is more insulated from threat.

3. *Accurate estimation of threat of loss or actual loss* if it occurs is the next critical step of fitting resources. Acting too soon, too late, or inappropriately can translate to undue waste of resources and greater ultimate loss. In order to shape and employ resources, individuals must first understand the nature of the stressor.

4. *Assessment of the adequacy of the resources that may be employed to offset loss or increase gain of resources* is the next critical step. It is possible to assess the situation correctly but inaccurately to understand resources that can be utilized directly, altered, or offered in combination from internal or external sources.

5. *Deciding whether internal resources are adequate to address situational demands or whether external resources are warranted.* Individuals calling on external resources must consider that these often come with attendant obligations, and they should consider the implied costs of both coping or not coping through such means (Schönpflug, 1985). This is a question that is further complicated by the fact that not asking for help from colleagues or loved ones can not only be a strategic error but also a social affront that leads to further isolation and social stress (Hobfoll & Stokes, 1988). In more communal cultures, this could result in an irreparable rip in the social fabric.

> Being unconquerable lies with yourself; being conquerable lies with the enemy ...
> Thus one who excels at warfare first establishes himself in a position where he cannot be defeated while not losing [any opportunity] to defeat the enemy.
> For this reason, the victorious army first realizes the conditions for victory, and then seeks to engage in battle. The vanquished army fights first, and then seeks victory (Sun Tzu, 6th Century B.C.E. pp. 183–184).

ADAPTATION

Despite years of research on coping, we know little about the process of adaptation. Coping has been conceptualized in terms of the things that people do when stressful circumstances occur and, in particular, what they do in the midst of stress. Surely, this is one stage of the adaptation process, but it is a narrow band of behavior over an even narrower time span. This has led to findings that show coping to have a limited influence. Indeed, emotion-focused coping is repeatedly found to be associated with negative psychological and health sequelae (Aldwin, 1994). Emotion-focused coping is the private, internal coping that people use to blunt threatening and painful thoughts and feelings. Clearly, if coping is what we do to try to overcome difficulties around the time of their occurrence, this is either a poor choice of efforts or a later-stage effort that people select when they are already experiencing more serious sequelae of stressful circumstances. Seen this way, the positive association with psychological distress and illness stems from emotion-focused coping efforts being made following unsuccessful adaptation, rather than a sign of mobilization of coping effort aimed at stress resolution, problem solving, or resource conservation.

What Lazarus and Folkman (1984) termed *problem-focused coping* is more clearly a potentially successful strategy. Although narrow in some respects in the way it is usually measured (Aldwin, 1994; Stone, Greenberg, Kennedy-Moore, & Newman, 1991), it is, as a general class of behaviors, more of what adaptation is about. People adjust and adapt by doing things to solve their problems. A major limitation, however, is that coping is almost exclusively measured and conceived as what people do in the midst of their problems. Hence, although more closely aligned with the adaptation process, it is still a very limited concept.

Vitaliano and his colleagues (Vitaliano, DeWolfe, Maiuro, Russo, & Katon, 1990; Vitaliano, Russo, & Maiuro, 1987) more broadly addressed the process of adaptation in their investigations. By examining the combination of kinds of coping and, for example, the ratio of emotion to problem-focused coping, they began to unravel the complicated dance of coping. Their work further suggests that the time frame and target of efforts be looked at more broadly and that we avoid seeing coping as what people do in response to a particular problem once that problem is known. Although emotion-focused efforts on their own may be detrimental to people's adaptation, used in combination with problem-solving efforts, emotion-focused coping allows the individual to regroup, reanalyze adaptational strategy, and communicate with others for advice, to replenish emotional and instrumental resources, and to reenter the fray.

My meaning might be better revealed by way of two examples. In chess, as a poor-playing aficionado, I tend to consider how I might respond to an imposing threat of my opponent's pieces. Her knight advances and I find myself boxed in. I parry the threat of her knight, only to find that she has developed the board to isolate and destroy my seemingly valueless pawns.

This, in turn, is a ploy to allow her to threaten my king from an entirely different direction in a swift move of the game to the opposite side of the board. The problem is that I was coping with her threats as they occurred. She was, on the other hand, playing chess. She was implementing a strategy that offered the board (and my pieces) to serve her strengths and minimize the jeopardy of her few weaknesses. She applied pressure to force my moves where she wanted my pieces to be and directed my attention away from where it might actually benefit me. The adaptation is in the overall nature of her strategy, not her individual moves. Nor did it begin when we sat down to play, but rather includes her preparation for the game and her analysis in its aftermath.

Likewise, those less knowledgeable watching soccer think that the game is boring because the goal is not attacked. Experienced observers are aware that the players are adjusting their game to tire their opponent, looking for an inroad at the point of their opponent's weakness, feigning pressure left while hoping for a crossover opportunity to the right, and conserving their resources for the optimal moment of attack. They wish to appear soft where they are strong, and strong where they are soft. They hope to expend their opponent's resources while theirs are still reasonably in tact. And again, their adaptation includes all that went on prior to their arriving at the game, their training, their strategizing, their development, as well as their postgame analysis of victory or defeat and their preparation for the inevitable next game in their schedule.

Broadening the Time Frame and the Processes of Adaptation

To draw the analogy then, coping has been conceptualized as the response to individual moves in chess, addressing the threat on a moment by moment basis. It has what the players do on the field after a play is set in motion and, at most, their personal reanalysis after a play is over. Adaptation is the overall behavior that I perform poorly at chess, my opponent performs well, and professional athletes perform in the larger sense of "the game." I move my knight, bishop, and pawn in the exact same way as my opponent given what I see in front of me, just as coping is measured as what people do in reaction to their circumstances.

This may be precisely why coping research seldom finds major differences in the outcomes of the kinds of coping people select. Play by play coping is rather common across people; it is in the complexity of broadly conceived and implemented strategies where major differences emerge. Our approach has been too immediate and the kinds of included behaviors are too individualized and isolated from the overall "game." My chess coping should include a design that is ever-altering and projecting behind and ahead to adjust strategy. Certainly, some people cope in the narrow band equivalent to how I play chess, but even this is their general strategy.

Optimization and Compensation in the Service of Adaptation

Margret and Paul Baltes (1982, 1990; Baltes, 1987, 1994) have developed a model of adaptation that provides an unusually insightful view of this fuller coping process. The richness of the Baltes model begins with their life-span perspective. During development, they emphasize that there are cumulative and discontinuous processes at work. Life is characterized by constant gains and losses, which they equate with growth and decline, perspectively. Moreover, both development and gains and losses fit into a particular historical space. This historical embeddedness is almost always treated in psychology on a superficial level, if it is considered whatsoever, whereas the Baltes model places historical context as a primary ingredient in adaptation as it dictates what broad social challenges are omnipresent.

A thick contextual paradigm emerges, in contrast, in the sense that development, loss and gain cycles, and history are understood to interact to create a specific panorama that is both broadly shared by others in some sense and individual in another. This perspective demands an interdisciplinary posture, because "a 'purist' psychological view offers but a partial representation of behavioral development from conception to death" (Baltes, 1987, p. 613).

For the Baltes model, the process of adaptation may be described by what they term *selective optimization with compensation* (or SOC model; Baltes, 1987). This process is viewed as both largely prototypical and general to those sharing social and historical context, and specific to the individual's life history and personal development.

> The process of selective optimization with compensation has three features, each indicative of a gain/loss relation: (a) continual evolution of specialized forms of adaptation as a general feature of life-span development; (b) adaptation to the conditions of biological and social aging with its increasing limitation of plasticity; and (c) individual selective and compensatory efforts dealing with evolving deficits for the purpose of life mastery and effective aging. (p. 616)

Optimization involves the process by which individuals, groups, or organizations strategize to select into and out of circumstances that match or do not match their strengths and weaknesses accordingly. This stage is part of the fitting of resources whereby the organism, individual, or group attempts to shape their resources to meet demands and both selects and seeks to mold external circumstances to provide optimal matches. A single father may choose a flexible job close to home so as to optimize his strengths for the task of raising his children. His ability to nurture, care for, chauffeur, and feed three children could be entirely marginalized by the time and energy limitations if he does not select into circumstances that help him realize his potential.

Compensation entails the process of readjusting, changing, increasing, and honing resources to meet changed environmental circumstances or personal resources. For example, Salthouse (1984) found that older typists compensate for their slower reaction time by developing more forward processing of letters and word sequences. Given their decreased personal abilities, they adopt a new strategy that countervails this loss. If optimization is a process of seeking and selecting the situation that best matches an individual or group's talents and capacities, compensation is the process of accepting certain deficits and implementing extra or alternative effort to substitute for nonoptimal approaches.

However, compensation is also the process by which creativity and perhaps wisdom may be generated. Rather than viewing usual paths as optimal, they are in fact often just ordinary status quo. Because adaptation to stress is likely to follow culturally sanctioned and practiced scripts (Cantor, 1990; Nisbett, 1993), obstacles do not necessary impede the true optimum choice as much as they do the standard choice. That is to say, since creative choices may not have been tried, there may not be impediments blocking their application. As women enter executive positions in larger numbers, they may bring fewer dominance-seeking styles to solve problems, which may compensate for their "lack" of inappropriate but standard, overly aggressive behavior. This may aid team building, provide more nurturant management, and, in turn, increase worker morale (Dunahoo, Geller, & Hobfoll, 1996; Martin, 1993).

An excellent illustration of the point of compensation that is optimal to usual practice comes from early American football. Until this time, and before the standard use of helmets, players simply ran the ball and smashed forward yard by yard in blistering carnage. Although legal for a few years, no one had really considered the option of passing the ball forward until

> ... on the plains of West Point, Novermber 1, 1913 ... [Gus] Dorais, the Notre Dame quarterback, tucked the ball under his arm and started a dash around his right end. But he stopped, cocked his arm and passed diagonally across the field to Rockne. The end and captain caught the pass over his left shoulder and easily ran the remaining 10 yards to complete a 30-yard touchdown play.... The Cadets [opposing players] were shocked. The football-proud East was amazed, and before it was all over Notre Dame, the little college from Indiana, had blasted respected Army 35–13.... It was the confusion bred by the pass ... as much as the passes themselves, that wrecked the Cadets. (Claassen, 1960, p. 15)

Although in the Baltes' terms this is a compensatory adaptation, it is actually preferable to the normative approach; the compensation is actually the optimum.

To the extent that we emphasize the commerce of resources, given the Baltes SOC model or COR theory's resource approaches, the process of adaptation takes on greater centrality in understanding the stress process. Appraisal-based approaches to stress have depicted compensation as reframing, citing such examples as when elderly individuals deemphasize health problems (Aldwin, 1994). However, this is not only compensation but also the cognitive stage-setting that elderly adopt in order to aid selection of compensatory strategies of behavior (Brandstädter, 1989). If reframing is seen as a process of evaluation rather than an end point in coping, then the real strengths of Lazarus and Folkman's (1984) transactional model can take more center stage. Following reframing, people typically act by positioning themselves to use their resources more optimally, compensating for losses and weaknesses, and investing their resources to change the stage setting. Again, the emphasis must be placed to a greater degree on resource management, and the time frame must be moved away from the immediate period surrounding coping. According to Aspinwall and Taylor (1997), this entails a proactive stage that involves the accumulation of resources and the acquisition of skills that are not necessarily linked to any given stressor, but that focus instead on the range of possible resource challenges, threats, and losses. Following this proactive coping, individuals, families, and organizations scan for likely threats and may initiate anticipatory coping. Once a loss occurs, both reactive coping and a new sequence of proactive and anticipatory coping may be implemented to forestall the wake of threat and loss that often follows initial stress and to build new resource reserves and capacities for the future.

Historical Influences in Adaptation

Time frame must also be viewed historically. The skills, resources, and plasticity of individuals are partially a result of historical context (Nesselroade & Baltes, 1974). Major alteration of optimatization and coping patterns occurs when there is marked sociohistorical upheaval. Events such as the Vietnam War, the Great Depression, the breakdown of the Berlin Wall, and the famine of Biafra alter coping approaches because they generate different skills and resources, set limitations on jointly held reserve capacities, and create certain ways of viewing the world (e.g., fatalist, determinist, optimist). The introduction of computers and the Information Age makes some skills obsolete, demands accumulation and reward for a different variety of resources, and changes the work habits, fit of strengths and weakness to social, work, and family demands, and the nature of the physical workplace. Historical change alters the nature of what are resources and skills, and societies adapt as do individuals.

> The warfare is too bloody to last; the Christians killing every Indian, and the Indians doing the same by the Christians. It is melancholy to trace how the Indians have given way before the Spanish invaders.... In 1535, when Buenos Ayres was founded, there were villages containing two and three thousand inhabitants. Even in Falconer's time (1750) the Indians made inroads as far as Luxan, Areco, and Arrecife, but now they are driven beyond the Salado. Not only have whole tribes been exterminated, but the remaining Indians have become more barbarous: instead of living in large villages, and being employed in the arts of fishing, as well as of the chase, they now wander about the open plains, without home or fixed occupation. (Darwin, 1845, p. 110)

Although Darwin is underestimating the size and complexity of Indian cities of South and Central America by perhaps 50-fold, his point is well taken. When the access to resources and way of life is altered, cataclysmic change in resource–adaptation interactions occur and new patterns of behavior evolve for individuals, organizations, and societies. Given the frequency of major war, periods of economic decline or prosperity, social unrest, political takeover, and the swiftness of change in modern society due to technology, we cannot underestimate how much what we see as psychology and sociology is attached to history.

Moreover, historical adaptation must be conceptualized within the context of culture. Western European and American culture tends to identify adaptation as a process of acquiring and winning. Competitiveness is esteemed and the individual is the ultimate unit of analysis. Buddhist cultures strive instead for adaptation via the middle road that avoids the extremes of hedonism and luxury or of self-mortification and extreme denial (DeSilva, 1993). Hsu (1963) proposes that the Chinese world is both situation-centered and relational. Adaptation takes the form of knowing one's place and the place of one's group, and understanding the relationships among people in this situational nexus. Whereas this nexus in China is primarily familial, it extends to broader social groups in Japan (Fukuyama, 1995). Yet, these cultures are also evolving with marked changes in global communication and commerce, technology, and spreading of Western culture through television, music, and film.

MODEL OF ECOLOGICAL CONGRUENCE

The model of ecological congruence (Hobfoll, 1985, 1988) offers a roadmap for understanding the interplay of development, history, stress occurrence, and resource application to the process of optimization and compensation. As illustrated in Figure 4.1, resources may fit, be fitted to, or

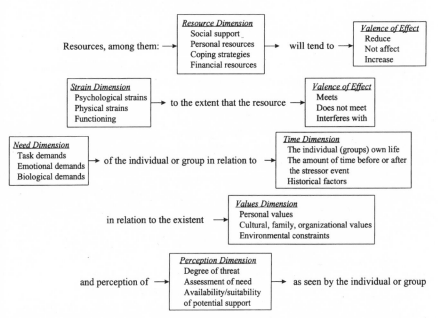

Figure 4.1. Revised model of ecological congruence. (*Source*: Hobfoll (1988). Reprinted with permission.)

not fit stress demands dependent on individual, social, historical, and maturational factors. The model of ecological congruence illustrates that resources may act to aid adaptation to the extent they complement task, emotional, and biological demands placed on the individual or group. This suitability of resources and their match to demands is always dependent on the individual, familial, group, and cultural values system. Values dictate whether resources are appropriate for use, the acceptability and social ramifications of adopting a certain adaptational posture, and the sanctions that may be imposed that prevent or demand certain response courses. For example, thrashing a colleague at work may be tempting, but the consequences based on current values systems make it an unacceptable alternative. Values channel the choice of adaptation more than we might think; because we often do not consider alternative courses, values are such powerful stage setters. Even such purely emotional responses as renting of one's clothing upon hearing of a death are now ritualized in the wearing of a torn cloth or black ribbon. In the Middle East, hearing of a death is responded to with loud wailing and keening; in New England, it might more likely be met with stoic silence.

Although perception also plays a role here, I would again emphasize that these include both socially dictated perceptions that are generally shared and idiographic appraisals that are personal to the individual but that must answer to social and ecological feedback (Shore, 1996). Many of our appraisals are based on culturally developed metaphors, scripts, and images. Following a fatal car accident in the Middle East, it is the nature of the metaphors created by the *Koran* to require a blood revenge of the offending party, even if not at fault. To assuage the grief, a brother or a son would feel obligated to murder the offender. A complicated intermediary process is required with many parties interceding to arrange a ritual, nonviolent intercession prior to the revenge that preserves honor for the victim and his family. If not, a vicious cycle of violence may be created. In Western Europe or the United States, if there were no reported fault, there might be no script for revenge perceptions. If fault were judged, revenge would probably be perceived as a matter for the courts. Individual differences would emerge, but still as products of cultural dictates. Hence, although Moslems would differ as to their postaccident perceptions, their departure point would be from the revenge metaphor. The West European and American response might also be individualized, but its departure point from socially prescribed perceptions would be from an entirely different metaphor.

We often see Western European and North American society as more ritual-free than traditional societies; however, this is probably more a matter of losing perspective from being so enmeshed inside our own culture. We have major scripts for nearly every major stressor, be they in the arenas of health, death, abortion, rape, victimization, work, or finances. In some cases, our traditions have become nontraditions. In contrast to the wakes, mourning periods, and masses of a generation ago, our tradition of death has become to almost ignore it. There is limited visitation, keening, drunkenness, and ritual. But this evolves as a scripted norm, and it becomes unusual to respond otherwise. In other domains, because of the relative lack of socially-based traditions in the United States, we have created them by becoming a nation of laws and lawyers, and have substituted legal regulations for social ones. For example, Japanese workers' rights tend to be fostered through nonwritten social traditions, whereas in the United States, the United Auto Workers' agreement with General Motors is a multivolume, encyclopedic document (Fukuyama, 1995). If anything, the regulations for the shop floor at GM concerning worker grievances, certainly a major source of stress for those involved, are more specifically scripted than at Honda, Japan.

Maturational, Event-Unfolding, and Historical Time

As emphasized earlier, time is also a key factor. There are three time sequences that are relevant. Time in the maturational sense indicates the stage of personal or organizational development of the individual or group. Just-marrieds will have a different sense of themselves and may not yet have even formed a psychological dyad but still essentially be two individuals who happen to share a domicile. Likewise, an older woman who has successfully raised her children and is no longer employed will have a different view of the threat of breast cancer than a young woman with children and for whom her breast is a more central dimension of her self-image (Hobfoll & Walfisch, 1984). Being at different maturational stages, people are likely to set different goals for adaptation.

Time is also measured in relation to the event or event unfolding. Different adaptational processes are demanded in anticipation of stress, during a stressful episode, and in recovery and readjustment of resources (Aspinwall & Taylor, 1997). Because research has often either lumped people together who are at many different stages or looked only at the imminent stress stage, this time line has been blurred. Finally, as suggested earlier, time is a historical account where events, proximal and distal, exert their influence. In his work on later-life Holocaust survivors, Lomranz (1990, 1994) illustrates how these three time lines interact. Hence, for Lomranz, we are instructed to think of how an older woman (personal maturation) who is postmastectomy (time in relation to the event), and who is a Holocaust survivor (historical time), will react and what resources she will require to adapt to this threat and loss.

Lomranz (1990, 1994) makes another point about the interaction of the stress and coping process with history. Using the case of Israel, he illustrates how the coping of Holocaust survivors shaped the history of Israel. These re-creationist copers embarked on the task of building a new life out of the ashes of the Nazi concentration camps. Most came without families, possessions or, even in many cases, true childhoods. They greatly influenced Israeli society both in how they reacted to it and how it reacted to them. Similarly, the Great Depression shaped a kind of stress responder who may have been more cautious, looked to find permanent work, and thought the United States should take care of itself in isolation of other nations. Hence, how individuals cope with major historical events, in turn, shapes the society.

Applying the Model of Ecological Congruence

Rizzo and Cosaro (1995) adopted the model of ecological congruence in their examination of the friendship formation and purposiveness of young children's social support processes in addressing the everyday stress and challenges in preschool. They term their investigative process, that is, how they analyze their data, *abductory induction and indefinite triangulation*, which consists of offering several culturally based interpretations of behavior by persons culturally knowledgeable. These interpretations are then expanded to auxiliary hypotheses and these, in turn, are tested. If the auxiliary hypotheses spring from the first-order interpretations that spring from "correct" interpretation of the data, then the auxiliary hypotheses should also be confirmable in the said environment.

Rizzo and Cosaro (1995) studied a university preschool environment, where sharing and individual rights were offered by teachers as core values, and, in response, the children's play reflected these principles. For example, they developed nonintrusive strategies for entering a play group that circumvented resistance to new members. In contrast, for the African American children they studied in an inner-city Head Start program, a similar set of preschool demands was described as having simultaneously to encompass a harsher adaptive reality of inner-city life. Thus, these two ecologies (home and school) were seen as creating demands to balance conflict with community. Children responded by verbally aggressive play that was generally not interpreted by other children as aggressive. The teacher's role was more indirect and encouraged independent conflict resolution by the group with minimal intrusion. For example, a child might say, "Give me up that big old shovel," to which the other child would respond, "You're too weak to handle this shovel." Rather than escalating, however, the children would just go on with their play, as if no challenge and retort were proffered. These competitive but supportive kinds of social relations have been noted many times among African American children where verbal opposition and conflict are used as strategies to quell physical escalation of violence that might otherwise be more endemic in a high-stress, materially poor segment of society (see also Abrahams, 1975).

Paradoxical or Noncongruent Person–Ecology Fit

Finally, the model of ecological congruence cautions that resources may become not only nonadaptive, but also maladaptive given the mix of task, emotional, and biological demands and the value concordance with the system. Aggressiveness toward outgroups may be deemed perfectly appropriate in Japan, but modesty, humility, and submissiveness may be the appropriate in-group resources. Having one set of resources in the wrong ecological niche can spell disaster. For aggregates of individuals in families, groups, or organizations, resource complementation is vital. Resource redundancy within any social group limits its ability to respond to multiple demands. Intercoordination of these resources is a delicate dance that further calls on management resources to systematically match, shape, and apply resources in the evolving adaptational process. Most importantly, resources are always maladaptive if exhausted, suggesting that more attention be paid to reserve capacity and the need to conserve resources for future stress responding (Baltes, 1987; Hobfoll, 1988; Schönpflug, 1985). Although nonresponding is seen in coping research as passive and maladaptive, when viewed in context, it may in some instances actually be an energy and resource conservation strategy aimed at garnering resources for later action or to preserve the minimal resources required of subsistence.

LIMITATIONS: OBSTACLES TO RESOURCE FITTING

The next aspect of the FALL model is *limitations*. Resource-based models are subject to the distortion that merely by knowing someone's resources and knowing objective demands, we can predict the fitting of resources to demands. This proposition is challenged by the fact that social structures are biased by shared and individual perceptions, especially concerning race, class, color, gender, age, and sexual preference. These social perceptions create biases that profoundly influence the fitting of resources to demands in the process of adaptation.

A concrete example serves to clarify the essence of limitations of resource utilization. The purchase of a home to move to a better neighborhood and to enable one's children to attend better schools should be a matter of having the financial resources. The purchase price and the availability of credit for a mortgage are the demands and a family's finances are the key resource. However, in much of the United States, an African American family will need a greater amount of capital to purchase a home, because to obtain a mortgage, they will require more money than the comparable white family. One hundred thousand dollars becomes a relative, not an absolute, amount as a resource, and its character is altered by the degree to which bias is present. At a greater extreme, although far from an unusual case, no amount of money will purchase a home for an African American in many neighborhoods (Myers & Chan, 1995; Vanderhart, 1993). When recently looking for a home, I was informed by a realtor that a privately maintained street on which an ideal house sat was governed by the local "street maintenance" association and that in the past they had used this loophole to prevent Jews from purchasing one of the properties. These examples provide insights into an important principle: Not only does bias itself create stressful demands in the form of prejudice, but it also limits the application of resources.

This is a complicated dynamic. Most Western societies since the American and French Revolutions are founded on the principle of citizens' rights and equality under the law. Of course, this is an unfolding process, and the generalization of equality is a struggle within all societies, even those that proclaim it as their central belief. Although political scientists are aware of this reality, stress theorists and mental health clinicians have been taught to ignore inequality of resources and to concentrate on personal perceptions under the assumption that all are equal (Levine & Perkins, 1997).

Women often face this dilemma in the workplace. If they want to retain co-workers' and management's approval, they are pressed to demonstrate female sex-role qualities of warmth and expressiveness. They are asked to provide a nurturant role, not display anger, and not to be aggressive. However, professional success dictates that they behave assertively, competitively, and firmly (Bhatnagar, 1988; Grant, 1988). If women adapt the former female sex-role model, they are likely to find workplace support and positive feedback, but not success, promotion, and higher pay. If they adapt the more traditionally male role, they are likely both to lose support and receive only limited advancement. This is because social stereotypes may place them on either the mommy-track, despite their aggressive, hardworking demeanor, or rejection because of acting inappropriately for their gender (Geller & Hobfoll, 1993, 1994). Furthermore, they are often excluded from Old Boys networks that involve afterwork activities that are so critical for acceptance, recognition, and advancement in most organizations. Stress research, to the extent it has considered sexism at all, has viewed it as a stressor, which is most certainly the case. However, it is also a resource-limiting factor, indicating that bias both creates additional demand and curtails the latitude or plasticity of resource fit.

Goffman's (1963) classic work on stigma provides many insights about how resource limitation transpires. The stigmatized individual is invalidated in terms of both the self and the possessions, resources, and attributes associated with that self. Stigma can be placed as a matter of a natural class (e.g., race, sex, AIDS infected), or as a matter of assignation, such as when we label someone mentally ill, criminal, or lower class. One's accent not only prevented the ascent of Eliza Doolittle in *My Fair Lady* in Victorian England, but also it is a cornerstone for success in today's England, where an Oxbridge accent is required for entrée to any corridor of esteemed white-collar employment. Although we no longer brand (stigmata) slaves, criminals, or adulterers, widespread biases serve to preserve the limitations society wishes to place on those of lower or spoiled status.

Limitation also serves in a more relative sense. Assistant professors or junior executives are hardly stigmatized individuals in Goffman's sense of the term. However, the lack of tenure is a reminder that their opinion might be better held than rendered at a meeting with their seniors. Of course, this depends on the overt and covert rules governing their status at that setting. But that is the very point. Where such limitations are placed, the resources of having the right answers become less relevant than the limitation factors placed on that resource. Within any social unit, there is a relative ordering of bias against certain members. Children are more limited in their ability to enact and apply their resources than parents, junior employees are more limited than senior employees, and high school freshman are more limited than seniors. Our society is stratified and hierarchical, and this plays into the plasticity and value that resources possess.

LENIENCY: BENDING THE ECOLOGICAL RULES
TO BENEFIT THE ENNOBLED

Although there has been great interest in the influence of bias in sociology, political science, and psychology, I have argued that it has seldom been applied to the study of how obstacles are placed in the path of resource utilization in the stress process. In contrast, the study of bias's opposite, which I call ennoblement, has seldom even been studied in any sense. The study of impediments to women and blacks in the workplace, for example, is always conceived as a negative bias against a baseline, white, male standard. The supposition is that there is a base standard that signifies a fair playing field, and that those who are stigmatized are treated unfairly. This concept stems from Goffman's (1963) spoiled identity and the social processes that are used to maintain the social systems that offer privileges to some and sanctions to others. The concept of ennoblement, in contrast, suggests that there is conferred dominance and privilege by being a member of the ennobled group (McIntosh, 1988).

This conferred dominance and privilege represents the last "L" in the FALL model, standing for Leniency. I define *leniency* as a positive bending of the rules either to lower obstacles in the environment or artificially overevaluate resources (i.e., to makes resources worth more than they are, not just to think they are so). Either or both of these actions benefit the ennobled self or organization in a manner that is different than bias. As stated in this chapter's title, the concept of ennoblement is embodied in the tradition of majesty. Those who are esteemed by birthright were traditionally subject to different laws in practice, if not in fact. The local lord had rights to dispose of land, persons, and peasant women at his pleasure. This right was accorded to slaveowners in the South, and this tradition was tragically continued in many ways until modern times for any white Southerner. Thus, a white male could rape a black woman with virtual impunity, despite secular laws to the contrary. Moreover, he could avoid religious sanction within his spiritual community, despite clear outlawing of rape and adultery in the Old and New Testament. Note how this is not the same as bias and discrimination in which many black males were wrongly accused of rape or lynched for even being seen with a white woman (National Association for the Advancement of Colored People, 1969).

Ennoblement is for most part the opposite of bias, but not its direct opposite. Discrimination is used against someone compared to the fair play of common ground. Ennoblement is used in favor of someone compared to the fair play of common ground, and to this extent they are opposites. However, ennoblement is actively denied by those who are ennobled because it undermines the concept of meritocracy that they esteem and infer as the mechanism for their obtaining higher status. Discrimination explains why someone else perhaps did not achieve but does not threaten those who have attained status, position, and are part of a privileged class. Accepting the concept of ennoblement says something else—that you may have achieved what you did unfairly. If one accepts the process of ennoblement, one may also need to relinquish "the myth of meritocracy. If these things are true, this is not such a free country; one's life is not what one makes it, many doors open for certain people through no virutres of their own. These perceptions mean also that my moral condition is not what I have been led to believe" (McIntosh, 1988, p. 81).

The theme of enoblement is a frequent subject of protest-oriented folk music found in union organizing, antiwar, freedom, and sufferage movements.

William Zanzinger killed poor Hattie Carroll with a cane that he
twirled round his diamond ringed finger ...
With rich, wealthy parents who provide and protect him
And high office relations in the politics of Maryland.
In a matter of minutes on bail was out walking ...

Hattie Carroll was a maid of the kitchen.
She was 51 years old and gave birth to ten children
Who carried the dishes and took out the garbage
And never sat once at the head of the table
And didn't even talk once to the people at the table ...
And emptied the ashtrays on a whole other level.

In the courtroom of honor, the judge pounded his gavel
To show that all's equal and the courts are on the level
And that the strings in the books ain't pulled and pursuaded
And that even the nobles get properly handled ...
And that the ladder of law has no top and no bottom,
stared at the person who killed for no reason ...
And he spoke through his cloak, most deep and distinguished,
And handed out strongly, for penalty and repentance,
[and gave] William Zanzinger with a six-month sentence.*

*Lonesome Death of Hattie Carroll, by Bob Dylan. Copyright © 1964 by Warner Bros. Music renewed 1992 by Special Rider Music. All rights reserved. International copyright secured. Reprinted by permission.

Ennoblement eases much of the strain on the fitting of resources to environmental demands. Given the fixed, lock-and-key concept of fit (French et al., 1982) there is little room for maneuvering. However, by loosening the constraints of fit to the more active fitting or shaping of resources and of the environmental demands, the value of ennoblement becomes manifest. Given that the process of shaping resources or optimizing environments is both directly demanding of resources and requires that resources may need to be depleted from other arenas of demand, by lowering the obstacles to resource implementation or the stressful demands of the environment, individuals receive treble benefit. First, by answering demand, there are fewer stress sequelae, and avenues of resource gain are opened. Second, fewer resources have had to be expended to answer the stressful demand. Third, the individual or group did not need to weaken its stance in other stress and adaptation domains by borrowing or calling on resources from these arenas.

One of the central ironies of the process of ennoblement is that ennobled individuals and groups are typically the rulemakers and powerbrokers in society and social settings, but yet deny that they either hold privilege or break the rules. In the familial example, parents make rules for the household to which they hold their children but often themselves transgress. This may be forgivable because parents and children are seen as actually having different status, authority, judgment, and rights. However, a similar process occurs on a social level when the police are involved in corruption, or in everyday work and legal practice, whereby privileged status receives its attendant awards. These processes are centrally involved with stress and coping because they influence access to preferred medical care, investment opportunities, job advancement, tenure, seniority, and almost every facet of what is either potentially stressful in our lives or the resources we are accorded to answer stress.

The difference in ennoblement versus bias can be seen in the differential prosecution of crack cocaine and cocaine, the former being an inexpensive drug used disproportionately by inner-city African Americans and the latter an expensive drug used disproportionately by wealthier, white Americans. The differential application of the law results in the stress of imprisonment of black men due to recent laws that demand jail time for nonviolent drug-related crime. Yet the same laws have resulted in limited prosecution of white cocaine users, who, when prosecuted, are more likely to receive suspended sentences rather than jail time (Lewis, 1996). This imprisonment of black men is the application of the law judiciously. They are not necessarily treated unfairly, but rather to the true letter of the law. However, a differential investigation, arrest, prosecution, and imprisonment rate occurs because of the ennoblement of white, upper-middle-class cocaine users. The stress differential is felt by black men, their families, and their communities, who have been rocked by this differential application of law. Unlike the case of parents, whites and blacks have exactly equivalent status in the eyes of the written law, and again, it was white politicians who created the law and then chose not to enforce it on their own class.

On a less macrosocial level, ennoblement is often practiced in the workplace in the form of preferences for gender, class, and ethnicity among employees. These individuals are placed on the fast track and their worklife is structured for rapid advancement. While consulting with businesses, I have been struck by the fact that these individuals were at times excused from participation in the competitive process. One young man I recall seemed to earn his stripes more on the tennis court than in the boardroom, yet no matter what mistakes he made (and this individual made many), they were excused by the senior executives who were grooming him "in their own image."

In general, the process of leniency is afforded to persons or groups who are in some way privileged. Their subsequent task of matching resources with environmental demand is eased. The range for optimization processes is broadened and the amount that they need to compensate when resource-demand fitting is not optimum is lessened. This has multiple influences, because it not only limits stress reactions in an immediate sense, but also it allows them to garner resources for other use and to reduce resource loss and enhance resource gain in other domains. By not having to invest resources as fully in the immediate demand, other areas of loss are less likely to develop and a less defensive, more gain-oriented posture is nurtured.

RESOURCE FITTING, ADAPTATION, LIMITATIONS, AND LENIENCY OVER TIME AND WITHIN CULTURES

Given the greater weight of resource loss compared to gain, and the notion of loss and gain cycles, the process of FALL takes on the status of an ongoing film rather than a set of still-frame photographs. Fitting of resources occurs whether or not resource loss is present, but is accelerated when losses to key resources are threatened or occur (Hobfoll et al., 1991). The process of adaptation, with its optimization and compensation co-phases, in turn, becomes more frenzied when multiple losses occur or major chronic losses transpire. Returning to the metaphor of battle, drawing board strategy can be calm, metered, and well thought. Field action, once the battle is engaged, is chaotic, often difficult to interpret, and factors change even as decisions are being made based on quickly irrelevant facts. This metaphor suits stress as a process quite well.

Change Processes over Time

In the case of persons or groups that are resource enriched, there may also be the luxury of greater thoughtfulness and preparation. Where resource reserves are lacking, or where they become depleted, decisions will be more haphazard because of the effects of strain on cognition. Stress, in this regard, increases the use of magical thinking and an illusory sense of control (Friedland, Keinan, & Regev, 1992; Keinan, 1994). Rather than thinking out their options and ramifications of action, people paradoxically come to premature closure on decisions when stress is high (Kahneman, 1973; Keinan, 1987). Because people will make judgments based on resource and demand combinations that are so greatly changed from their prestress standard, they will also be subject to influences that are outside of the involved individuals' or group's experience. Coping and adaptational habits will have been based on one set of resources, but a different combination of resources will be available at the point of crisis.

Crisis teams practice responding to unusual, high-stress combinations of demands and available resources by planning and implementing crisis action given possible combinations of resources and stress demands that might occur in different scenarios (e.g., tornado, flood, terrorist attack). Individuals are less likely to project forward to crisis states because they are more myriad and less predictable for the individual or family. A family may have an adaptational plan for financial setbacks, but will be less likely to have a plan for the emotional strain that might accompany job loss or the relational conflict that might emerge. Because couples and families are unlikely to develop a plan for serious conflict or hardship when things are going well, they will be unlikely to have crisis strategies prepared. Of course, when the threat of such crises becomes more likely, families might begin to plan (Aspinwall & Taylor, 1997) and mental health professionals may be especially potent resources at this stage because of their experience with other families or individuals in similar situations (Caplan, 1964).

Major stress sequences seldom change a person's or group's status to a more ennobled state. However, they often stigmatize individuals and groups, and change the degree to which limitations are placed on their resources, or forgiveness is no longer extended from their environmental demands. Illness, divorce, old age, and poverty all involve stigmatized roles and this means that the equations of matching resources and adaptational processes will be altered. In the United States, it is common for middle-class women to fall below the poverty line when they divorce, women dropping in their standard of living by an average of 73% in the first year after divorce (men rise an average of 42%) (Weitzman, 1988). This means that not only will they have a set of many diminished resources and greater environmental demands, but also that their resources and demands will be subject to different rules. They, their children, and the resources they bring to the table will be accorded different status, feedback, potential, and worth (Weitzman, 1988). This in part comes from the caravan of resources that cotravel, as money, self-worth, insurance, quality health care, vacation time, security, hope, and sense of mastery are intertwined. But it also stems from the fact that limitations are placed on resources by schools, courts, and banks that interact in a less favorable, more disempowering fashion with the poor than with the middle class (Goffman, 1963, Rappaport, 1981).

Moreover, as these processes are moving cycles, it is difficult to adjust to any given set of rules, resources, or demands. The entire constellation is in motion. In our study of mothers of severely ill children, we found, for example, that social support had a positive effect initially for mothers of chronically ill children and for mothers of acutely ill children, because the process of resource drain had not yet changed their constellation of resources and demands. In time, however, social support became a burden, because mothers' sense of social obligation seemed to increase with all the favors they owed and felt they could never return.

Baltes (1987, 1994) outlines how culture also plays a role in this mobile, adaptational process. Culture has a relative influence in support of adaptation, being better matched to some problems for some kinds of people and poorly matched for other combinations. For example, for the young-old (approximately ages 60–70 years), he cites that many institutions have been created by society to support their coping efforts. Special insurance, state-operated programs, housing communities, and health care have advanced with the great increase of young-old in the society. The culture for old-old (perhaps 90 years and older), in contrast, is a younger culture, as the percentage of old-old is only recently increasing in marked numbers. With a young culture, there are few supports for the old-old, and they must either adapt using their own diminished resources or depend on their families for care. Their families, in turn, have few social institutions to turn to for assistance in their care. Similarly, despite enormous changes in the number of dual-career families in the United States, child care for young children and afterschool care for older children has not kept pace. Here again, we see how culture and its ambivalence about women working may have failed to create a support net for working families (Hobfoll & Hobfoll, 1994; Hochschild, 1989).

Culture also deeply influences resources more directly. In her book, *The Second Shift*, Hochschild (1989) finds that although many women have entered the workforce, their husbands have not entered the realm of household labor. This means that a disproportionate amount of the overall family labor falls on women's shoulders, even when they are working outside the home. The widespread nature of this phenomenon clearly indicates its cultural basis. This, in turn, interacts with workplace support that women often lack, again culturally constituted, and a cycle of potential resource loss obtains fertile ground to flourish. The culturally interwoven nature of these phenomena are further illustrated in the case of older working women, who disproportionately must leave work to support the old-old, even if they are the parents of their husband (Brody, 1990). Now they must operate within a social–cultural system that undermines both their coping and that of their elderly loved one.

Research and Clinical Implications of Time and Culture

Although combining all these factors is daunting, by recognizing the multiple influences and factors in the stress and coping process it is possible to conduct both sophisticated and careful research. Investigations by Schwarzer, Jerusalem, and Hahn (1994b) and Schwarzer, Hahn, and Schröeder (1994a) concerning migrants from East Berlin at the time of the demise of the Berlin Wall are cases in point. By carefully capturing samples of migrants in the early days of the Wall's demise and understanding their culture of origin and the demands of the new culture, they were able to examine how stress and adaptation influenced this first generation in flight. Not surprisingly, they found housing, work, and social losses were critical in adjustment, affecting both mental and physical well-being. To the extent that refugees reconnected with work and social attachments, their distress was attenuated and their adjustment enhanced. Moreover, based in part on COR theory, they hypothesized that successful adaptation would involve recreating the lost social support network that they left behind in the former East Germany. Those who were able to recreate a new social support system clearly had the most successful overall adaptation in terms of physical and psychological health and general social adaptation. Furthermore, as COR theory predicts, those who did not adjust well psychologically experienced a downward spiral in terms of their social support. This, in turn, made them more vulnerable to the stress of migration and the corresponding social demands. As presented in Figure 4.2, possessing a major condition resource—employment—contributed to lower levels of psychological distress (i.e., anxiety, depression) and greater social support resources. Support, in turn, contributed to later support and ongoing ability to limit negative psychological sequelae. However, to the extent that negative psychological sequalae developed, they also diminished social support. In this way, we can see the clear interweaving of resources to resources, resources to adjustment, and adjustment to resources.

The FALLS perspective has significant implications for mental health

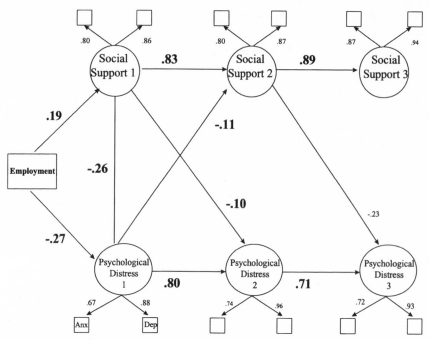

Figure 4.2. The reciprocal relationship between social support and psychological distress among East German migrants. (*Source*: Adapted from R. Schwarzer, A. Hahn, and M. Jerusalem (1993). "Negative Affect in East German Migrants: Longitudinal Effects of Unemployment and Social Support." *Anxiety, Stress, and Coping: An International Journal, 6,* 66. Copyright 1993 by Harwood Academic Publishers. Reprinted with permission of the authors.)

professionals' approach to intervention with individuals, families, and groups. Certainly, clinicians are already likely to be attuned to the need to help people shape their resources to the stressful demands that they encounter, and indeed the process of therapy is often one of shaping new resources and a recognition that current resources are inadequate, overtaxed, or diminished. However, clinicians are not always sensitive to resources that are not traditionally considered psychological. Hence, they might be more likely to address self-esteem than job skills, economic viability, or social support at work. The process of optimization and compensation is also probably commonly practiced by clinicians on some level, but perhaps not within the kind of clear theoretical model that Baltes (1987) outlines. Instead, it is my impression from the literature that the two distinct processes are mixed. Distilling them may help both the clinician and the client in the adaptation process.

I was almost entirely unable to find references to the process of limitations in the stress and coping process outside of the distinct literature on the
psychology of women (cf. Fagenson, 1993; Greenglass, 1993) and limited
writing on intervention with ethnic minority populations (Allen & Britt,
1983; Moritsugu & Sue, 1983). The pervasive effects of bias are not well
represented in the mainstream clinical literature. By ignoring sociocultural
limitations, clinicians potentially confuse clients by either implying that it is
all just a matter of their cognitive framing or causing them to feel at fault.

If there was a relative lack of clinical literature on sociocultural limitations exercised against people's resources, I could find no intervention
literature whatsoever on the process of leniency and how this influenced the
stress and coping process. This might be because those who receive the
privilege of leniency are less likely therefore to experience psychological
distress. However, one coping strategy that clinicians may encourage is
alignment with an ennobled group through entrée to new social networks.
Indeed, the involvment with a mental health professional is an alignment
with a relatively ennobled figure that may have special access to other resources, may facilitate court or social service leniency (e.g., not having
children removed from a home), and use professional resources in someone's favor. Also, the process of lost ennoblement, where senior executives
find themselves subject to job layoff, is an increasingly common stress
experience and one that deserves more attention.

CONCLUSIONS

In the next chapters, COR theory and the FALL model are analyzed as
they speak to major kinds of stress experiences. Both prior research and
intervention strategies and possible new avenues for research and intervention will be explored. Throughout these chapters, it is important to keep in
mind that culture plays a key role that we will try to draw out of its blurry
background in order to better understand its influence. There is a danger of
COR theory leading us to too macrosocial a perspective to expect that
intervention, outside of major government policy changes, will be viable.
However, by remaining on a social level of analysis that includes the person-
nested-in families-nested-in organizations, we enlarge the social perspective
of psychological stress theory and intervention but do not exceed the
reasonable limits of intervention.

Moreover, if my thesis is correct, by perpetuating only a microsocial
understanding of stress and not including the mesosocial level of the marketplace and village, we lose the richness that such work as that of Baltes
(1987), Schwarzer and his colleagues (1994a, 1994b), and those who have

explored stress and coping among women and ethnic minority groups offers. Even where someone or some group is a member of the majority culture, we cannot drop culture out of the equation. We are all influenced by sociocultural processes, and our resources operate subject to, and tempered by, the same laws and properties, taken within the boundaries of the FALL model.

NOTE

1. By modern social structures, I refer here to communism, capitalism, mixed social structures (e.g., Sweden), and current monarchies. Differential treatment by class was more overt in earlier societies. Vestiges of this, for example, in England include tipping one's hat to one's "better" and the use of the term *governer* or *lord* when addressing someone of a higher or aristocratic class. In the United States, similar behaviors were expected along racial lines. Although class distinctions that this chapter addresses still exist, they are no longer socially sanctioned in overt social behavior. Structurally, these distinctions nevertheless continue to operate and influence behavior, or so this chapter argues.

5

Our Coping as Individuals within Families and Tribes

I have been discussing stress and stress resistance, highlighting the role of resources. The question arises as to how people put their resources to work for themselves, their families, and the social networks to which they belong in the process of adaptation. Having resources and the ability to use them effectively are related but are far from one and the same. Stress researchers almost uniformly have examined whether people possess a resource, or how much of it they possess. However, with few exceptions (Bandura, 1997; Pearlin & Schooler, 1978; Sarason, Pierce, & Sarason, 1990) have the mechanisms by which resources operate in service of the self, family, or social system been explored. Consequently, there is a folklore of how a given resource works that stems from our cultural beliefs, but little actual empirical validation of whether these are myths or social insights. This chapter explores some central myths concerning the question of how people employ key resources in the service of coping.

The behavior of people in the face of stress has been conceptualized under the rubric of coping. Lazarus and Folkman (1984) in their pioneering work defined coping as "constantly changing cognitive and behavioral efforts to manage specific external and/or internal demands that are appraised as taxing or exceeding the resources of the person" (p. 141). In this framework, coping focuses on the process of overcoming stress, linking it with appraisal. In so doing, Lazarus and Folkman rely on the individual as the arbiter of these perceptions. A critical point of further direction is added by Kaplan (1983, 1996), who theorized that people's social identities provide a compass by which they judge what is threatening and how to respond. According to Kaplan, "Behaviors, events, or ongoing experiences that impinge on identify-related values" or "cherished values" (1996, p. 12) will be emotionally significant.

Thus, Kaplan provides the necessary roadmap to assess how people respond in the larger realm of adaptation developed in the prior chapter; that is, people respond according to their social identities and their place within social structures (e.g., family, work, society) and, more specifically, conserve and protect their resources in these keystone domains. Moreover, because most of our roles and social identities are shared with others like us (e.g., our family, coreligionists, Americans), shared perceptions will predominate and individual perceptions will be largely derived from these broader social structures. Once again, individualized (i.e., idiographic) appraisals will also be important but secondary to those derived from broad cultural standards.

As in the case of stress, the study of coping emphasized the self, as if the individual is unattached to a social network. Aldwin (1994) insightfully writes that the construct of coping is founded in mythopoetic roots of hero sagas. These figures, most of them men, include princes fighting dragons, as well as historical and contemporary figures such as Abraham Lincoln or Martin Luther King. They embody model individuals who withstood physical, psychological, or emotional tests in the face of adversity. The critical point underlying the hero myth is that they stood alone. That stress often occurs in interpersonal contexts and that, even when it does not, it often involves interpersonal solutions is virtually incompatible with these myths and consequently has not been the focus of theory or research. Moreover, the idea that coping behavior has consequences beyond the individual copers, impacting others around them has generally been ignored (Coyne & Smith, 1991). This contrasts with Japanese and Chinese hero myths in which sacrifice for family or the social group are the moral undertone of the legends. For example, the *samurai* ideal is bound to a complex web of social relationships and obligations, and it is his allegiance to these that esteems him (Downs, 1970; Nitobe, 1905a,b; Masatsugu, 1982).

This chapter discusses how coping has traditionally been studied and how we might develop a more balanced view of coping by *individuals-nested-in families-nested-in social settings.* After all, in every culture, we cope as individuals who are in some form of family and in conjunction with members of some form of tribe that has certain rules and guidelines for thoughts and behaviors. As Kaplan (1983, 1996) instructs, the linking tissue of individuals and social settings is the values that are shared by individuals within settings and that in many ways describe what we mean by culture (Schwartz & Bilsky, 1990). By coping, I am referring here to the things that people do to combat stress, their thought and behavioral reactions, and particularly their guarding, investing, and building of resources. I hope to follow Kaniasty and Norris's (1997) seminal theorizing that links people's personal and social coping effort within the complex ecology of the kind of stressor that they are confronting, which in turn, makes individual and shared demands upon them and their resources. This, I hope, will move us closer to the broader concept of adaptation developed in Chapter 4.

I begin by examining cultural and historical factors that contributed to the schism between the self and the community, leading to psychology's focus on the individual coping agent. After reviewing a traditional, individualized study of coping, I offer an alternative *individual-in social context* perspective. I hope to illustrate that theory and research have attended well but to only half of the gestalt of coping, being both individualistic and mentalistic, but avoiding the social, interdependent nature of coping. In so doing, it has followed a "human as controlling agent" bias that fits a masculine, Northern European and American model. This model obfuscates the interwoven nature of resources that are intertwined between individuals, families, and social organizations (Trickett, 1995). Again, we must move between the individual, family, and village and neighborhood levels to disentangle this web.

EARLY RELIGIOUS AND CULTURAL INFLUENCES ON INDIVIDUAL VERSUS COLLECTIVIST COPING

Individualism and collectivism actually lie on a continuum. Attempts to separate the concepts as *either–or* mistake this crucial point and the dialectics represented here, because social contingencies define the self and the *self-in-collective* comprises the community. As the concept of the self emerged during the late Middle Ages in Europe (Baumeister, 1987; Sampson, 1988) it replaced a collectivist model but never entirely extinguished those underpinnings. Individualism and collectivism always coexisted, even where individualism has predominated. Nor can it be concluded that the ages that preceded the emergence of a strong sense of self in literature, the arts, and philosophy were devoid of the concept of self. Nevertheless, from about the eleventh through the fifteenth century, it can be said that the concept of a single, separable self crystallized in Europe. With this crystallization emerged notions of individual salvation, self-related concepts of honor, glory and virtue, and identification other than in set roles such as serf, lord, or landowner (Baumeister, 1987). Even in eating, people moved from the bench and shared bowl to personal chair and individual utensils (Tuan, 1982).

The concept of individual acting as a unified self, separated from others, is illustrated in a common religious theme of prophet or man (and occasionally woman) meeting God the Father. Moses at Mount Sinai, Jesus's temptation in the desert, and Mary acting as intermediary replay this theme. In each case, they are central metaphors that define the nature of the parameters and sanctity of the unified self. After all, in each of these cases, an individual, not a committee, approached God. But again, even in these "self as worthy of facing God" themes, a communal component is meant in the metaphor as well. The more social theme, however, has been lost in the championing of individualism. This dialectic of individual self as stand-in for our collective society is clear in that Christ is said to have died for mankind's sins and Mary is the symbolic mother of all. Moses was, for all his virtues, ordinary—the everyman. The story tells of a pauper prince, found in the reeds with a tattered blanket, a stutterer, filled with self-doubt and angst, "slow of speech, and of a slow tongue."

The self as collectivist representation is deftly illustrated in the story of Abraham (the name literally meaning "father of a nation") and the sacrifice of Isaac. One rabbinical interpretation of this event suggests that Abraham never intended to slay Isaac because he knew that God would never ask this of him. Instead, he goes along with the charade to do to God what God is doing to him: exact future promises. Abraham was a consummate trader, a classic desert nomad whose life revolved around a system of barter still central today to this region's mentality. For the price of Isaac's life, as it were, Abraham receives guarantees from God for the future of the Jewish people.

> By Myself have I sworn, saith the Lord, because thou hast done this thing, and hast not withheld thy son, thine only son, that in blessing I will bless thee, and in multiplying I will multiply thy seed as the stars of the heaven, and as the sand which is upon the seashore; and thy seed shall possess the gate of his enemies; and in thy seed shall all the nations of the earth be blessed; because thou hast hearkened to My voice. Genesis (22:16–19)

That is, if we accept that he knew that God would not allow the sacrifice of a human and the seed of the new covenant, then all that God exacted from Abraham, promises for a chosen people, is actually being manipulated by Abraham of God. Indeed, on a number of occasions, Abraham, the individual, barters outright with God for better conditions for Israel, for his people, and for future generations. Says Abraham to God:

> "That be far from Thee to slay the righteous with the wicked, that so the righteous of the earth shall be like the wicked; that be far from Thee; shall not the Judge of all the earth do justly?" And the Lord said: "If I find fifty righteous within the city [Sodom], then I will forgive all the place for their sake." And Abraham answered and said: "... who am I but dust and ashes. [If] there shall lack five of the fifty righteous; wilt Thou

destroy all the city for lack of five?" And the Lord said, "I will not destroy it if I find there forty and five." And [Abraham] spoke unto Him yet again.... "[If] there shall be forty there." And He said, "I will not do it for forty's sake." "Oh let not the Lord be angry ... [If] there shall thirty be found there." [With God twice more agreeing to terms, Abraham continues] ... "Oh let not the Lord be angry, and I will speak yet but this once. [If] ten shall be found...." Genesis (18:23–30)

So effective was his negotiation that it created two of the world's prominent religions and cultures, as both Islam and Judaism evolved from its seed. Along the road to individualism, the common interpretation has lost that we are asked by this text to identify with a single *individual as a nation*, the inseparable self and community.

Based largely on this religious heritage, neither Jewish nor Christian Europe saw a possible separation between the self and the community in the process of facing adversity. Antagonism between self and collective actually emerged during fairly recent times and may have been responsible, in part, for the schism between the individualistic and communal perspective in Western thought within psychology. Earlier Judeo-Christian viewpoint had no conflict between a concept of individual and a concept of collective. Puritanism, however, began to sow a departure between the individual and collectively linked self, as Puritanism placed a greater emphasis on individual action than had earlier Christian or Jewish ideals. Historians suggest that concepts central to Protestantism highlighted human self-consciousness to a new height and allowed individual accomplishment to stand as a marker for self-worth. Yet, still, at this departure point, the underlying philosophy also valued community relations and people's ties with each other (Weintraub, 1978; Whyte, 1960).

SECULAR AND RECENT HISTORICAL INFLUENCES AND THE EMERGENCE OF SELF-RELIANCE

The self as inconsistent with the collective is actually a more secular notion that evolved during the Romantic period in the late eighteenth to early nineteenth century. Romanticism searched for a place for the self outside of religious salvation alone. Romanticism especially esteemed individualism in terms of its love for creative work. Human potential came to be viewed in terms of personal fulfillment, rather than fulfillment of predestined social roles. Romanticism also placed an ideal on individual isolation. Here, we have Thoreau's image of the individual living in the woods, separated from society at Walden Pond. Thoreau was said to have no profession, he never married, he lived alone, he never attended Church, he abstained from both the privileges and duties of citizenship, he refused to pay taxes, and he abstained from flesh, wine, and tobacco (Eliot, 1989). Within this image, however, lies a paradox or absurdity. If we are all to leave society and live in the woods, society empties and the woods become crowded. It is a sustainable reality for only a few, a romanticization of the individualized self.

Romanticism began to reveal a hostility toward society. Wrote Emerson in his famous essay *Self Reliance* (1841).

> Society never advances. It recedes as fast on one side as it gains on the other. Its progress is only apparent like the workers of a treadmill. It undergoes continual changes; it is barbarous, it is civilized, it is christianized, it is rich, it is scientific; but this change is not an amelioration. (p. 80)

Moreover, Emerson associated creativity and nonconformity with isolationism.

> We must go alone. Isolation must precede true society. I like the silent church before the service begins.... How far off, how cool, how chaste the persons look, begirt each one with a precinct or sanctuary. So let us always sit. Why should we assume the faults of our friend, or wife, or father, or child, because they sit around our hearth, or are said to have the same blood?... The whole world seems to be in conspiracy to importune you with emphatic trifles. Friend, client, child, sickness, fear, want, charity, all knock at once at thy closet door and say, "Come out unto us."—Do not spill thy soul; do not all descend; keep thy state; stay at home in thine own heaven; come not for a moment into their facts. (p. 73)

It may be in choosing Emerson's *Self Reliance* as the piece that is so often taught that we have selected only half his ideas, as Emerson was, in fact, an ardent abolitionist, believed in "access of the young and the poor to the sources of wealth and power" (p. 245), and advanced a rather collectivist ideology toward the immigrant, Native American, and the operation of the State in support of the people. However, it is self-reliance that is the predominant theme that we take from this most influential of American thinkers. In importuning people to follow their own path in a crusade against "foolish consistency," he may have inadvertently created a philosophy of isolationist coping wherewith individuals face their demons alone.

Romanticism in Emerson, and for other philosophers of his time, still saw the individual and the self as sustainable in face of society, in "peaceful coexistence" (Baumeister, 1987). Indeed, some feel that Romanticism led the way to Victorian notions of progressivism and a hope for a utopian society (Baumeister, 1987). However, the late nineteenth and early twentieth century increasingly saw society as an outright evil. This thinking is apparent in academic themes of alienation (Durkheim, 1897/1952), literary themes of society as devouring the individual (e.g., Kafka), and muckraker journalism of Sinclair (see Klein, 1964). In part, this may have stemmed from the omnipresent march of machines and the ever-widening factory floor and city tenement, and the ever-diminishing contact with bucolic rural farms and village life. Urbanization acted to disengage individuals from communal access to resources as they became increasingly mechanized. Indeed, the great architect of American industrial philosophy, Taylor (1911) created a workplace based on the supposition that maximum efficiency could be achieved by treating individuals as replaceable cogs and divorcing them from attachment to the whole product, avoiding the need for individuals to demonstrate initiative, judgment, or skill. Given work's centrality as a defining contact between people and society, the success of this doctrine was tantamount to a dissolution of any semblance of social contract between the self and the greater commune.

> ... for the woman worked so fast that the eye could literally not follow her, and there was only a mist of motion, and tangle after tangle of sausages appearing. In the midst of the mist, however, the visitor would suddenly notice the tense set face, with the two wrinkles graven in the forehead, and the ghastly pallor of the cheeks; and then he would suddenly recollect that it was time he was going on. The woman did not go on; she stayed right there—hour after hour, day after day, year and year, twisting sausage links and racing with death. It was piece-work, and she was apt to have a family to keep alive; and stern and ruthless economic laws had arranged it that she could only do this by working just as she did, with all her soul upon her work, and with never an instant for a glance at the well-dressed ladies and gentlemen who came to stare at her, as at some wild beast in a menagerie. (Sinclair, 1878, p. 160)

Many historians feel that this alienation schema was codified by the death and destruction wrought by World War I. This "war to end all wars" created an image of the State as hateful and utterly disregarding of the individual that has remained etched on Western consciousness even as few know the issues that led to the Great War. French, German, and, later, American generals sent millions to their deaths in battles that continued for months and won little or no territory. Even the serfs were more highly regarded, as without them the lord had no workers. Soldiers were not resources, but cannon fodder. Indeed, Soviet Russia was created over the fervor against government that grew among the Russian troops who withdrew in the middle of the war and overthrew their government (Golovine, 1931). The anarchist movement was also strong in the United States at this time, and its theme was that no government represents the people (De-Leon, 1978). The art of dadaism personified this theme, which turned against culture and society having any logic worthy of more than comic derision (Greenberg, 1979; Verkauf, 1975). The individualism of psychology may stem in large part from this post–World War I *zeitgeist*, because in this period psychology defined itself. As far apart as Freud and Skinner stood on the individual, they stood on the individual as the linchpin of psychology. Although both imagined a role for society, they were deeply critical of the society as it then stood (Freud, 1915/1961; Skinner, 1948). How, then, is the individual to cope with the stress that the environment offers? The themes that emerge in response are self-reliance, pitting oneself against social influences, isolationism, and control of both one's inner forces (Freud) and social contingencies (Skinner).

The individual becomes the isolated, self-contained individual, "a sense of self with a sharp boundary that stops at one's skin and clearly demarks self from nonself" (Spence, 1985, p. 1288). If this is psychology's model, then it would be expected that the study of coping would encompass individual action that focuses on the self and has clear boundaries between self-action and the action of others. It is very different than the ensembled individualism that other cultural models may have offered (Sampson, 1988). Ensembled individualism is personified by fluid interaction with others, lack of clear self–other boundaries, and sharing of control between the self, others, and the environment. Self-reliance instead led us according to Max Weber to a "rational–legal" approach to coping (see Gerth & Mills, 1946). Rational–legal coping deemphasizes collective bonds between people or deep connections that set forth people's common enterprise (Sampson, 1988). Any coping in association with others is contractual rather than based on shared bonds (see also, Mills & Clark, 1982). Self-reliance demands a clearly defined self that demarcates the individual from his or her social ties (Perloff, 1987). It is not that self-reliance does not consider others; rather, it views relationships in terms of exchange and reciprocity rather than obligations and mutuality (Clark, Mills, & Powell, 1986).

As Riger (1993) writes, "A great deal of research in psychology rests on the assumption that the healthy individual is one who is self-contained, independent, and self-reliant, capable of asserting himself and influencing his environment" (p. 280).

My argument could easily be turned on itself as well. For if our society is individualistic, then it is fit and proper that coping be conceptualized individualistically. This thinking holds to no small extent. However, if I am correct that individualism has only recently left more collectivist roots, there is a great deal of collectivism contained even in American individualism. Sampson (1988) and Baumeister (1987) both make this point as well in concluding that individualistic models overstate European and American culture's personification of individual ideals. Moreover, individualism may operate as the dominant system for men of Northern European descent. It is not necessarily the predominant worldview for Italian-Americans, American Jews, African Americans, Hispanic Americans, Asian Americans or American women (Riger, 1993; Sampson, 1988). As such, it would seem that what is called for is a balance between individual and collectivist notions when considering coping, as cultural roots have probably instilled both individual-based and collectively oriented models for our thinking, behavior, and emotional responding. A collectivist approach may be more true of women than men and of African Americans than WASPS, but these modes are in fact often blended and encompass aspects of each source. Moreover, when Turks move to Germany, Mollocans to the Netherlands, and Asians to the United States, they are likely to incorporate their more communal mother-culture with the more individualistic bases of their adopted culture in a complicated amalgam. They may enter the new culture seeing resources as shared and having obligations to others but will naturally adopt a more individualized resource and adaptation viewpoint and coping repertoire.

TRADITIONAL MODELS OF COPING

Following Lazarus and Folkman's (1984) pioneering theoretical contribution and empirical advances, most research and theory have divided coping into two types, problem-focused coping versus emotion-focused coping. Problem-focused coping addresses the source of the stress or its solution. Emotion-focused coping addresses the stress-induced emotions that accompany stress. Most stressors elicit both problem- and emotion-focused coping, but problem-focused coping may both predominate and be more effective when the sources of stress or its solution are within individuals' control. Emotion-focused coping may more likely be elicited and be more effective when the stressor is something that must be endured, at least until a solution is possible (Lazarus & Folkman, 1984).

In general, research based on Lazarus and Folkman's model found that problem-focused coping is more effective than emotion-focused coping (Aldwin, 1994). Indeed, studies repeatedly find that emotion-focused coping has decidedly negative correlates (see also Amirkhian, 1990; Endler & Parker, 1990). This is troubling, because although we should not presuppose that coping is only coping if it proves successful, we would nevertheless expect that efforts to ameliorate stress's negative impact should generally lower psychological distress, improve or protect health, and enhance functioning. Aldwin (1994) suggests that emotion-focused coping may have other functional correlates and that because research mainly addressed emotional outcomes, we may have limited our potential understanding of coping. Her point is a good one, but when more functional outcomes are considered, emotion-focused coping fares no better (Taylor & Aspinwall, 1996). Moreover, emotion-focused coping is potentially confounded with psychological outcomes, such that rather than preceding coping efforts it may actually reflect psychological sequelae of stress (Dohrenwend et al., 1984). Because coping research has not done well at denoting the actual time that coping takes place, it is difficult to tease out answers to these questions (Stone, Greenberg, Kennedy-Moore, & Neuman, 1991, Chapter 4).

TRANSITIONAL MODELS OF COPING

Problem-focused and emotion-focused coping are not exact opposites, but they generally lie on either side of a continuum between active and passive responding. Carver, Scheier, and Weintraub (1989) suggested that coping might be profitably divided further than this two-part distinction. Carver et al. integrated their thinking on self-regulation of sustained behavior with the coping construct, such that coping could be conceived as operating effectively either to sustain effort at goal-directed ends or fail to do so in varying degrees. Given this addition, a richer model evolves. Most problem-focused coping is still conceived as healthy because it acts to help achieve goals. This includes active coping, planning, seeking support on tasks, and restraint coping to wait for proper timing. However, emotion-focused coping becomes divided into efforts that help sustain motivation or problem-solving versus emotion-focused coping that limits goal-directed effort. Helpful emotion-focused coping might include acceptance and positive reinterpretation. Negative emotion-focused coping, in turn, involves avoidance, dwelling on negative emotions, or denial. This more theoretical perspective differs from earlier coping formulations because it states *a priori* what kinds of coping are likely to be effective. This moves us away from Lazarus and Folkman's thesis that coping is neither an individual style nor given to be more or less effective across contexts. It also challenges the premise that coping effectiveness could only be predicted for individuals in specific circumstances.

Carver et al.'s (1989) position would predict that coping style should be characteristic of people, even if they might display a wide range of coping behaviors in any given context and across contexts. Coping as a style, as opposed to a personality trait, supposes that given individuals will display a characteristic mode of coping in certain types of situations, especially where their goal achievement is at stake, because in such instances their tendency to self-regulate will be evoked. Herein may also lie the link between coping and resources. An increasing amount of research suggests that more goal-directed coping is related to possessing or sustaining a stronger resource armamentarium (Hobfoll, 1988; Taylor & Aspinwall, 1996). Those who retain an active coping style in the face of stressors tend to have greater object resources, personal resources, condition resources, and energy resources (Holahan & Moos, 1987). Among these, personal resources have received the most intensive study. In particular, more effective, goal-oriented coping is seen in those with greater hardiness, optimism, inter-nalized control, self-esteem, self-efficacy, mastery, and lower neuroticism (Aspinwall & Taylor, 1992; Bolger, 1990; Edwards, Baglioni, & Cooper, 1990; Jerusalem, 1993). However, it stands to reason that those with more educa-tion, financial resources, and condition resources (e.g., employment, good marriage) will also be more likely to sustain more goal-directed behavior in the face of adversity.

Cozzarelli (1993) conducted one of the more inclusive studies of per-sonal resources, coping efficacy, and psychological outcomes, focusing on women undergoing abortions. Consistent with both Carver et al.'s (1989) view of self-regulation and COR theory, she found that self-esteem, optim-ism, and sense of control were more or less exchangeable resources. More-over, possessing these personal resources led to greater coping efficacy in addressing the stress that women felt when confronting abortion and its aftermath. Women who felt more able to cope, in turn, had better immedi-ate and 3-week adjustment. Jerusalem (1993) similarly found that higher levels of personal resources predicted less negative emotional coping, more positive stress appraisals, and better subjective health outcomes.

In a study that employed an intervention aimed at enhancing resource levels in a controlled experimental design, we noted lower burnout levels in nurses who gained mastery and social support resources (Freedy & Hobfoll, 1994). Nurses were given group and individual exercises and homework designed to increase their coping through mastery and more effective help seeking. Greatest gain was apparent in groups that focused on personal and social aspects of coping simultaneously, and just addressing personal coping was not found to be as effective. Nurses who were in "control" intervention groups that did not seek to raise both their personal and social resources experienced less resource change and worse outcomes in turn.

The clear trend across these studies suggests that those who lack per-sonal, social, and perhaps other resources are more likely to disengage from goal-directed coping and seek emotional solace or dwell on their negative emotions (Holahan, Moos, Holahan, & Brennan, 1997). Those who possess resources use emotion-focused coping to strategize, conserve resources, and redirect effort in service of their problem-solving efforts. Taylor (1983) had earlier viewed coping efforts as likely to be successful to the extent that they allowed individuals to reframe circumstances in a positive manner, or at least one in which they could find an avenue of control. In more recent work, she has appeared to revise this model, tying it to resources (Taylor & Aspinwall, 1992; Aspinwall & Taylor, 1997). More specifically, self-regulation is more closely tied to possessing resources and using them to shape chal-lenging and stressful contexts so that successful coping efforts can be exer-cised. Similarly, Baumeister, Heatherton, and Tice (1993) theorized that those low in personal resources may adopt self-protective modes in order to preserve the already-diminished state of the self. By considering their resources and environmental stress more in terms of what they stand to lose than gain, they defer to a defensive posture.

These more integrated coping-resource models move us to a more person–environment balance, as opposed to the more purely appraisal-based earlier model. Recalling back to the iceberg metaphor, by tying adaptation to the orchestration of resources, this theoretical approach includes more of what is below the water's surface and addresses more of the objective aspects of people's resources and challenges. This shift occurs without losing the importance of some of these same resources in influencing appraisal as a means of sustaining self-regulatory behavior. By expanding the time element, Aspinwall and Taylor (1997) are simultaneously moving coping closer to the basic notions of COR theory and Baltes's (1987) life-span adaptation model, which posits that adaptation involves the overall struggle to protect against resource loss and enhance resource gain (see Chapters 3 and 4).

THE ILLUSION OF SELF-RELIANCE

A self-regulatory view is valuable to the extent that we are to understand achievement of individual goals. An individualized, self-regulatory view is consistent with a philosophy of self-reliance and an outlook that presupposes that the individual is the sole or, at least, central agent of concern. It rests on the assumption that individuals have power over acquisition and protection of their resources with minimal dependence on others. However, because stress is largely a product of people's overall value system, stress will encompass challenges or losses to those things they value (Kaplan, 1996). Thus, given the importance people place on social connectedness in terms of both emotional and instrumental ties, we need to widen the social aspects of coping efforts and move from self-regulation to *self-in social setting* regulation. Individuals' goals are interlaced with family, organizational, group, and societal goals, and they are accomplished through interpersonal behavior. This is not to say that coping scales have entirely ignored social aspects of coping, as they have considered social support seeking as one coping option. However, even where social support coping is considered, it is in the context of achievement of individual goals and efforts.

I would argue that the concept of self-reliance, both as Emerson and Thoreau advanced it, and as modern psychology portrays it, is largely an illusion. It is the *primum mobile* of the modern stress literature (Bandura,

1982, 1997) and one of the principle mechanisms of coping that we have mytholigized. Individualized coping is the heart of "rugged individualism." It was imported to America by Protestant German, British, and Scandinavian settlers, and honed by the pioneer spirit. Rural Americans were indeed separated from the more advanced culture and support of the city and its offerings, and needed to be more self-sufficient (Fukuyama, 1995). Even so, it was really familial reliance that was practiced, with husbands, wives, and children working together to manage their farms and create usable commodities from raw materials, the resources necessary for their survival. Only in the cowboy culture did individuals practice *self*-reliance, and the cowboys seldom married and produced few progeny (Atherton, Frantz, & Choate, 1955). They died with their culture. Moreover, the cowboy culture was parasitic on the ranch and town cultures of the West, as most individuals in the West were not cowboys, and the cowboy was dependent on these others for his livelihood.

Even in the culture of men in the mining town, miners formed coalitions to work claims together because it was vital both to get the work accomplished and to protect themselves (Caughey, 1948). Adaptation demanded dependence on others to create a defendable resource system. Interestingly, Asian-American miners formed even more powerful mining collectives during the days of the California Gold Rush. To counteract the superiority of these Asian mining communes, white miners pressed local authorities to disenfranchise the Asian miners, enacted mischief and special taxes against them, and managed to have many Asians deported or pressed back into manual labor for others.

In our study of patients with life-threatening pulmonary disorders, we witnessed the modern reification of this myth, with men frequently reporting that they depended on no one. This despite their needing constant care from their wives to eat, dress, travel, and, in many cases, bathe (Lane & Hobfoll, 1992). They maintained the societal myth of self-reliance to sustain their self-esteem, because their actual dependent state was abhorrent to them within our dominant cultural models. In this and some prior studies, we had to invalidate our social support scales because men left items unanswered or gave responses that our interviewers coded as improbable based on the overall interview and what they observed in the respondent's home. In the course of the study, one woman was propping her ill husband's pillow, serving him lunch, adjusting his oxygen, giving him his medication, reminding him of our appointment, and casually straightening the room with few wasted motions, while her husband boldly told the interviewer, "I don't receive help from others. I believe you should get things done on your own. There's too much of that kind of stuff in America. That's our problem."

Because most studies rely on self-report alone, these false reports are coded as real. Women do a disproportionate amount of the housework and child-related labor. In many ways, they make possible their husband's perceived self-reliance by the sweat of their brow (Hochschild, 1989). Similarly, the sense of mastery and self-reliance at work is incorporated in the executive myth, which holds that executives need to think for themselves and act boldly, ignoring both that each position is dependent on a web of other positions and that most decisions have consequences for others as well.

GENDER DIFFERENCES IN COPING

Given that coping has been placed within this mythopoetic hero schema, it is small wonder that gender differences on coping have been found. Although there is sizable overlap, men have been found to practice more problem-focused coping than women (Billings & Moos, 1984; Endler & Parker, 1990; Stone & Neale, 1984). Women have been found, in turn, to use more emotion-focused coping and avoidance than men. Despite social support's clear value, seeking social support is both more common for women and has negative mental and physical health correlates when examined within coping research (Endler & Parker, 1990). In other words, even the health-protective influence of social support is masked and reversed within the study of coping. This strongly suggests that the model underlying scale usage that has been theoretically advanced has some flaw. That is to say, although we would expect some gender differences in coping, they should be consistent with the broader body of research on gender differences in stress resistance. This added disadvantage for women within coping models implies that this domain of stress research may be more seriously biased on the individual versus communal dimension than studies of personal and social resources and stress resistance. The portrait of male versus female differences in coping makes suspect not the studies themselves, but the underlying assumptions or paradigm that has driven the research.

Part of the gender differences found for coping is structural in that men and women are often in different settings or have different demands on them within settings (Folkman & Lazarus, 1980; Roth & Cohen, 1989). Men are more likely to have control over solutions, which has better fit with problem-focused coping, and women are more likely to have fewer control opportunities, making emotion-focused coping more suitable. However, this fails to explain the paradoxical influence of support seeking. Endler and Parker (1990) found support seeking to be related to avoidance. Yet this only partially corresponds to what we know about support seeking, or as Carver et al. (1989) have pointed out, it relates to one dimension of support seeking. The healthier dimensions of support seeking, more common for women than men, however, do not seem to surface in this area of investigation. Indeed, although Endler and Parker found that social support seeking was related to avoidance, its negative correlates were only apparent for men and not for women. Again, it would seem that the individualistic bias may have resulted in a misrepresentation of the benefit of more social coping, at least for the more collectivist gender, women.

The negative findings for support seeking as a coping alternative may also be related to the costs of social coping. By being more involved in a social network, individuals are exposed to the difficulties, frustrations, pain, and suffering of others (Kessler, McLeod, & Wethington, 1985). By being connected to these others and making them more central, there is added risk of *stress contagion* (Riley & Eckenrode, 1986), such that the borders that protect the self-reliant individual break down and crossover of stress occurs. Together with Perry London, we (Hobfoll & London, 1986) also noted what we called the *pressure cooker effect* in our study of Israeli women during the Israel–Lebanon War. Specifically, because many stressors communally tax a group, both potential supporters and supportees are often experiencing the same crisis. In our investigation, we found that women who sought and received more social support experienced a greater degree of psychological distress. As such, their resources were taxed as a group, and by seeking one another for help, they added further burden to the already overtaxed system. Thus, this added burden may undermine the benefits of social support coping.

Men and women may have different experiences with seeking social support as well. Men are socialized to be more self-reliant and to "pick themselves up by their own bootstraps." This tendency might be inadvertently encouraged by men's female partners, as they may be expected to be the "rock of Gibraltar" for their family. Consistent with this premise, Weiss (1990) found that men whose wives did not work outside the home could not bring their work problems home because it was too stressful to their wives. Not knowing the work culture and being dependent on one salary, wives would catastrophize about more or less everyday problems. This may have encouraged men to follow their already-learned tendency of self-reliance after some initial tests of their wive's ability to offer them support.

Women, in turn, may be burdened because they are expected to be the conduits of support. Being the resident social experts in the family, they may have extra stress placed on them to be the handlers of emotionally charged material. This division of social labor, so to speak, seems natural if women are better at the emotional and interpersonal side of stress, but it places them at added risk for stress contagion and the pressure cooker effect. Studies of social support have repeatedly found that the commerce in social support is more women's than men's mode (Kessler et al., 1985; Hobfoll & Stokes, 1988), perhaps because they are more comfortable with intimacy and place greater value on social attachments. Still, if we understand that families are social systems, then we see that men are utilizing women to promote their self-reliance, but at the same time remain socially connected through their wives' actions. Men cannot, in other words, preserve their self-reliant illusion without women taking responsibility for the work of social obligations and role patterns that families, businesses, and organizations require. They perform agenic tasks and delegate social tasks.

Acitelli and Antonucci (1994) suggest that although men and women may both use social support, men may utilize support for achievement of instrumental goals rather than to meet relational needs. Women, in turn, are utilizing men to allow themselves to continue in their socially connected role. With men performing the more agenic responsibilities of the family, women are freed to address the more social roles. Women, then, are performing more social coping responsibilities in the name of the family and delegating agenic tasks more to men, as well.

SOCIAL RELATEDNESS SEEN AS WEAKNESS

Our society, and psychology, when it studies this domain, has forced a schism between communal and agenic roles due to the value placed on self-reliance and its believed association with men's way of coping. Communality and social support become equated with weakness and ineffectiveness, because by being more interdependent, they are *de facto* linked with a less esteemed form of adaptation. However, if we for a moment devalue self-reliance as an ideal, we see the fallacy of this viewpoint, as effectiveness is really a matter of product, not method. Whether the individual is self-reliant or jointly reliant is a matter of method and is not of necessity related to the advantages of either coping style. Consider the power and strength noted in the classic "Woman of Valor" found in Proverbs (31:10), paying special attention to the strength of the metaphors and efficacy associated with nurturance, sharing, and caring:

> A woman of valor who can find. For her price is far above rubies.... She is like the merchant ships; she bringeth her food from afar. She riseth also while it is yet night, And giveth food to her household... She considereth a field and buyeth it; With the fruit of her hands she planteth a vineyard. She girdeth her loins with strength, And Maketh strong her arms.... She stretcheth out her hand to the poor, Yea, she reacheth forth her hand to the needy.... Strength and dignity are her clothing. And she laugheth at the time to come. She openeth her mouth with wisdom; and the law of kindness is on her tongue.... She looketh well to the ways of her household, and eateth not the bread

of idleness. Her children rise up and call her blessed; Her husband also and he praiseth her.

So pervasive has been this bias against communal coping that this very passage has been slightly altered and used to indicate women's subjugation to men, although the opposite is found here in the original text.[1] To the extent that women are being reconnected to the family and village economy in today's society, I would expect that we will experience increased value being placed on more collectivist means of adaptation and resource acquisition and protection. Because post–World War II economy saw fit to banish women from the active economic network, there may have been an associated mistaken tendency to equate men's way of coping with agency. With the rise once again of "women of valor" who are mixing communal approaches to the home and workplace (Hoschchild, 1989), effectiveness is being reinserted in association with this style of coping.

Surely, this division of social labor is less apparent in less sex-role-traditional families, but research suggests that despite some attitude change, actual family behavioral patterns have not changed so greatly for most families (Hoschchild, 1989). Thoits (1991) suggests that men's and women's way of addressing problems continues to differ by virtue of women's more social approach. Moreover, although research has tended to deemphasize these gender differences in coping, Eagly (1995) suggests that gender differences in this domain are marked and that the decision to deemphasize them may be more political than scientific. Indeed, Eagly's precise point is that whenever male–female differences are found, they have been interpreted as signs of female deficiency, and hence more feminist researchers have been reticent to highlight areas of difference.

CULTURAL DIFFERENCES IN COPING PATTERNS

Gender differences in coping have often been equated with East–West differences in coping patterns, but Kashima et al. (1995) suggest that this is an oversimplification. Specifically, given that women are more communally oriented than men and that Asia and Africa are more communally oriented than America or Europe, gender and cultural differences have frequently been equated. There is indeed some overlap if we look at the level of social connections. Women in the West are more socially connected than men in close relationships and use social means for coping more.

However, on other levels, the nascent research suggests that Western women are not collective in the same ways as Asiacentric or Africentric approaches would be. Gender differences in collectivism are likely to have arisen from gender-based division of labor within a given society (Eagly,

1987). Cultural differences could not have these same evolutionary pressures and develop due to different ecological pressures within each disparate culture and environment. Gender differences, in other words, have developed *within* an ecosystem and cultural differences develop *between* ecosystems (Kashima et al., 1995).

Obligation Orientation

Africentric and Asiacentric models of collectivism are more obligation-oriented and structurally determined than Western women's collectivist patterns (Kashima et al., 1995). Such concepts as conducting oneself for the sake of nation, emperor, or for social demands themselves are not Western concepts, and are probably not shared by Western women (Fukuyama, 1995; Schwartz & Bilsky, 1990). That is, men's and women's values in the West do not vary greatly on these dimensions (Kashima et al., 1995). Consider Confucius (Eliot, 1980) on obligation as to its lack of fit to what has been called "women's collectivism" in the West:

> ... to family.
> The Master said: "A father or mother may be gently chiden. If they will not bend, be the more lowly, but persevere; not murmur if trouble follow." (IV, 18)
>   The Master said: "If for three years a son does not forsake his father's way, he may be called dutiful." (V, 20)
>
>   ... to others.
> The Master said: "Good is no hermit. It has ever neighbours."
> The Master said: "To be respectful at home, painstaking at work, faithful to all. Even among savages none of this may be dropped." (XIII, 19)
>
>   ... to one's emperor, clan, and own self.
> Fan Ch'ih asked, When can a man be called a good crown servant?
> The Master said: "In private life he wants a sense of shame: if sent to the four corners of the earth he must not disgrace the king's commands ...
> A man who his clansmen call dutiful.
> A man who clings to his word and sticks to his course, a flinty little fellow. (XIII, 20)"

Said another way, Western women, although more socially enmeshed and interconnected with others than men, still have a strong sense of self, self-esteem, and self-oriented goal direction (Gilligan, 1982). They are not collectivist in a Confucian sense. Hence, although men and women differ within each culture, they tend to hold the same values and differ as to means of social interaction.

Indirect Coping, Stage Setting

More similarity between non-Western and Western women's approach to coping may exist on the dimension of coping directness. Self-reliant models and rugged individualism in particular tend to disdain subtlety.

Being straightforward, honest, and forthright are primary rules for the self in social context within a system that values self-reliant coping. Indeed, being other than straightforward and forthright in psychology is equated with manipulativeness, passive–aggressive behavior, and psychological disorder (American Psychiatric Association, 1994; Brosliman, Clarkson, Rosenkrantz, & Vogel, 1970). Similarly, being indirect is linguistically equated in the thesaurus with being devious, deceitful, dishonest, and passive. The only positive synonym I could find for behavioral indirectness, in contrast, was judicious, but judicious is often used as a euphemism for weak-kneed or overly cautious.

The direct opposite meaning for directness is held in the East. In Japan, being straightforward and direct is viewed as boorish and lower class. This is not because the Japanese believe that "fools rush in" and are likely by so doing to encounter personal failure. Rather, indirectness is called for because one must preserve the honor of others and the self simultaneously. Direct action is likely to risk either personal or social disaster. Instead, one must be indirect, and the emphasis for coping here is placed on stage setting rather than direct action. Hence, if the individual or group sets the stage for certain desired ends, no one will lose face if they do not succeed. Being confrontational risks placing people on the spot and embarrassing them or highlighting their inadequacy. This indirect route is hardly passive, as stage setting demands a great deal of activity in order to ensure the desired outcome.

> The Master said: "Listen much, keep silent when in doubt, and always take heed of the tongue; thou wilt make few mistakes. See much, beware of pitfalls, and always give heed to thy walk; thou wilt have little to rue. If thy words are seldom wrong, thy deeds leave little to rue, pay will follow." (II, 18)

> The Master said: "Men of old were loth to speak; lest a word that they could not make good should shame them." (IV, 22)

> The Master said: "Who contains himself goes seldom wrong." (IV, 23)

> The Master said: "A gentleman wishes to be slow to speak and quick to act." (V, 24)

> The Master said: "In my first dealings with men, I hearkened to their words, and took their deeds on trust. Now, in dealing with men, I hearken to their words, and watch their deeds." (V, 9)

Western women have a similar task in that much of what they do socially has to be indirect in order to preserve its prosocial character. Studies in business, for example, find that women work more for group consensus and are less confrontational than men (Martin, 1993). This indirectness in part has been attributed to their having less power in the family and in the workplace (Martin, 1993). Having less power, direct action is less a viable option. Their lack of power demanded that they achieve their goals more by stage setting than by direct action.

A 1939 Chrysler ad in the *Ladies' Home Journal* shows a pretty woman with the following text:

So-oo ... I'm a wonderful little wife!
There was Jim telling Randy how *he* picked out our new Chrysler Royal ... that I—his wonderful little wife!—leave such things to him! As if I hadn't been working on getting that Chrysler for months! As if I hadn't left magazines around opened up to the Chrysler ads ... sighed wistfully every time we passed a Chrysler on the road ... primed Dad to say the right thing at the right time! And, of course, the Chrysler salesman just *happened* to stop in at our house!*

Clearly, this ad speaks of a time when women were not empowered to purchase cars or even, it seems, to enter the exclusively men's world of large financial commitments for anything mechanical. Although psychology has tended to vilify her approach as manipulative, channels of direct action were closed to her. She was not only getting her needs met, but also having to preserve her husband's fragile sense of self that demanded that he have a "good little wife." Moreover, seen this way, the connection to collectivist cultures is more obvious. Indirect social action serves to protect others from being openly undermined and preserves their self-esteem. In raising children, it is an essential strategy for building self-esteem, such that parents practice stage setting to create an environment wherein the child is challenged with the next developmental or academic step and sheltered from overly advanced challenges (Erikson, 1968). The idea here is the same: to create settings indirectly in order to preserve the positive sense of self of the individuals involved. Of course, this said, in the preceding example and in other cases where power is not equitably distributed, those who must be indirect must often deny themselves in order to help others.

Hence, the dimension of coping directness versus indirectness may be a critical and less obvious dimension by which we are to understand collectivist coping. Moreover, it may be a dimension that holds for both traditional collectivist cultures and for Western women. In contrast, East versus West (and Africentric vs. West) divisions may differ more in terms of social obligations and fixed social roles within those obligated structures (Triandis, 1995a,b). Women within Western societies seem to differ less on this social dimension.

Cultural Change

Finally, it is important to underscore historical factors that influence these cultural and gender differences and similarities. Japanese culture has reduced its sense of interpersonal obligation since World War II due to the

---

*Used by permission of the Chrysler Corporation.

perception that this tendency was linked to earlier ultranationalism (Hamaguchi, 1977). Koreans placed their relatedness in more emotional terms and were the occupied rather than the occupier, resulting in a different interaction between cultural and historical ingredients (Choi, 1994). Women in the West, in contrast, may have felt that self-sacrifice, which is essential to communalism, resulted in their lower status and have thus worked in recent years to be more self-assertive and less demure (Eagly, 1987, 1995). In one of the only studies with a long enough follow-up period, Roberts and Helson (1997) found that from 1958 to 1989, a sample of educated American women increased in individualism and narcissism and decreased in norm adherence. Hence, communalism, relatedness, directness, and concepts pertaining to the self should be seen as in flux. These changes will be especially dynamic as we enter a period in which there is greater international mixing and more common aspirations toward liberal democracy and the individualism that often goes with this part and parcel, perhaps because it is inherent in it, and perhaps because this form of society is so linked with Americanism (Fukuyama, 1992).

CONCLUSIONS

I intended in this chapter to offer a more balanced view of coping and adaptation that addresses the individual-nested-in families-nested-in social setting. Both individual and collectivist notions of coping not only have certain strengths; they are also both represented in some form in every culture. No society is so individualized as not to have a collective sense, and no collective culture is entirely deindividualized. Societies such as the United States, which represent an amalgam of peoples bringing their disparate culture, and where women are achieving an ever greater voice, are especially likely to reflect elements of both individualism and collectivism in people's behavior and consistency with social norms.

As I have underscored in earlier chapters, we may be tempted to adopt communal coping over individualistic coping wholesale if we become intellectually infatuated with its more prosocial nature and in so doing fail to appreciate that both concepts are multidimensional. Communal and individualistic coping should really be understood as differing on several subcomponents. When seen this way, Americans are actually more communal than Japanese on the dimension of acting because one cares about others (Kashima et al., 1995). Communal and individualistic coping styles subsume dimensions of control, orientation toward the group, directness of action, social obligations, social attachments, and in-group versus out-group standards. The Japanese may have been able to commit atrocities of war toward women during World War II because they could distance Koreans as an out-group more easily than an individualistically framed culture might have. Similarly, the Nazi's increased communal notions in order to enhance obligation to Fatherland and party. We need to take care not to romanticize one mode or another, but to understand strengths and weaknesses simultaneously.

Returning to the theme of self-reliance, American and some European cultures may have been shaped to fit individualistic and mentalistic approaches to problems. Hence, even if we might intellectually prefer some elements of communalism, they may have poor fit with social pressures and adopted metaphors within these cultures. Self-reliance allows greatest independence of action and personal freedom, which are particularly idealized notions within these societies. Self-reliance also eschews the need to disclose weaknesses, a foundation for sustaining rugged individualism. Fisher, Nadler, and Whitcher-Alagna (1982), in an insightful line of research, found that those who are high in self-esteem may act more independently because help seeking places them in a potentially weak situation. The feelings of helplessness attendant with relying on others may actually be easier for low self-esteem individuals to tolerate. Swann (Swann & Read, 1981; Swann, Stein-Seroussi, & Giesler, 1992) similarly finds that those high in self-esteem act to shape their environment to receive high self-esteem messages. Given the Western penchant for self-reliance as a prerequisite for self-esteem, having to rely on the collective may put a negative strain on the self. Hence, although I have asserted a need to balance coping with collectivist notions and to lessen emphasis on control and self-promotion, it seems clear that each cultural system has advantages and disadvantages, and that all cultures have both individualistic and collectivist components. Within a given culture, predominant cultural themes must be acknowledged.

NOTE

1. It is important not to confuse one Biblical text with another, and more importantly one Bible with another. The "Woman of Valor" text could not be more different from Peter (3) in the New Testament. "Wives, in the same way be submissive to your husbands so that, if any of them do not believe the word, they may be won over without words by the behavior of their wives.... Husbands in the same way be considerate as you live with your wives, and treat them with respect as the weaker partner." The woman of valor talks of a woman who independently purchases fields, acts as a merchant, runs her household, buys and sells, and does all of this for her family's sake, but without consult, let alone subservience to her husband.

6

Marching to a Different Drum, Singing the Same Song

In the last chapter, I discussed aspects of coping by individuals, emphasizing that we are always connected to families and tribes, and subject to the social roles and values that these social links create. When we act, the results ripple like the proverbial pebble thrown in a pool. Our coping actions influence our own resources, but because so many of our resources are shared, this impacts others, and more often in a dramatic than an incidental fashion (Lyons, Mickelson, Sullivan, & Coyne, 1998). We are constantly acting in concert with others, against others, or in isolation of others, from cradle to the grave (Horney, 1937, 1950). We are prevailed upon by the culture of self-reliance to march to our own drum, but as members of families and villages and tribes, we must sing in concert with others.

This view of the self as interdependent contrasts to principles of *rational self-interest* or *economic man* that traditional psychological theory assumes to underpin human motivation (Kelley, 1979; Luce & Raiffa, 1957; Von Neuman & Morgenstern, 1947). Rather than solely acting independently of others according to one's own self-interest, people act in their own self-interest, in cooperation with others, and against others (Van Lange, De Bruin, Otten, Lotten, & Joireman, 1997). In fact, a collectivist orientation implies that people will often act in a self-sacrificing manner if it will benefit their families, social group, or society.

There has been nascent interest in the social aspects of coping and adaptation, beginning with examination of social support seeking (cf. Carver et al., 1989). Indeed, Coyne and Smith (1991) argued that social interaction underlies coping processes and is a basis for development of coping strategies. Eckenrode (1991) similarly suggested that social environments influence how we cope by cuing certain behaviors. The settings in which we exist facilitate and constrain our behavior depending on the fit of coping demands conceived within the social ecology of the setting. Each of these theorists also concludes that current coping theories and scales do not adequately address this domain.

Lyons et al. (1998) underscores that traditional coping models offer a pale representation of the richness of people's actual array of potential adaptive behaviors, and tend to be still-framed rather than interactive. I would add that even where social aspects of coping have been addressed (Carver et al., 1989; Endler & Parker, 1990), it has been from an individualistic model and support seeking is typically the only dimension studied. Further, studying social coping has been problematic because support seeking may reflect a rather late stage in the adaptation process, confounding coping with outcomes. This occurs because people are generally reticent to seek help in a self-reliant culture, and as a result tend to do so when they are already experiencing particularly high levels of distress (Schwarzer & Leppin, 1989).

Coping has generally been an area that lacks overarching theories. Attempts to add theory have tended to be piecemeal, looking at theoretical underpinnings of individual scales (Carver et al., 1989). In the current chapter, I present our rather imperfect attempt to develop both a general model of coping and a coping instrument that reflects a midpoint between individualistic and communal coping, or perhaps more accurately, that allows for representation of both. This seems reasonable given that individualism and communalism are not as much distinct as continuous, and given that they are not necessarily orthogonal or unidimensional. Kashima et al. (1995), for example, noted that although Japanese were high on collectivism in terms of willingness to stick to and sacrifice for their group, they were low on what Hamaguchi (1977) called *Kanjin-shugi*, which might be translated as relatedness to others (e.g., "I often do what I feel like doing without paying attention to others' feelings"). This suggests that the Japanese may be high on elements of both communalism and individualism, challenging a unitary conceptualization of these concepts.

Throughout this chapter, I highlight how a multicultural model of coping can successfully capture individual and collectivist notions. Adventuring in this new domain, within which so little is yet known, has been the most exciting stage in my career. Because it is so unexplored, we are constantly uncovering new knowledge and are fascinated with our findings. However, I also underscore the difficulty of doing so and the nascent nature of our own pioneering, one might say, primitive efforts. Because, I believe, we are treading on unchartered territory, we frequently have stumbled.

Even from the very aspect of language, it is difficult to capture many more collectivist concepts succinctly. Where language served, other biases emerged. For example, some aspects of indirectness are difficult to translate to English. Other concepts are translatable but have opposite meaning. Although we are all dependent on others, there are few words that are more negatively emotionally charged than dependency, with its decidedly negative interpretation in English and as a way of coping (Hobfoll & Lerman, 1988; Fisher et al., 1982). Because some cultures have a crystallized self and others a porous self interconnected with others (Sampson, 1988), coping actions that address the self and others take on different meanings. Factory solutions that worked so well for Swedish automakers failed when transported to the United States because sharing initiative was rejected on the American shop floor, where only individual initiative was valued (Fukuyama, 1995). The following, then, is our imperfect attempt to chart new territory; like any explorer, please allow for a map that I hope will be helpful to others but has many gaps and more than a few miscues.

THE MULTIAXIAL MODEL OF COPING

Separating Activity Level from Sociability

The Multiaxial Model of Coping begins with two axes (Hobfoll, Dunahoo, Ben-Porath, & Monnier, 1994), and we had originally thought of it as a dual-axis model. The two original axes were (1) active versus passive coping and (2) prosocial versus antisocial coping.

The Active–Passive Axis

This first axis denotes the level or extent of coping activity. It separates being action-oriented from the way the coping behavior interfaces the self with others. Persons from any culture or gender may be placed somewhere on this continuum depending on how active they are in addressing the problems confronting them. They may be active in response to their assessment that a stressor might occur, they might be active in building resources, or they might be reactive once a stressor has occurred or in reconstituting a diminished resource reservoir.

To the extent that current scales operated from the self-reliance, or individual-in-control model, our active–passive dimension is distinguishable from what has been called problem-focused coping. Specifically, problem-focused coping, as it has been studied (Lazarus & Folkman, 1984;

Endler & Parker, 1990), implies self-reliance, going it alone, or being in control of others in accomplishing tasks. These are potentially active ways of coping, but they have vast implications beyond just the level of coping activity. In this way, how stress researchers have conceptualized problem-focused coping, and perhaps how Western individualism denotes this mode of adaptation, emphasizes individualized, controlled action, whereas activity per se is not constrained in this manner.

The Social Axis

The second axis of the multiaxial model is the social dimension. Coping action differs in the degree in which it considers and interfaces the self with others. It underscores that our coping often occurs through a process of social interaction. The midpoint of this scale denotes an *a*social posture. At this level, individuals act fairly independently of social surroundings. Coping in response to an examination might exist on this level, whereby individuals might accept the challenge of the test and study on their own. They would be active, but *a*social.

At the two end points of this scale are prosocial and antisocial coping postures, respectively. Prosocial coping involves adaptive acts whose intent is to care for others, seek their care, or behave in a way that involves positive social interaction. Prosocial coping would include seeking support and attempting to build coalitions with others. It can be quite active, but it might also be reflected in a certain activity level denoted by cautiousness. Although often viewed negatively within our culture that so values aggressive action and being assertive, when others are involved, being cautious may represent a tendency to feel out others, understand their needs, and act in a way that others can support and that will not cause them to lose face. Japanese silence in conversation comes from the social demand to consider carefully one's words and to act cautiously so as to not infringe on societal injunctions.

When involved in the investigation of a psychological claim following a plane crash, I was with a group on St. Lawrence Island in the Bering Sea, near the coast of Siberia. Many were killed and injured in the crash and there was much work to be done in our investigation. We were advised by the anthropologist on our team, however, to speak little, keep our heads down, and avoid eye contact in our initial contacts—acts that would be interpreted as overly aggressive. It felt unnatural sitting through a long meeting where few words were spoken and little accomplished. We later received feedback that the whaling captains, our esteemed hosts, felt that we were unusually well cultured (meaning socially sensitive) for whites! The most silent in our group was referred to as wise. Most important, our initial respect for others was rewarded by affording us positive social sanction that allowed us to proceed effectively with our work (Hobfoll, Morgan, & Lehrman, 1980).

Antisocial coping, in contrast, includes coping activities that either are directly meant to harm others or that display general disregard for the likely harm they will cause. This includes outright antisocial coping, which is used in order to gain advantage over others through exploiting their weaknesses or attacking them to better position oneself in terms of achieving goals and objectives. "Alls fair in love and war," and the means are often seen as justifying the ends. The strict social boundaries and prizing of competition between people in our society allow for people justifying antisocial acts as a socially permissible coping pattern. Stricter in-group versus out-group distinctions in Japan and China, in contrast, inhibit antisocial coping and open competition within in-group structures, such as among coworkers and extended family, but allow for antisocial acts against others who constitute the outgroup.

Other antisocial coping is nested in certain kinds of activity that are more inadvertently antisocial. To act instinctively is often called "shooting from the hip" and is not intended to cause others harm. A "shoot from the hip" response is literally a style of coping derived from a cowboy metaphor. Gunslingers became so good that they fired their six-guns from the hip without taking aim. This kind of coping has many positive connotations, however, and is often used as a metaphor for honesty and forthrightness, even though it blatantly disregards others. Harking back to Emerson, who more than any other defined and shaped the American philosophy of self-reliance, the "shoot from the hip" style can be equated with having little regard for social protocol. In his essay on heroism (1841), Emerson appeals to the hero notion of coping as follows:

> There is somewhat not philosophical in heroism; there is somewhat not holy in it; it seems not to know that other souls are of one texture with it; it hath pride; it is the extreme of individual nature. Nevertheless we must profoundly revere it.... Heroism feels and never reasons, and therefore is always right....
> Heroism works in contradiction to the voice of mankind. (p. 124)

Emerson's hero is almost the diametrical opposite of the Eastern champion, who is philosophical to the point of having evolved into the intellectual class, who is devoted to his liege lord and his culture, and who reasons carefully before taking action (Downs, 1970; Nitobe, 1905a,b; Masatsugu, 1982).

Within a culture that values an aggressive self-reliance, a more modified form of antisocial coping may nevertheless prove adaptive. What we might call aggressive coping, which seeks to be dominant and enterprising, is esteemed in American and Australian culture, for example (Kashima et al., 1995). This same posture is viewed as blustering, even by most Western

European standards, where a more humble, less aggressive stance is considered more socially acceptable. Still, this means that an active, aggressive stance could have good ecological fit within some Western cultures and would be rewarded and not socially sanctioned. I take care here to distinguish the aggressive coping stance from one that is either outright antisocial or "shoot from the hip," as an aggressive stance implies that the protagonist is socially aware enough not to cross certain boundaries that result in social censure.

Placing the active–passive and antisocial–prosocial axes together in Cartesian space (see Figure 6.1), we can place individuals at the point that is defined by how high they are on activity and sociability. It should also be noted that the two axes are not entirely independent. If one is aggressive or building social coalitions, one must be active. If one becomes extremely inactive, there may be little or no social action whatsoever. This follows from early work of Alfred Adler (1927, 1933), who defined the healthy personality as being active and having high "social interest" (see also Allport, 1937, 1961; Erikson, 1968; Horney, 1937). Adler and Erikson both theorized that passivity tended to obviate either positive social interest or social aggressiveness. Antisocial and prosocial behavior can, however, be sustained at relatively low levels of activity, and I would add that although we imagine passivity in absolute terms, few people ever become entirely inactive. As such, for most individuals, in most circumstances, the low end of activity still

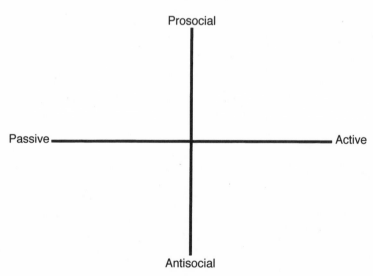

Figure 6.1. The Dual-Axis Model of Coping.

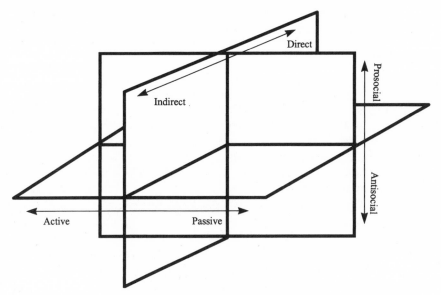

Figure 6.2. The Multiaxial Model of Coping.

implies some degree of action, and probably enough to maintain a positive or negative social posture vis-à-vis others.

Distinguishing Directness from Activity Level

A more communal understanding of coping is created by adding a third coping axis, *directness*, as presented in Figure 6.2. As discussed earlier, directness is very different from activity, and indirectness cannot be equated with passivity or inaction. In fact, indirectness often demands an active social coping strategy, because stage setting is less efficient than acting directly on objects or persons. In stage setting, coping is aimed at creating an ecology or setting where a certain desired behavior or outcome will be likely.

> The location where we will engage the enemy must not become known to them. If it is not known, then the positions they must prepare to defend will be numerous. If the positions the enemy prepares to defend are numerous, then the forces we will engage will be few. (p. 192)
>
> Thus the army is established by deceit, moves for advantage, and changes through segmenting and reuniting. Thus its speed is like the wind, its slowness like the forest.... It is as difficult to know as the darkness; in movement it is like thunder.

Thus the strategy for employing the military: Do not approach high mountains; do not confront those who have hills behind them. Do not pursue feigned retreats. Do not obstruct an army retreating homeward. If you besiege an army you must leave an outlet. Do not press an exhausted invader. These are the strategies for employing the military. (Sun Tzu, 5th Century B.C.E., p. 199)

The words of Sun Tzu translate to a kind of indirectness that is an important ingredient of collectivism and one that Western psychology is just beginning to appreciate. Borrowing from items on various measures of collectivism, it entails "not saying anything when dissatisfied with decisions of the group," "pretending to agree with the majority opinion in the group" (Kashima et al., 1995), not "having frank talks with others to clear the air" (Triandis, 1994), and not "telling your parents when you disagree with them" (Yamaguchi scale in Triandis, 1994). In general, it means acting to maintain harmony rather than assert self-needs. The indirectness that is implied in this is that one is still supposed to remain true to one's ideals, even if these are socially derived ideals. Hence, one must often appear one way and act another. Rather than being straightforward, the ideal is being "difficult to know."

Creation of the Strategic Approach to Coping Scale (SACS)

In order to assess the multiaxial model of coping, a new instrument was devised, the Strategic Approach to Coping Scale (SACS). We selected items that reflected both individual and collectivist coping strategies, focusing on how people approached problems and utilized their personal, social, condition, and object resources. The items for the SACS were collected from a variety of sources that dealt with coping strategies in individual and social settings. Items were adopted from Sun Tzu's *Art of War*, chess strategy books, and modern texts on gaming and business strategies. We also reviewed books containing common sayings that refer to coping that we could identify conceptually in a number of different languages, albeit sometimes in different forms (e.g., "Don't give up, even when things look their worst" or "Take the bull by the horns"). We also created items that fit the multiaxial model.[1]

Our research identified nine subscales (Hobfoll, Dunahoo, Ben-Porath, & Monnier, 1994; Dunahoo, Hobfoll, Monnier, Hulhizer, & Johnson, 1998):

1. Assertive action
2. Avoidance
3. Seeking social support
4. Cautious action
5. Social joining

6. Instinctive action
7. Aggressive action
8. Antisocial action
9. Indirect action

Reliability of the subscales was as good or better than subscale properties of comparative multisubscale coping instruments. Items from a preliminary version were altered where reliability information suggested they should be, and additional items were added to relatively weak subscales (Dunahoo et al., 1998).

In order to assess whether our measure actually reflected the theoretical structure upon which it was based, we subjected the subscales to analyses that revealed three replicable associated sets[2] (associated subscales) across samples: (1) active-antisocial/aggressive, (2) prosocial–cautious, and (3) a pure active–passive set. Directness–indirectness, interestingly was associated with different sets in various samples, sometimes appearing with greater weight on one set than another, suggesting that degree of directness could be applied to both active and passive and pro- and antisocial styles. Items of the SACS are presented in Table 6.1 for each subscale.

Figure 6.3 presents a schematic representation of the sets superimposed on the heuristic multiaxial model. By examining the set structure, we can judge to what extent the SACS represents the theoretical model that underlay its construction, responding to Carver et al.'s (1989) criticism that coping scales generally fail to follow a theoretical plan.

Active-Prosocial Coping

Examining our findings (see Figure 6.3), it became apparent that the active, prosocial profile that emerged actually may be better called judicious-prosocial, as it is linked to cautious action more than assertive action. Active-prosocial coping thus includes the following kinds of adaptive strategies. By viewing them together as an associated set, rather than scale by scale, a sense of an overall composite strategy begins to emerge: (1) cautious action, (2) social joining, (3) support seeking, and (4) assertive action (in some samples). This linkage is consistent with collectivist models of behavior that demand careful attention to environmental cues before action is taken. Self-reliant models might see this cautiousness as a sign of weakness, but Eastern cultural models suggest that by assessing the environment, one is more likely to act correctly for all those concerned. If social action considers the consequence to others, it is more complicated and time-consuming than individualistic action that only considers self-referent consequences. To the extent that honor is more crucial in collectivist coping, increased emphasis on

Table 6.1. Strategic Approach to Coping Scale (SACS) Subscales

Assertive Action

1. Don't give up, even when things look their worst, because you can often turn things around.
10. Move on to other things; ther's little hope for such situations getting better $(-)$
15. Retreat; avoid contact until the problem blows over. $(-)$
25. You'll probably feel bad, but there is not much you can do about this sort of thing. $(-)$
26. Just work harder; apply yourself.
33. Get out of the situation; when problems arise, its ususally a good sign of worse to come. $(-)$
50. Be asserive and get needs met.
51. Be strong and forceful, but avoid harming others.
52. Directly address the situation; don't back away from problems.

Social Joining

17. Join together with others to deal with the situation together.
23. Try to help out others involved, as giving of yourself usually helps solve problems like this.
24. Think carefully about how others feel before deciding what to do.
30. Try hard to meet other's wishes, as this will really help the situation.
41. Try to meet the needs of others who are involved.

Seeking Social Support

2. Check with friends about what they would do.
9. Check with family about what they would do.
13. Turn to others for help.
18. Depend on yourself, but at the same time rely on others who are close to you.
28. Go to someone for emotional support.
38. Talk to others to get out your frustrations.
46. Ask friends or family for their opinions about your plan of action.

Cautious Action

12. Be very cautious and look very hard at your options (better safe than sorry).
14. Go forward, but don't use all you resources until you know full well what you're up against.
29. Move very cautiously; there may be a hidden agenda.
40. Break up the problem into smaller parts and deal with them one at a time.
43. Do something to help you calm down and, only then, start problem solving.

Instinctive Action

5. Depend on yourself and your personal strengths; its not a good idea to depend on others.
6. Trust your instincts, not your thoughts.
11. Depend on your own gut-level reaction.
35. Go with your intuition.
42. Follow your first impulse; things usually work out best that way.
48. Rely on your own judgment, because only you have your best interests at heart.

Avoidance

7. Avoid dealing with the problem; things like this often go away on their own.
20. Do something to help you avoid thinking about the problem.

Table 6.1. (*Continued*)

Avoidance

22. Back off and just let the smoke clear.
27. Hold back, as it is better to wait until the smoke clears before any action is taken.
32. If it doesn't get worse, just avoid the whole thing.
47. Focus on something else and let the situation resolve itself.

Indirect Action

4. Try to be in control, but let others think they are still in charge.
21. Others often need to feel they are the boss, so you have to work around them to get things done.
34. Let others think they are in control, but keep your own hands firmly ont the wheel.
37. Sometimes your only choice is to be a little manipulative and work around people.

Antisocial Action

16. Counterattack and catch others off guard.
19. Look out for your own best interests, even if it means hurting others that are involved.
36. Assert your dominance quickly.
39. Act quickly to put others at a disadvantage.
44. Look for other's weaknesses and use them to your advantage.

Aggressive Action

3. Act fast; it is better to throw yourself right into the problem.
8. Mount an all-out attack; be aggressive.
31. Move aggressively; often if you get another off guard, things will work to your advantage.
45. Take the bull by the horns; adopt a take-charge attitude.
49. Be firm; hold your ground.

(−) = negatively keyed items.

cautious action may also be required in order to ensure that some *faux pas* is not made.

Social joining represents attempts at coalition building, acting in concert with others, and seeking strength in numbers. Support seeking is also part of this grouping and represents attempts to rely on others for emotional and instrumental support and advice. When seeking support in response to stress, people often did so through indirect action, whereas social joining was associated with a more direct style.

In some of our studies, we found people to tie assertive action to the other coping behaviors in the active-prosocial set, suggesting that prosocial coping can be associated with a more clearly active coping style (see Figure 6.4) (Hobfoll et al., 1994). Whether prosocial coping takes a more assertive or a more cautious direction may hinge on protagonists' personal styles or, alternatively, to varying social demands of different circumstances. The fact

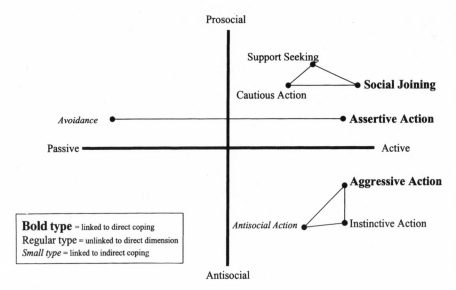

Figure 6.3. Schematic of SACS Subscales on Multiaxial Model of Coping: Primary Patterns. The direct–indirect axis is indicated by bold, regular, and italic letters.

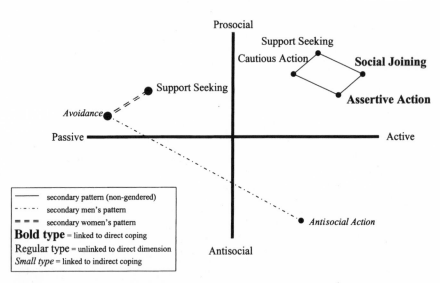

Figure 6.4. Schematic of SACS Subscales on Multiaxial Model of Coping: Secondary Patterns. The direct–indirect axis is indicated by bold, regular, and italic letters.

that cautious action is consistently, positively related to assertive action suggests that it may reflect two variations of approaches that are used by many of the same individuals, where they sometimes tread more carefully and sometimes more forcefully. This would be puzzling if we merely assumed as fact the cultural imperatives that esteem assertiveness but are more ambivalent about cautiousness. But how society wishes to stereotype us, and even how we imagine we adapt, may not always be veridical with how we are. Instead, the coappearance of the two styles—assertiveness and cautiousness—fits with a culture that actually is best traversed by incorporating one style or the other dependent on the demands of the setting (Wheaton, 1983).

The correlates of the judicious-prosocial style are consistent with the multiaxial model as well. Women have been depicted as more communal in their coping than men (see Chapter 5) and were consistently more judicious-prosocial than men across samples tested in college, general community, inner-city samples, and in a German version of the SACS (Monnier, Hobfoll, Dunahoo, Hulsizer, & Johnson, in press; Starke & Schwarzer, in press). Prior coping research has found more prosocial coping to be counterproductive and to lead to poor stress resistance (Endler & Parker, 1990). By beginning with a more collectivist model that portrayed questions in a form that allowed for assessment of prosocial action in a strong and active manner, rather than limited to a weak and passive style, we uncovered a very different set of results. Adopting judicious-prosocial coping effectively limited psychological distress for men and women (Dunahoo et al., 1998; Wells, Hobfoll, & Lavin, 1997). Specifically, loss of resources was found in community and university samples to be related to greater depression and greater feelings and expression of anger. However, individuals who employed more judicious-prosocial and active-prosocial strategies were much less negatively influenced by resource loss than were those who did not employ prosocial strategies.

As the multiaxial model predicts, an active, prosocial profile is a protective coping style. This set fits theoretically in the upper right quadrant of the multiaxial model and straddles the direct–indirect axis as would be expected. Its correlates also offer clear support for the expected positive influence of this kind of coping.

Active-Antisocial Coping

The active, antisocial set falls in the more active region of the active–passive axis than does the judicious-prosocial set. It is also clearly more socially aggressive (see Figure 6.3). The active-antisocial set is theoretically consistent with the lower right quadrant of the multiaxial model and again bridges the directness axis (i.e., foreground and background in the diagram). It is represented by (1) aggressive action, (2) instinctive action, and (3) antisocial action.

It is important to note that although we have found aggressive action to be employed in tandem by the same people who employ antisocial action, we have repeatedly found no association between assertive and antisocial action. Those who adapt to coping demands antisocially do not often choose an assertive stance. This is a critical finding and it suggests that being antisocial is quite distinguishable from an assertive coping strategy.

Aggressive and antisocial coping are less easily differentiated, but they are not one and the same either. Those who use aggressive action tend to use direct action, but those who employ antisocial action somewhat surprisingly combine it with indirectness. Antisocial coping emerges as more conspiratorial, underhanded, and backstabbing. Aggressive action implies a more frontal assault at problems that is more dominance seeking than it is intentionally socially destructive. However, the fact that they appear as a set means that they are often used by the same individuals.

The multiaxial model would predict that aggressive and antisocial coping would be more common among men and that it would be less effective than active-prosocial coping. In fact, we have repeatedly found an active-antisocial strategy to be higher among men than women. This buttresses our premise that what has masqueraded as problem solving and an action orientation among men may often be linked to an antisocial coping posture. Further confirmation of this premise was found when we correlated our active-antisocial subscales with what others have called active coping (Dunahoo et al., 1998). In these analyses, we consistently found that what individualistic, self-regulatory models call active coping is mixed in large measure with antisocial coping. Again, the traditional view of problem-focused coping is acted out in some individuals through a more pernicious underside.

The aggressive-antisocial posture not only ignores others, but also often aggresses against them. At times, this aggression is inadvertent, as when people act instinctively and "shoot from the hip." However, at other times, it is a planned, decisive strategy to achieve one's goals—to self-regulate—over the backs of others and at their expense, as when people "Look for other's weakness and use them to your advantage," or "Counterattack and catch others off guard." In a number of studies, we have found that antisocial coping is related to greater anger, greater depression, and lower levels of social support. Those who employ antisocial coping tend to alienate others and isolate themselves (Lane & Hobfoll, 1992; Monnier, Hobfoll, & Stone, 1996).

[Jones] is at the top of his special breed in American business. His skills encompass every conceivable attribute of the compleat [*sic*] corporate executive, save those in the subjective area of sentimentality, the appearance of kindness, or an inherent willingness to give a man in error a second chance. It is not that he couldn't, if he cared, acquire the polish of gentleness, but rather that he regards it as superfluous characteristic.... [His] favorite phrase is, "I'll cut his balls off." (Rodgers, 1969, pp. 249–250)

Although aggressive and antisocial actions are frequently employed by the same people, they are not necessarily tied together. Some individuals seem to employ aggressive action in concert with assertive action, rather than with antisocial action. These individuals experience lower depression and do not experience the negative social consequences of antisocial coping (Monnier et al., in press). In fact, they often have the most favorable stress outcomes. This suggests that within the U.S. samples that we have studied, aggressive action may be tolerated, whereas when it crosses a threshold to a more antisocial style, both the self and others are negatively affected. As men are higher than women on aggressive action, this may offer men an advantage in settings where more aggressive action may not only be tolerated, but also encouraged, such as in competitive sports (Stoll, 1997) and business (Dunahoo et al., 1996).

Still another group of men display the unusual pairing of antisocial action with avoidance (see Figure 6.4). It is possible that in the socialization process, some men overstep social demands that press them to be aggressive and slip into a kind of coping posture that is a decidedly negative version of the "strong" male stereotype. This, in turn, is met with rejection and social sanction, which may force them to become more masked in their coping behavior.

Historically, this slippage from aggressive to antisocial coping has been discussed in terms of the slippery slope between Nietzsche's man and superman, and the Nazi and white supremist adaptation of this image into the "superior-super man" *Übermensch* (Gambino, 1968). Hall and Barongan (1997) suggested similarly that the individualistic, male ideal may at its extreme be responsible for men's higher levels of violence and sexual aggression. Although such conjecture must be viewed cautiously from our available data, a Polish version of the SACS found very high antisocial coping patterns among a sample of incarcerated criminals (Zabielski & Politynska, 1996), suggesting some foundation for these extrapolations to wider sociohistorical issues.

Your enemy shall ye seek; you war shall ye wage, and for the sake of your thoughts!... Ye shall love peace as a means to new wars—and the short peace more than the long.

You I advise not to work but to fight. You I advise not to peace, but to victory. Let your work be a fight, let your peace be a victory!

Ye say it is the good cause which halloweth even war? I say unto you: it is the good war which halloweth every cause.

War and courage have done more great things than charity. Noth your sympathy, but your bravery hath hitherto saved the victims. "What is good?" ye ask. To be brave is good. (I, X)

"Man must become better and eviler"—so do I teach. The evilest is necessary for the Superman's best.

It may have been well for the preacher of the petty people to suffer and be burdened by men's sin. I, however, rejoice in great sin as my great *consolation*. (Nietzsche, 1896, IV, LXXIII)

Active–Passive, Asocial Coping

The third set that our research has uncovered is a pure active–passive set, which does not associate with the prosocial or antisocial subscales. It suggests a style of coping that is independent of social interactions (see Figure 6.3). This kind of coping may be especially appropriate in settings that are more individualistic or on more individualized tasks. Many work, academic, and even family tasks are done alone and can be performed in such a way with greatest efficiency and without harming others, and even benefiting them by ultimately adding to communal resources. A mechanic working on a car may bring home more money for his family, and an executive may work more efficiently on her own than in committee.

In most of our samples, and very much unlike findings of others with various coping measures, we have found no gender differences on this set. Women are neither less assertive nor more avoidant than men. This suggests that by including agenic and collectivist models in our original formulation, we may have succeeded in creating a less gender-biased coping measure.

This said, in one sample of older individuals, women were less assertive and more avoidant than men, suggesting a possible generational change. In these older cohorts of women, there may be more of a tendency to use social support as a means of avoiding problems as well (see Figure 6.4). This suggests that some women fall into a more socially demure profile.[3]

Preliminary Multicultural and Social Status Findings

We have also examined the SACS with inner-city and public-service samples of African Americans and European Americans. Subscales tended to be supported as to their reliability and validity across samples (Monnier & Hobfoll, 1997; Monnier, Stone, Hobfoll, & Johnson, in press). Among inner-city samples, we noted that antisocial action did not have the negative social ramifications on partners that it did among other samples. However, we failed to ask about the target of people's aggression, and their antisocial action may have been directed at nonfamily and out-group members. Consistent with this interpretation, we found that individuals who tended to use antisocial and aggressive strategies were more likely to employ these approaches in work than in family or romantic circumstances (Hobfoll et al., 1994). Nevertheless, our failure to find negative ramifications for antisocial coping in this sample is inconsistent with the multiaxial model and may indicate either a partial failure of the model or the SACS instrument that will have to be examined in more depth in future research.

Some work on translations of the SACS and testing of the multiaxial model has been conducted. German (Starke & Schwarzer, in press) and Polish (Zabielski & Politynska, 1996) versions of the SACS have been adapted and support the structural breakdown found in the English version. In a Russian version (Vodopyanova & Starchenkova, 1997), managers who were more active-prosocial were found to be more successful in making the transition to a free, open economy than active-antisocial managers. Preliminary work with a Hebrew version (Westman, personal communication, 1997) is also progressing. These studies are at early stages, but their findings suggest the transportability of the SACS and its underlying multiaxial model across Western countries and cultures.[4] The suitability of the SACS to the Polish and Russian contexts, which for over 50 years have emphasized collectivist notions embodied in communism despite recent political changes, is encouraging, but, again, the data are only preliminary.

Although we had truly not thought much about children's coping in formulating the multiaxial model, a children's version of the SACS (the BISC) was developed by Lopez and Little (1996). Children in grades 2 to 6 who were associated with American military families were being dispersed from their communities due to the drastic troop reductions subsequent to the fall of the Berlin Wall, resulting in the disbanding of entire communities. The prospect of this kind of move can be particularly stressful for young children, owing to their resources being friendship and school tied (Raviv, Keinan, Abazon, & Raviv, 1990).

Children who were higher in self-related sense of agency were more likely to use prosocial coping, had reduced antisocial coping, and reduced anxiety. These associations are similar to the stress and coping profile pattern found in adult samples using the SACS. Boys were also more likely to rely on antisocial coping than girls, as found in adult samples. Furthermore, as found for adults, antisocial coping was linked to hostility, which in turn was associated with greater anxiety. As suggested by the COR model and the work of Baltes (1987) discussed in detail in earlier chapters, loss of resources resulted in attempts to adapt to the new challenge. However, only those children with a prosocial adaptive style enjoyed coping benefits. Children who tended to adapt relying on more socially exploitive means experienced detrimental coping sequelae. In addition, consistent with COR theory, those who experienced more anxiety also sought less emotional support, indicating that stressful circumstances not only have negative psychological influences, but also deplete resources. Although only one study, the ecological context of this investigation and its thoroughness point to early developmental patterns consistent with the multiaxial model.

Costs of Collectivist Coping

It is tempting to embrace new models and scientific iconoclasm, and the constant search for new models and need to advance science could lead to idealization of the communal models of coping that I have been suggesting. However, the results and even the basis of the multiaxial model of coping suggest that a balance between individualistic and collectivist coping may be advantageous. Our findings further attest to positive relationships for both active-prosocial coping and more purely active-asocial coping postures. This said, more antisocial coping clearly tends to backfire against individuals, both by nature of their own psychological outcomes and the outcomes of those around them.

COR theory also suggests another potential insight into the cost of a communal coping orientation. Specifically, because prosocial coping must weigh the consequences for others, it is likely to demand more resources and hence be a more resource-depleting strategy. Despite the way coping is discussed in the literature, people are neither free agents in making coping choices, nor can their coping efforts be implemented without expending resources. As I discussed earlier, this results in women's greater cost of coping (Kessler et al., 1985). When one relies on and offers social support, one is vulnerable to stress contagion (Riley & Eckenrode, 1986) and pressure cooker effects (Hobfoll & London, 1986). This occurs because social support also translates to sharing stress exposure among others for whom consequences may be jointly experienced or empathically shared (Hirsch, 1980). In this way, individuals could feel greater stress because their supportee or member of their group is experiencing negative consequences and by caring for that person, they care about their pain and suffering.

In addition to greater risk of resource loss and exposure to stress, communal coping efforts are relatively inefficient. They demand greater cautiousness, increased communication, more patience, and consideration of others' needs (Lyons et al., 1998). One's personal goals are much more efficiently known and acted upon. In comparison, when interacting with others, any miscommunication or falsely based intuition is likely to lead to some resource waste. For example, a man may believe he is acting to meet his wife's needs, but in fact may poorly understand her circumstances or her desires for the role she wishes him to play. These misunderstandings may indeed increase psychological distress for those involved, as they may be interpreted as testimony to poor understanding and lack of empathy (Chapman, Hobfoll, & Ritter, 1997).

Wethington and Kessler (1991) examined the coordinated coping of couples who were confronted with a shared stressor. They noted that couples at times coordinated their strategies and complemented each other's coping, for example, where one handled the finances and the other handled the emotional issues, usually in a gender-typed pattern. However, they also noted many kinds of miscommunications and how trying to be empathic might interfere with coping. Pearlin and McCall (1990) suggested that this leads marital partners not to share occupational troubles in order to avoid the risk of inviting inappropriate responding.

Imagine a chess game in which two players share the same side and play against another, single player. The duo has the advantage of two heads, but much greater responsibility for coordination. Moreover, the choices made by one member of the team limit the choices of the other. The more individuals that are involved and must be considered in a collective, the more cautious and inefficient the system. Or in the words of Lewis Carroll (1866), in *Alice's Adventures in Wonderland*, "If everybody minded their own business," said the Duchess in a hoarse growl, "the world would go round a deal faster than it does."

Focusing on resources, which in turn becomes more social in part, and more proactive (Aspinwall & Taylor, 1997) also means there will be a likely cost due to miscues and misjudgments. Waiting until stress occurs may be a dangerous course, but it at least allows people to know what they are up against. Proactive coping, especially in social contexts, demands a good deal of forecasting based on current circumstances and past experiences. Proactive coping strategies have to cast a broad net in order to forestall multiple possible threats. Many of these actions will be misdirected and the amount of resources that must be invested will, in large part, determine the nature of proactive people's stance. People cannot safely invest resources in the service of coping with projected future resource loss past a juncture that leaves their resource reservoir vulnerable to some major loss sequence that may strike from another quarter.

Still another potential limitation of a collectivist view of coping is that it is gendered and more descriptive of women than men's course of action and that each gender is culturally set into a certain style for which it has particular prerequisite skills. Research suggests that Western men may not be as well socialized as women to attend to the social cues necessary to enact a more collectivist coping strategy. Cronkite and Moos (1984) found that men were less responsive to environmental influences than women, whether these influences were beneficial or detrimental. They found women's depressive mood to be impacted by their husband's alcohol consumption, whereas men were primarily influenced by their own life experiences. Wheaton (1990), studying divorce, similarly noted that women were more context dependent than men. Extrapolating across cultures, Western men and women may not be socialized to attend to the subtle environmental cues that are readily apparent to those raised in Japan, China, or Korea. Hence, to expect a fully collectivist coping to emerge in the West, or among men, without major changes in developmental socialization experiences first transpiring, would be naive.

CONCLUSIONS

Finally, changing coping may not change outcomes in expected ways, because social conditions allow, encourage, or disallow some kinds of coping from some classes of people (e.g., women vs. men, blacks vs. whites). Women, for example, might not receive the benefits of more aggressive coping if they were to adopt this style. In the prior chapter, I introduced the concepts of limitations and leniency in adaptation. Specifically, resources or coping style does not merely fit or not fit with environmental demand. Rather, environments act by imposing limitations or leniency on coping efforts and utilization of resources in accordance with cultural imperatives.

Individuals who have higher status are treated with greater leniency, implying a threefold advantage. They tend to have more resources, use them more effectively, and their coping is treated with greater acceptance. Those with very high status may be forgiven any behavior, and those with somewhat high status may be offered partial leniency. In contrast, those of low status are *persona non grata*, no matter what they have or how they behave.

Given the emphasis on self-reliance and the status advantage of men, it may not be that the way men cope is more effective as much as it has been treated with leniency, hence artificially inflating its effectiveness. The negative ramifications of self-reliant coping actions such as social isolation, antisocial action, and lack of group promotion may be overlooked when self-reliance is heavily favored. For example, because we culturally favor self-reliance, self-reliant workers may be rewarded more for their efforts and forgiven any negative spinoffs of their behavior. In contrast, others who behave more collectively may be disfavored despite their success, and their transgressions may be treated more severely. As Baltes's (1987) life-span development model illustrates, the cultural backdrop influences the acceptability of certain coping responses and not others.

A more balanced view of coping reveals how individual and collectivist efforts, control and the giving up of control, and direct influence and stage setting, all play a role in obtaining, retaining, protecting, and advancing people's own and shared resources. The multiaxial model of coping and its companion measure, the SACS, may provide some insights into this process.[5] Our research and discussion also underscore the complexity of a model that involves the commerce of resources among individuals nested-in families, nested-in organizations, nested-in communities. But once self-reliance and personal agency are exposed as facets of *relational reliance* and shared agency, we have little alternative but to accept the task of seeing the coping process as a woven fabric. Individualism attempts to demarcate the self and justify this as a necessary scientific step, whereas there is overwhelming evidence that the self can also be seen as interconnected with others. This, in turn, demands that the self be reinserted into the social process and that these multiple levels of understanding be reintegrated.

NOTES

1. Others, in composing coping scales, have avoided two-part questions such as, "Follow your own first impulse; things will usually work out best that way." However, we included such items because common aphorisms across languages typically take this two-part format, identifying a behavior (e.g., follow your first impulse) and a strategic reason behind it (e.g., things will work out best). Later statistical examination of the questionnaire indeed showed no problems with these items.

2. The statistical term here is *factors*, but since factor analysis is not widely understood outside of psychology, I will use the more general term *sets*. Readers interested in actual statistical analyses can refer to the published articles referenced in the text.

3. A question that has plagued the literature concerns whether coping should be viewed as a strategic style or a situational response (Compas, Forsyth, & Wagner, 1988). Lazarus and Folkman (1984) argued that coping was a situationally determined construct, and that it was too variant across situations to be considered a style. Compas et al. (1988) found, however, that coping styles were fairly stable for people within similar situations, but that individuals varied in how they chose to cope across situations.

    The multiaxial model of coping suggests that people approach situations with a stylistic strategy, but they adopt that situation to circumstances, settings, and context. Factors that may affect how people cope in a given situation include the importance of the situation, the risk of resource loss, the opportunity of resource gain, and their relative status vis-à-vis others in terms of their power, control, and social relationships. We developed a situational version of the SACS that asked the same questions referring to a specific recent event or context. For example, the general item, "Just work harder; apply yourself," translates situationally to "I just worked harder and applied myself." The full version of the Situational SACS is presented in Table 6.2.

Table 6.2. Strategic Approach to Coping Scale (SACS) (Situational Form)

Respond to the following questions as they pertain to the stressful event(s) you just mentioned. Indicate how much your reactions are described by each statement from 1, *Didn't do this at all* to 5, *Did this a lot.*

1. I didn't give up, even when things look their worst, because you can often turn things around.	1 2 3 4 5
2. I checked with friends about what they would do.	1 2 3 4 5
3. I acted fast; it is better to throw myself right into the problem.	1 2 3 4 5
4. I tried to be in control, but I let others think they were still in charge.	1 2 3 4 5
5. I depended on myself and my personal strengths; it's not a good idea to depend on others.	1 2 3 4 5
6. I trusted my instincts, not my thoughts.	1 2 3 4 5
7. I avoided dealing with the problem; things like this often go away on their own.	1 2 3 4 5
8. I mounted an all-out attack; I was aggressive.	1 2 3 4 5
9. I checked with family about what they would do.	1 2 3 4 5
10. I moved on to other things; there's little hope for such situations getting better.	1 2 3 4 5
11. I depended on my gut-level reaction.	1 2 3 4 5
12. I was very cautious and look very hard at my options (better safe than sorry).	1 2 3 4 5
13. I turned to others for help.	1 2 3 4 5
14. I went forward but didn't use all my resources until I knew full well what I was up against.	1 2 3 4 5
15. I retreated; I avoided contact until the problem blew over.	1 2 3 4 5
16. I counterattacked and caught others off guard.	1 2 3 4 5
17. I joined together with others to deal with the situation together.	1 2 3 4 5
18. I depended on myself but at the same time relied on others who are close to me.	1 2 3 4 5
19. I looked out for my own best interests, even if it means hurting others.	1 2 3 4 5
20. I did something to help avoid thinking about the problem.	1 2 3 4 5
21. Others needed to feel they are the boss, so I worked around them to get things done.	1 2 3 4 5
22. I backed off and just let the smoke clear.	1 2 3 4 5
23. I tried to held out others involved in the situation, as giving of yourself usually helps solve problems like this.	1 2 3 4 5
24. I thought carefully about how others felt before deciding what to do.	1 2 3 4 5
25. I thought I'd probably feel bad, but there is not much you can do about this sort of thing.	1 2 3 4 5
26. I just worked harder; I applied myself.	1 2 3 4 5
27. I held back, as it was better to wait until the smoke cleared before any action was taken.	1 2 3 4 5
28. I went to someone for emotional support.	1 2 3 4 5
29. I moved very cautiously, because I thought there may have been a hidden agenda.	1 2 3 4 5

Table 6.2. (*Continued*)

Respond to the following questions as they pertain to the stressful event(s) you just mentioned. Indicate how much your reactions are described by each statement from 1, *Didn't do this at all* to 5, *Did this a lot.*

30. I tried hard to meet other's wishes, as this will really help the situation.   1 2 3 4 5
31. I moved aggressively; often if you get another off guard, things will work to your advantage.   1 2 3 4 5
32. It wasn't getting worse, so I avoided the whole thing.   1 2 3 4 5
33. I got out of the situation; when problems arise, it's usually a sign of worse to come.   1 2 3 4 5
34. I let others think they are in control, but kept my own hands firmly on the wheel.   1 2 3 4 5
35. I went with my intuition.   1 2 3 4 5
36. I quickly asserted my dominance.   1 2 3 4 5
37. My only choice was to be a little manipulative and work around people.   1 2 3 4 5
38. I talked to others get out my frustrations.   1 2 3 4 5
39. I acted quickly to put others at a disadvantage.   1 2 3 4 5
40. I broke up the problem into smaller parts and deal with them one at a time.   1 2 3 4 5
41. I tried to meet the needs of others who were involved.   1 2 3 4 5
42. I followed my first impulse; things usually work out best that way.   1 2 3 4 5
43. I did something to help calm down and, only then, started problem solving.   1 2 3 4 5
44. I looked for others' weaknesses and used them to my advantage.   1 2 3 4 5
45. I took the bull by the horns; adopted a take-charge attitude.   1 2 3 4 5
46. I asked friends or family for their opinions about my plan of action.   1 2 3 4 5
47. I focused on something else and let the situation resolve itself.   1 2 3 4 5
48. I relied on my own judgment, because only I have my best interests at heart.   1 2 3 4 5
49. I was firm; I held my ground.   1 2 3 4 5
50. I was assertive and got my needs met.   1 2 3 4 5
51. I was strong and forceful, but avoided harming others.   1 2 3 4 5
52. I directly addressed the situation, and didn't back away from the problem.   1 2 3 4 5

Note: Questions 10, 15, 25, and 33 are reverse scored on the assertive action subscale.

Our research (Dunahoo et al., 1998; Monnier et al., in press) indicated that the situational SACS produced similar subscale reliability and factor patterns to those found for the general SACS. The general SACS was predictive of psychological distress over time, but the situational version only predicted immediate outcomes. Furthermore, as we had hoped, the situational measure was the best predictor of immediate outcomes, as it most closely captures actual behavior surrounding the particular stressful circumstances. General coping was also predictive of situational coping 12 weeks later across a variety of situations. This partially corroborates the notion that the concept of a general coping style has validity, as otherwise, a general measure would not predict later situational reports. In fact, these correlations ranged from .43 to .71, indicating rather robust associations. Overall, this is the pattern of findings that would be expected from a general strategic and a situation version of the instrument.

4. Not too much should be made of this point, as individualistic concepts have been found to be transportable across cultures as well, because cultures are psychologically multifaceted. This is only a first step in judging the model or measure's cross-cultural meaning and viability. It is most critical that the measure seems to have similar correlates with gender and other personality and psychological distress measures across cultures.

5. Our most recent work finds that self-mastery is most closely related with active coping, but that communal mastery is more strongly related to active-prosocial coping. Communal mastery is the sense that one will be successful because of "one's self in conjunction with others"—*the self-nested in family-nested in tribe.*

Items for the Communal Mastery Scale are scored from 1–2, strongly disagree to strongly agree.

1. By joining with friends and family, I have a great deal of control over the things that happen to me.
2. Working together with friends and family I can solve many of the problems I have.
3. There is little I can do to change many of the important things in my life, even with the help of my family and friends.
4. Working together with people close to me I can overcome most of the problems I have.
5. What happens to me in the future mostly depends on my ability to to work well with others.
6. I can do just about anything I set my mind to because I have the support of those close to me.
7. With the help of those close to me I have more control over my life.
8. What happens to me in the future mostly depends on my being supported by friends, family or colleagues.
9. I can meet my goals by helping others meet their goals.
10. Friends, family, and colleagues mainly get in the way of my accomplishing goals.

7

Turbulent Spiral
or Graceful Pirouette
Cycles of Resource Loss and Gain

In this chapter, I illustrate how resource cycles and spirals occur, that is, identify and describe the movement and mobility of resources during the stress process. I examine how loss and the threat of loss trigger loss and gain cycles, how they gather momentum, and how they impact people. As in prior chapters, I bridge between the individual, family, and group to the level of the village or neighborhood, because the resource rules and operations that I have identified and the coping strategies I have described operate at each of these levels interactively. Higher order social structures, such as state and nation, certainly interact with lower level social structures such as family and community as well, but the sharing of resource reservoirs becomes looser at this point, and perhaps less tightly connected to the purview of psychology. For more macrolevel social structures, the concepts that might be true of the village and its members begin to break down, and COR theory and the companion ideas that I have set forth become less applicable. To illustrate the concepts of resource cycles and spirals, I focus on how major life crises, on one end of the continuum, and the slow bleeding of burnout at work, on the other end, act to diminish resources and well-being, and how individuals, families, and communities react to retain their resource integrity.

REGULATION OF RESOURCES AS THE KEY
TO SUSTAINED FUNCTIONING

In earlier chapters I have presented Conservation of Resource (COR) theory and its central tenet that *individuals strive to obtain, retain, protect, and foster that which they value—these valued entities being termed resources.* Based on this tenet, I have argued that stress will occur when this keystone goal is threatened or blocked. Hence, *stress follows circumstances where people's resources are threatened with loss, when resources are lost, or where there is failure to gain resources following resource investment.* I have outlined how people also rely on these very same resources to protect other resources. People rely on social support resources to provide safe harbor to their self-esteem when they turn to friends to boost their lagging sense of self after experiencing personal failure. They rely on financial resources to protect their health when they purchase insurance, vacations away from stressful work, or safer housing. Similarly, sense of self-efficacy is used to sustain effort in the face of adversity, so that sense of self-efficacy itself can be preserved. In this way, those high in self-efficacy can rely on it when their sense of mastery is being challenged in any of life's vicissitudes (Bandura, 1997).

Conservation of resources, then, emphasizes our striving to regulate our resource reserves in order to support survival, preserve well-being, avoid illness, and retain the fabric of our social ties. As such, successful resource cycling represents a standard of functioning and the basis for motivation of behavior. That is to say that people are motivated to remain with sufficient resources to sustain themselves and their core social groups, and ideally to help themselves to prosper physically, spiritually, and functionally. This chapter focuses on these cycles of resource loss and gains, with an emphasis on transactional rather than static stress processes.

Stress research has seldom looked at conservation of resources, or any other standard of functioning, as a focal point. Rather, research and theory has concentrated on physical or mental health outcomes, and more precisely, physical and mental illness. Interest has been directed at the association between stress and physical or biological dysfunction or breakdown. Hence, what is studied is stress and heart disease, stress and cancer, stress and colds, stress and depression, and stress and anxiety. On one hand, the choice of outcome variables is inconsequential if it is understood that stress is a cycle that is iterative, repetitive, and transactional, a point upon which almost all stress theorists agree (Aspinwall & Taylor, 1997; Holahan & Moos, 1991; Lazarus & Folkman, 1984). As such, any point may be taken to be an outcome variable for the purpose of obtaining a sense of causal patterns and cotravelers that illuminate important insights about the process. If stress is transactional, we can choose any point as the predictor and any point as the outcome, and with equal justification reverse them, as long as we state that we are only spotlighting one step of the process.

Mental and physical illness or dysfunction are indeed particularly good candidates for study and deserve careful attention for a number of reasons. First, physical and mental illness are important in their own right because they suggest breakdown of functioning on biological, psychological, or behavioral planes. It is critical that we recognize and predict when breakdown occurs, because breakdown limits functioning, interferes with well-being, and often leads to yet worse consequences. Second, they are significant because they are experienced as painful and discomforting, and insights may contribute to reversing or restricting such pain and suffering. However, indicators of lack of well-being are clearly not the only outcomes of interest and, from a functional viewpoint, are not even the major concern.

By focusing on illness, we accept dysfunction as the end point and treat the stress picture as static. The individual is ill, depressed, or anxious, and that is that. As Maslow (1962) suggested, by focusing on pathological outcomes, we end up with a "crippled psychology." By turning our attention instead to people's resources, we learn about the strengths people bring to bear on problems—not mythological heroics, but management of threats ranging from the mundane to the most serious (Antonovsky, 1979; Maslow, 1962). Moreover, functioning is more closely related to individuals' social actions than illness models typically reflect. How people behave as parents, spouses, colleagues, and citizens preserves the social fabric and allows individuals the privileges and connections of ongoing membership in the very social groups that define them.

In 20 years of working with medical and psychiatric patients, I have been struck by how little diagnosis reveals, even about the course of illness, let alone functioning. Using depression as an example, every experienced clinician has seen slightly depressed individuals who are terribly dysfunctional and observed extremely depressed others who remain at work, father or mother their families, and remain involved in life's small and large battles. Likewise, even after opening an individual surgically and viewing an inoperable cancer firsthand, experienced surgeons are often unable to give more than a broad range of months, which sometimes lead to years, as to the person's survival, and are unable to predict the physical quality of that life during that time. Nor does this inability to predict emanate from clinicians' lack of knowledge; rather, it emerges from their having the knowledge to understand that illness and functioning, biologically and psychologically, are linked but not intimately tied.

Luckily, I received this lesson about the limitations of diagnosis early in my career. One day, I am conducting family therapy with a withdrawn, anxious man who could not begin emotionally or instrumentally to parent his children or nurture his wife. He was removed, detached, and almost interpersonally paralyzed. Some weeks later, I find myself an inexperienced expert witness, where as judge, the same man is nimbly protecting me from the onslaught of cross-examination by a seasoned attorney who not only knows more law than I, but has a psychologist and psychiatrist examining my testimony! The then patient, now judge, was sensitive, strong, attentive, protective, and focused on finding the closest possible approximation of the truth in a complicated murder case. Simply, our roles were reversed by the change in context—one in which his resources fit the call and I was the novice, one in which my resources could answer and his could not.

When we look at a person's life course, it becomes obvious how uninformative is any static account. A close family member, a diagnosed manic–depressive, was seldom manic and seldom depressed over her life. Most of the time she was happy, productive, creative, a musician, artist, career woman, mother, wife, and friend to many. Her illness at times weighed on her tragically, but it did not describe her typical functioning, or even her course of recovery. It related to her behavior and state of mind for a few months of her total life. Her diagnosis then could be seen as one possible choice for study, but not the most interesting one, not the most important one, and not one very descriptive of the cycles of resource gain and loss she experienced. It was not unimportant by any means, as it was at times painful for her and those around her, and at times threatened her very life, but even these episodes exist in a brief temporal space and interact with other more biographically relevant cycles of events in her life and among those around her. I recall visiting her during one of her hospitalizations for depression. Even at this juncture, she was counseling a young woman who was recently released from the ward and returning to continue to seek the advice and comfort of this middle-aged woman who had comforted her. She was providing solace and advice in her usual warm, resonant voice, holding the young woman's hand and making esteem-building eye contact. She was quite depressed at the time, certainly needed help, but this said little about her style, her spirit, and her constant reaching out to others. By placing our attention on illness outcomes, we overlook not only patterns of strength, but also avenues to recovery.

Finally, I submit that resource cycles are more important because here is where our motivation lies. We strive to obtain, retain, and protect our resources. Illness and dysfunction are what occurs when we fail on this journey or as warning signs that resources are dangerously weak. When we speak of illness, we really mean the symptoms of the underlying illness. Symptoms are signals of distress, but distress at what? They are signs that sleep, nourishment, shelter from cold, love, friendship, optimism, self-esteem, and other resources have been lacking and that the biological, psychological, or interpersonal systems have been rendered vulnerable to illness agents (Antonovsky, 1979). And these illness agents are omnipresent in the environment, pathogens are everywhere. The question is where are the resistance resources that are meant to combat them and contribute to well-being and health?

CONSERVATION OF RESOURCES, ECOLOGICAL CONGRUENCE, AND CYCLES OF LOSS AND GAIN

A resource perspective lends itself to viewing stress as a dynamic process and functioning as the central property of interest. This is pivotal to resource-based theories of Antonovsky (1979), Baltes (1987), Holahan and Moos (1991), and COR theory. In earlier chapters, I introduced COR theory and the model of ecological congruence implying a dynamical process, but not addressing those dynamics fully. In this chapter, I concentrate on how these two models are translated into cycles of resource transactions in the domain of stress and stress resistance. People are in a constant state of flux. Both individually and as members of various social groups, they are always coming from some past, in some present, and moving toward some future. If COR theory is correct in claiming that people are motivated to obtain, retain, foster, and protect resources, then people will be resource vigilant. They will be aware of their resources, aware of how their resources are being impacted by events, and will strategize about how to manipulate their world to better their resource standing.

Reviewing the principles and corollaries of COR theory developed earlier and how they relate specifically to loss and gain cycles might be helpful before looking at people's responses to crisis events and burnout as examples.

Principles and Dynamical Processes

Principle 1

The first principle, and perhaps the most important, is that resource loss is disproportionately more salient than resource gain. People place more weight on loss than gain and are more motivated to protect against loss than to obtain gain.

Resulting Dynamics.   When a major loss or chronic loss sequence occurs, people become increasingly loss vigilant and pay more attention to cues about loss than gain. Losses begin to influence them with ever greater negative impact and countermanding gains are seldom sufficient to offset the negative sequelae that follow major resource loss.

Principle 2

Principle 2 states that people invest resources to protect against resource loss, recover from losses, and gain resources. People rely on the resources they possess or that are available to them to limit resource loss or obtain gain.

Resulting Dynamics. When people see a pattern of events that is likely to lead to ongoing loss, they map a strategy and act to protect themselves and their group following conservation of resource principles:

1. First act to stop losses when possible by investing resources.
2. Act to minimize the negative impact of loss—damage control.
3. Keep some resources in reserve if possible.
4. Look to outside sources to complement or substitute for resources that the individual alone cannot bring to bear.
5. Attempt to replenish resources if possible—initiation of gain sequences.

As discussed in earlier chapters, these first two principles of COR theory lead to four corollaries that in turn expand the dynamic process that is set in motion when high demand circumstances occur.

Corollary 1

Because people rely on resources to obtain, retain, foster, and protect resources, the first corollary of COR theory posits that those with greater resources are less vulnerable to resource loss and more capable of orchestrating resource gain. Conversely, those with fewer resources are more vulnerable to resource loss and less capable of achieving resource gain.

Resultant Dynamics. Those with greater resources will be less negatively affected by initial resource loss and will be more likely to create gain cycles, because they can invest resources that are not required for everyday functioning or reserve capacity. Those with few resources will be more deeply impacted by the initial blow of major crisis or by chronic demands and will have few reserves to rally. If very low in resources, initial setbacks will be particularly devastating and result in immediate and rapid loss spirals.

Corollary 2

Those who lack resources are more vulnerable to resource loss, *and* initial loss begets future loss.

Resultant Dynamics. If individuals, groups, and organizations rely on resources to counter losses, and since stress results from resource loss, at each iteration of the cycle, there are fewer resources available for mobilization in defense or to invest in gain cycles that might countervalence stress's impact. This results in depleted resource reservoirs that are decreasingly capable of mobilizing to defend against future challenges. This further suggests that loss cycles will have initially higher velocity for resource-poor individuals or groups, as they are from the outset in a resource-challenged state characterized by their resources being already stretched in protection of the self, family, or social system. Hence, Corollary 2 predicts that loss cycles will have advancing momentum and strength (i.e., speed and impact).

Corollary 3

Those who possess resources are both more capable of gain, *and* resource gain begets further gain.

Resultant Dynamics. Corollary 3 mirrors Corollary 2, but pertains to resource gains and gain cycles. Because loss and gain are inequivalent, however, they differ significantly. Specifically, the need for gain is not as imminent as the demand to act to offset loss. When initial gains are achieved, additional resources thereby become available for investment, as with resource surpluses, individuals and social systems are less vulnerable and so do not necessarily need to rely on these resource surpluses for reserves. Because resource loss is more potent than resource gain, gain cycles will also have less momentum (e.g., speed) and less impact than loss cycles.

Corollary 4

Those who lack resources are likely to adopt a defensive posture to guard their resources. With few resources, the cost of resource investment quickly outstrips demands and renders the individual or organization vulnerable (Schönpflug, 1985).

Resultant Dynamics. A defensive posture holds a maximum of resources in reserve for the possibility of having to forestall the impact of a major loss sequence. This strategy can appear self-defeating because it seems to avoid problem solving, but is logically and experientially based on the need to hold some modicum of resource reserves.

Ecological Congruence

In prior chapters, I have also introduced the concept of *fitting*, rather than fit of resources. French and his colleagues, in introducing resource fit theory, postulated that resources will be capable of offsetting stress to the extent that they fit circumstantial demands (French et al., 1982; French et al., 1974). However, once again, this way of depicting fit is static. Rather, I have suggested that people and groups act by fitting their resources as part of the transactional process.

Resultant Dynamics. Resources are shaped, parlayed, traded, and sometimes corrupted (i.e., grossly misused) in order to meet demands that are themselves changing over time. Those who possess richer resource reservoirs are more likely to resist negative stress sequelae because they can shape and combine resources to counteract challenges, while still retaining adequate resource reserves for daily functioning and adequate resource stockpiles in case of emergencies. Moreover, by having greater resources of more varied types, they are less likely to have to corrupt resources, such as when people misuse friendship when in a bind, or have to sell badly needed transportation to purchase groceries. This transactional fitting can be conceptualized within the model of ecological congruence, such that people can shape, alter, and apply their resources to meet situational demands, within the limits that these resources are finite, tend to operate within broader social value systems, and are of consequence transformed in the process.

Hence, as Baltes (1987, 1997) has so aptly postulated, the life course inevitably presents people with resource losses. In response, individuals and social systems respond by attempting to optimize their position so as to make their current resources fit demands as best possible and by compensating through adapting and acquiring new resources to meet ongoing demands and address losses. This process, in turn, unfolds within a value structure that is socially determined and therefore common to individuals within cultures and subcultures (Kaplan, 1983, 1996). If COR theory can make more specific predictions about how these processes unfold, it might be a valuable tool for understanding stress and designing interventions to alter stress cycles and spirals, to limit their destructive potential, and even to help create resource-gain series in their place.

EXTREME STRESS: RAPID LOSS AND GAIN CYCLES

Disasters and War: Cases of Communal Stress and Rapid Resource Depletion

Extreme stress offers an important natural laboratory for testing COR theory because the loss cycles that follow extreme stress are likely to be rapid and marked (Hobfoll, 1991; McFarlane & deGirolamo, 1996). Extreme stress that confronts a large group of people is unfortunately quite common, even if any given individual may be spared such circumstances. Lifetime chance of exposure to a disaster has been estimated at 13 percent in the United States (Norris, 1992), and between 1967 and 1991, disasters were estimated to have affected 3 billion people worldwide (International Federation of Red Cross and Red Crescent Societies, 1993). Following such events, psychiatric disorder in the form of posttraumatic stress disorder (PTSD) and depression is quite common, with over 20 percent of those exposed likely to be seriously enough affected to display a diagnosable disorder and a much greater percentage showing deteriorated functioning (McFarlane & de-Girolamo, 1996). We can learn much about stress from such encounters, and this knowledge may also be applied to less severe circumstances because many of the same mechanisms occur whenever there is shared stress, albeit on a smaller scale and with less devastating consequences. By studying how people are affected by disasters and war, we can also learn more about the interaction between individuals' coping, group reactions, and broader social processes, because extreme community stressors influence all these systems simultaneously and transactionally.

The drought of 1930 developed slowly. As the disappointment of Spring grew into acute apprehension with the continued dryness of July, the field representative of the Red Cross began to report conditions that might later, if the weather did not change, call for Red Cross action. But there was no way of knowing yet how the resources and credit of the farmers had been exhausted by the depressed market for farm products in the several years preceding. If these farmers were bereft of resources, then the drought might result in famine. (p. 17)

The drought of 1930, which parched the fields of 1,057 counties in twenty-three states with severe reactions in the early months of 1931, was the greatest calamity of its kind in the country's history. Official records and preceding traditions reveal nothing comparable to it in extent. It brought famine to the doors of millions and created a national emergency....

Unfortunately for the country, the great drought of 1930 occurred at a time of world-wide economic depression, marked by unemployment in industries, stagnation in trade, and low prices for farm products—so low that in some instances the price did not cover production costs. The coincidence of this depression naturally brought the evil effects of the drought into greater prominence....

There was nothing spectacular about the drought. There was no one dramatic day, with its terror and anguish and supreme tests of courage. But its slow and insidious advance proved far more trying to human nerves in the long run than a sudden catastrophe.

Farmers stood by helplessly as ruin spread and intensified. Some times hopes of rain were raised by banks of clouds, which dissipated without a drop falling. Day by day they saw their young crops wilt and their fields turn into beds of dust and dead stalk, their pastures grown thin and brown, and the flow of wells, springs, and steams dwindle until the winds which swept across the river beds were polluted with the stench of dead fish.

The drought was a period of hope continuously deferred until no hope remained. And the sufferers faced the Winter with empty cupboards, lofts and cribs, and with exhausted credit (pp. 7–8).*

Since 1931, the American response to disaster has become increasingly sophisticated owing both to more advanced technological warning procedures, improved building materials, and better disaster-response planning, Nevertheless, the potential for severe loss of life and property continues to be real, and the aftermath of disasters continues to be devastating for victims. In less developed countries, disasters impact remains a major source of loss of life as well.

Freedy and his colleagues (Freedy, Resnick, & Kilpatrick, 1992; Freedy, Saladin, Kilpatrick, Resnick, & Saunders, 1994) applied COR theory to the study of the impact of Hurricane Hugo that hit the South Carolina coast in 1990 and the Sierra Madre earthquake that struck Los Angeles county in 1991. Specifically, they were interested in how resource loss influenced the mobilization of resources and how loss impacted mental health. These natural disasters resulted in sparingly little loss of life, but property damage was extensive and the threat to loss of life was enormous. Had the warnings been later in coming in South Carolina or had the earthquake struck a few hours later, the loss of life would have been enormous.

Paradoxically, COR theory predicts that although loss will have negative impact, if it is understood in terms of its survival origins, resource loss can also be seen as activating a biopsychosocial response system. Rather than viewing psychological distress as an end point, it is recognized as a painful warning system. Threat to the self, family, and prized social groupings results in a vigilance response (Leventhal, Leventhal, & Schaefer, 1991), appraisals of danger (Lazarus & Folkman, 1994), and decisions about how to combat the threat (Lazarus & Folkman, 1984). Freedy and his colleagues found that the greater the resource loss in the wake of disaster, the more coping that individuals initiated and the more psychologically distressed they became. Moreover, they found that the influence of resource loss was both independent of and of greater magnitude than the influence of posi-

*American Red Cross, *Relief Work in the Drought of 1930–1931: Official Report of Operations of the American Red Cross.* All rights reserved in all countries.

tive cognitive and behavioral coping responses. This clearly supports the COR premise that objective elements of events have central importance and that stress is not just a function of stress perceptions. On the other hand, cognitive coping mechanisms did have an impact that was independent of resource loss, as well, so the point should not be drawn that perceptions are inconsequential by any means.

It is of particular interest that Freedy and his colleagues found resource loss activated both constructive kinds of coping such as useful problem solving and self-defeating kinds of coping such as those that lead to denial and alcohol and drug use. Again, people employ the means of coping that they have, according to their strengths. If their remaining resources enable them actively to problem solve and a solution is viable, they will likely choose this route. However, if a problem-solving route is blocked, if they lack enabling resources, or if their history of resource utilization has been unsuccessful, they will still attempt to cope. But here enters the defensive postures predicted by COR theory when effective strategies are not available.

This sequence was carefully studied by Carver (1993). Carver examined the aftermath of Hurricane Andrew that struck south Florida in August of 1992. Andrew was a particularly powerful hurricane and it hit a major residential area, much of which was structurally ill-prepared for a hurricane, despite lying in a hurricane corridor. Winds of up to 145 miles per hour treated trailer homes, cars, and homes like so many leaves and twigs, and the subsequent scene looked like a bomb site. Some 25,000 homes were destroyed, another 50,000 were seriously damaged, and as many as 250,000 people were rendered homeless, with property loss and cleanup costs estimated at $40 billion. Carver and his colleagues were particularly interested in how loss of resources, on the one hand, and the central personal resource of optimism, on the other hand, influenced people's coping responses, psychological well-being, and physical health. They employed a powerful research design that included careful sampling, use of well-validated psychological measures, blood assays, and long-term follow-up of residents.

Comparing the impact of resource loss to other factors, resource loss was found to have the single most profound influence. The greater the resources lost by residents, the greater their psychological distress and the worse their immunological resistance (see Ironson, Wynings, Schneiderman, Baum, et al., 1997). Individuals' sense of optimism also played an important role, counterbalancing much of the negative influence of resource loss. Moreover, Carver et al. also found that coping and optimism both mobilized other kinds of coping. However, optimism–pessimism primarily activated negative emotion-focused coping that exacerbated people's plight: The less optimistic victims were, the more likely they were to turn to alcohol, deny their problems, or withdraw. Resource loss also resulted in these same reactions, but resource loss further activated problem-focused coping, an active orientation toward problem solving, and positive goal orientation. This mirrors Freedy et al.'s findings, but extends them to the physical health impact as well as the psychological impact of resource loss.

As in the case of Hurricane Hugo, the resource loss that Andrew created had a profound negative impact on victims, yet also mobilized their coping response. Those who had the resources, including optimism, were more likely to register a successful coping pattern. Those who lacked resources, including a more pessimistic orientation, were more likely to attempt more self-defeating responses that led to further distress and greater loss of resources, this being the defensive posture referred to in the fourth corollary of COR theory. From what we know from other research on coping, we can well predict that the victims who responded using active, goal-oriented efforts were more likely to halt or minimize loss spirals, and those who used denial, turned to alcohol, and withdrew from social contact were likely to exacerbate the loss spirals that were initiated by the disaster.

Communal Processes and Resource Loss

COR theory suggests that we do not stop at the level of individual responding, because individuals and communities are wed. McFarlane (1987) studied the Australian bush fires of 1983 that swept through the Australian landscape destroying towns, crops, and vegetation over 2,804 square kilometers of land. Twenty-eight people were killed and hundreds were injured, along with the loss of over 250,000 livestock. McFarlane found that firefighters who experienced greater loss from the fire to their own property were more deeply impacted by this factor than even their own exposure to danger. He also noted that communities' resources could combat major loss to the town or region, but that at a certain point of loss, a threshold seemed to be reached. After this threshold, resources became overwhelmed and the psychological impact multiplied (McFarlane, 1992). This observation suggests that, as in the individual case, communities may combine their resources to offset the negative psychological results of resource loss, but that at some juncture, resources are overly taxed and a watershed opens and becomes psychologically overwhelming and outstrips integrated community response.

It must also be underscored that even communities that are committed to offering their resources to victims in an ongoing manner, and who are fully empathic with victims, cannot entirely reverse the negative mental health sequelae of extreme stress. Studying Israeli combatants following the 1973 Yom Kippur War and the 1982 Lebanon War, Zahava Solomon has constructed the most complete, long-term data set on any extreme stressor. In Israel, I had served with the combat research unit under her command (she also drove me to the base), so I was truly able to obtain a firsthand look at her incisive work. Her unit found that soldiers who are in high-stress situations (even war offers a continuum of stressor levels) and who lack personal and social resources from their unit command and comrades are more likely to experience breakdown in combat (Solomon, Mikulincer, & Hobfoll, 1987).

Once breakdown occurs, the loss spiral for combatants shows its mark even 18 years after the Yom Kippur War, with significantly increased odds of continued diagnosable psychiatric disorder. Following the Lebanon War, Solomon found that more than 50 percent of those who experienced psychiatric breakdown during the period of combat continued to experience diagnosable PTSD one and two years after their breakdown experience (Solomon, 1995). Moreover, even after apparently complete recovery and evidence of full reintegration into family life and work, those who were reexposed to the traumatic stress of war, even years after their original breakdown or PTSD, were at increased risk for more severe clinical reactions, suggesting that the rebuilt personal and social resources for these men were still somehow fragile.

Solomon also notes another trend in her data that points to the need to halt resource loss cycles if recovery is to be accelerated. Specifically, she notes that as long as these men who experienced PTSD could potentially be called for duty in Lebanon due to the ongoing nature of Israeli reserve commitments, their levels of PTSD remained high. However, when the war ceased, there was a dramatic drop in PTSD levels among those formerly diagnosed with the disorder. Solomon suggests that with the war ended, not only was the continued threat of war removed, but also resources could be more fully dedicated to recovery. In particular, she concludes that self-esteem, self-efficacy, and social integration are key elements of this process. These resources are reduced by the trauma and must be reconstructed or otherwise increased to levels necessary for facilitating recovery on personal, social, and occupational levels, a scenario fully consistent with COR theory.

Major trauma cycles not only spiral for the individual in a personal sense with anxiety, depression, and loneliness, but also often result in reduced social involvement, diminished interest in life and family, feelings of social detachment, and a sense of alienation (Figley, 1978, Figley & Leventman, 1980). These reactions challenge the very social ties that are necessary to reweave the individual into normal family and social functioning. As in our study of severely ill individuals (Lane & Hobfoll, 1992), stress also produces anger and hostility, which are especially difficult reactions for loved ones who cannot understand why they are being punished when they are trying so desperately to help. This reduces supporters' ability to aid and succor the victim. Moreover, PTSD has a stress-contagion influence, producing psychological distress in loved ones who are challenged by the turbulent spirals that the combatant brings home, especially considering how long after the original incident war's shadows linger in family life (Solomon, Waysman, Avitzur, & Enoch, 1991; Waysman, Mikulincer, Solomon, & Weisenberg, 1993). Family members, reacting to the PTSD symptoms of the returning soldier, themselves display higher rates of social dysfunction in a broad range of contexts (feelings of loneliness, and impaired marital and family relations).

These examples from a diverse group of contexts, cultures, and stress levels clearly suggest that severe resource loss or major threats to resources have greatly increased negative impact on individuals and social systems. The very resources that are required for adjustment and readaptation are so fractured by events that recovery routes are undermined. Moreover, individual reactions are complicated by broader social reactions, as extreme stress often attacks the entire community and because those most deeply affected carry their psychological wounds for long durations. These loss spirals become difficult to interrupt and challenge the resources that are otherwise reserved for coping with everyday challenges.

Despite the enormous negative impact of severe stress, those endowed with greater resources are more likely to sustain the initial impact in good psychological stead. Likewise, communities and families that sustain the shock of extreme stress with reasonable resource reserves are more likely to aid communal recovery for the social group and its individual members. This latter process is now examined more closely.

Rallying of Resources Following Disaster and Extreme Stress

The 24th Division was responsible for the defense of Oahu at Pearl Harbor when the Japanese attacked in December 1941. Their defense was abysmal. They were unprepared, despite warning; many were away from their stations, and they felt largely to blame for the major sinking of U.S. ships and loss of American lives. What is most interesting, however, is not their initial response, which was understandably severe. Rather, throughout the war, this military unit, numbering thousands of men, was plagued with psychiatric breakdown, even of whole units, low morale, and poor military organization, despite attempts to replace officers and reintegrate and support troops (Marlowe, 1984). Their resources were devastated by their fundamental losses in their belief in their ability to serve and their shame in their initial defeat. I am quite sure that had they had that fateful day to do over, they would endeavor to respond effectively and, no doubt, many individuals acted bravely and with distinction in the face of the massive Japanese onslaught. However, once these losses were incurred, this community of men was plagued with an ongoing spiral of resource loss that was almost irreversible.

The fate of the 24th Army Division can be compared with the record of two American ethnic minority fighting groups during World War II, who each served with remarkable distinction and *esprit de corps.* The Tuskegee Airmen were a unit of the U.S. Army Air Corp, an all African American unit. Operating in the European theater, they were at first relegated to mundane assignments and restricted to "coloreds only" bases. Despite this discrimination, they were eventually assigned as a fighter group protecting the American fighter bombers who were being increasingly shot down on their missions by German fighters. The Tuskegee Airmen generated such high morale, support of each others' positions in terms of integrated defense, and individual heroism that they developed an unprecedented record of successful support of the bombers under their defense and became one of the most decorated air units in U.S. history (Francis, 1955).

Similarly, the 442nd Regimental Combat Team was composed of Nisei fighters (second-generation Japanese Americans). Many had come from concentration camps in the United States, where their families were still interned. Fighting in the Italian campaign against strong German forces, the 442nd Regimental Combat Team was consistently effective. They became the most decorated unit in U.S. fighting history, and in an era where psychiatric casualties ran at a rate as high as 10% of troop strength, they had few or no psychiatric breakdowns whatsoever (Marlowe, 1984). Both the Tuskegee Airmen and the 442nd attributed their record to the social support they derived from having others of their cultural background together. Furthermore, they felt that they must achieve their goal to prove that they were true Americans and deserving of respect (Francis, 1955).

How individual and communal resources can continue to be jointly mobilized even after major loss is further evidenced in the story of the Israeli Tank Corp. Being highly trained and having an almost superhuman belief in their joint efficacy, they withstood the Syrian attack on the eve of the 1973 Yom Kippur War. The Syrians fought bravely, well, and under good leadership. The Israelis fought at times with forces so low that they were reconstituting damaged tanks and injured crews in small groupings that nevertheless met, halted, and reversed the Syrian assault, with the finest weapons supplied by the Russian Army. Indeed, many of the key weapons held by the Syrians were unknown to the West and gave the Syrians a day and night advantage. Chaim Herzog (1984), the Israeli general, military historian, and later president, wrote:

A battalion commander, Lieutenant-Colonel Yossi, was caught on his honeymoon in the Himalayan Mountains when the war broke out. By superhuman efforts he managed to return to Israel, rushed to the battlefield and improvised a force of thirteen damaged tanks that had been towed back to the support echelons for repair. He organized crews (including many wounded who discharged themselves from hospital) and on the Tuesday afternoon, moved up into the 7th Brigade's sector just as the remnants of the 7th Brigade were about to withdraw. The seven remaining tanks of the brigade joined Lieutenant-Colonel Yossi's force and moved over to counterattack the Syrians. Taken by surprise, the Syrians, who had been extended, had been fought to a standstill, and who had lost some 500 tanks and armoured vehicles in the killing ground which came to be known as the "Valley of Tears," before the 7th Brigade's position, broke.... The Syrian attack was broken, and their forces withdrew before the 7th Brigade.

By midday on Wednesday 10 October, almost exactly four days after some 1,400 Syrian tanks had stormed across the "Purple Line" in a massive attack against Israel, not a single Syrian tank remained in fighting condition west of that line.

Against the most incredible odds, and to the indomitable spirit of the Israeli forces, which within a period of four days had suffered a crushing disaster, had recovered and, in one of the heroic battles in modern military history, had turned the tables and driven the invading force back to its starting line.*

After days of nonstop fighting, often so close-in that tanks could barely turn their turrets, the decision was made to enter Syrian territory. A psychiatrist who reviewed the tank crews that had fought 4 days and nights without sleep and suffered major casualties was intending to relieve these crews of duty so they could be medically treated and obtain rest, food, and sleep. He saw them as unfit for further service. They, however, had other plans, and they insisted on being part of the invasion of Syrian territory and the chasing of the Syrian Battalions beyond a corridor in which they could threaten Israeli territory.

The communal resources that characterized these troops were high-level-functioning individuals, thorough training, resilient leadership, high levels of shared-efficacy, strong sense of comradery and common purpose, and sophisticated equipment. In addition, a key ingredient of both individual and group functioning in the face of traumatic stress is the sense of a shared mission that deserves sacrifice. This can encompass the need for the family to survive, to return home to loved ones who need you, and more abstract notions such as the cause of freedom or national heritage (May, 1953, 1969). This sense of meaning follows once again, from perceptions that are jointly shared and consistent with the values fundamental to social connections and background. As Meichenbaum's (1995) work on traumatic stress suggests, this sense of meaning is paramount to individual and group narratives—the stories that people construct to define their lives and their

---

*Chaim Herzog, *The Arab-Israeli Wars: War and Peace in the Middle East from the War of Independence to Lebanon*, pp. 292–293 London: Cassell PLC. Used with permission.

purpose. At numerous junctures, Israeli troops were close to the threshold where loss spirals might have become insurmountable. In many instances where defeat seemed inevitable, an individual or a unit stepped up to fill the gap and allow time for replenishment of others' resources in materials, time, and spirit. Always, the sense that one's home and family were dependent on drawing some last measure of courage or strength rallied troops that might have otherwise faltered.

The battles should, however, not be romanticized. The cost to human life on both sides was staggering. For Israel, where such statistics are available, a sizable percentage of combatants also experienced PTSD, and many carry physical and psychological scars to this day (Solomon, 1995). Most troops were not professional soldiers, but civilian reserves who had families, businesses, and life to manage. But we can learn important lessons from them regarding communal resiliency in the face of extreme stress.

This ability of the group to rise above the individual and to rally collective resources is not reserved for military units, either, although the most scientific and well-documented information is, not surprisingly, based on military units. The following story told by Collins and Lapierre (1972) describes the rallying of a civilian group during the siege of Jerusalem during the War of Israeli Independence in 1948. Jerusalem had been cut off from the rest of Israel, and its inhabitants were being starved. Bombings produced five times the casualties of the worst period of the worst days of the bombing of London by German rockets. An Israeli officer, Bronislav Bar-Shemer, had kidnapped the trucks of Tel Aviv and a group of middle-aged Tel Aviv men for an extremely dangerous make-or-break mission.

> Most of them shared two characteristics. They were city dwellers and had rarely walked more than half a mile at a time. They were middle aged or older....
>
> A nervous silence prevailed in the buses. Like many of the men around him, Pinhas Bracker, the meter reader of the Palestine Electric Company who had promised his wife he would be back for dinner, wondered what anguish his prolonged absence was going to cause his family....
>
> It was midnight as the first buses started into the Judean foothills. A chill wind rolled down from the plateau, sending shivers through these men dressed in shirtsleeves for the humid sidewalks of Tel Aviv. Ahead, green, pink and yellow streaks of light danced across the dark skies, signal flares announcing, perhaps, their arrival to some hidden Arab gunner....
>
> The convoy struggled through cyclamen and lavender up to the village of Beit Susin.... There the men got down and slug their sacks on their backs.
>
> Bronislav Bar-Shemer, the officer who had kidnaped the trucks of Tel Aviv ... arranged them in single file. Each man was instructed to take hold of the shirttail of the man before him so that they would not get lost in the darkness. Then, Bar-Shemer at their head, they started forward into the night....
>
> After a slight decline, the track straightened out to assault the steep incline leading up to the first crest. It was there that the porters' martyrdom began. Without any light,

the men stumbled on hidden stones, slipped to the ground, grabbing a clump of wild carrots or a bush to keep themselves from rolling down the hillside. Felled by a heart attack, one man tumbled back down the ravine, bouncing helplessly from rock to rock. The men behind him stepped over his body to attack in their turn the slope that had killed him.

Some, too exhausted to go on, sank to the ground by the side of the path. The strongest struggled to the top, laid down their loads, then came back down to help them. To forget the pain of his ascent, Pinhas Bracker forced himself to remember a happy picnic had had in these hills as a young family man. Others remembered ... that they carried on their aching backs the ingredients of one hundred thousand Jews' survival. Still others thought only how to move one foot forward after the other. Mixed with the scraping and stumbling noise of their feet was a bizarre panting sound, the panting of their middle-aged lungs. At points the slope became so steep that the men literally had to pull themselves forward by tugging on stone ledges or grasping ... roots....

Some of the men crawled forward on hands and knees. On the reverse slopes, those who couldn't hold on slid down the hillside on their stomachs, moving like crabs from rock to rock so that the precious load on their backs would not be lost.

Without a word, without a cry, the column continued along its way. At its head, Bar-Shemer prayed that the guns of Latrun would remain silent and not turn their expedition into a disaster with a few mortar shells. Finally ... he saw ahead in the predawn grayness the silhouettes of a team of porters brought out from Jerusalem to load their sacks onto waiting trucks and jeeps. [Jerusalem's] desperate appeal had been heard. The efforts of Bar-Shemer's three hundred men from Tel Aviv would give ... Jerusalem ... food.*

THE SOCIAL SUPPORT DETERIORATION MODEL: COR THEORY APPLIED TO SOCIAL SUPPORT

Kaniasty and Norris, in a series of sophisticated studies, have developed the Social Support Deterioration Model by applying COR theory to the process of social support during disaster. Their careful methodology, replications of the model across different disasters, and ecological viewpoint make for a powerful case and help illuminate how resource loss and gain cycles operate during and following disasters. A number of authors have noted that stress may result in dramatic changes in available social support (Eckenrode & Gore, 1981; Rook & Dooley, 1985; Shinn, Lehmann, & Wong, 1984). Major stress events that involve resource loss such as divorce, death of a loved one, and serious illness often act to diminish social support availability (Lepore, Evans, & Schneider, 1991). At the same time, we know that stress often acts as an alarm system, calling for the mobilization of social support (Cohen & Hoberman, 1983; Dunkel-Schetter, Folkman, & Lazarus, 1987;

*Reprinted with the permission of Simon & Schuster from *O Jerusalem!* by Laury Collins and Dominique Lapierre, Copyright © 1972 by Laury Collins and Dominique Lapierre.

Hobfoll & Lerman, 1989). The question becomes how these antithetical processes co-occur.

People act to mobilize social support in times of stress in order to minimize the deleterious effects of threat and loss (Wheaton, 1985; Barrera, 1986). However, mobilization may be interrupted by a number of factors. First, the loss event may involve the very loved one who has been traditionally called upon for support, thus breaking down the primary supportive chain. Second, the actual support needed may prove ambiguous, even for major stressors. People may wish to help but not know how to proceed (Wortman & Lehman, 1985). Third, highly stressful conditions often exacerbate or create interpersonal conflict, thus short-circuiting potential avenues of support (Taylor & Shumaker, 1990; Vinokur, Schul, & Caplan, 1987). Fourth, severe stressors often become chronic or lead to chronically stressful conditions, diminishing resources, and creating burnout among caregivers (Eckenrode & Wethington, 1990; Schulz & Tompkins, 1990). Finally, disasters or other major communal stressors, such as factory closings, may disrupt entire indigenous networks, such that the fundamental linkage of relationships, communications, places to meet, and opportunities for meeting are lost (Giel, 1990).

Kaniasty and Norris (1993; Norris & Kaniasty, 1996; Kaniasty, Norris, & Murrell, 1990) applied COR theory to test the support deterioration deterrence model.

> Our interests were in applying these theoretical models to understanding the consequences of natural disasters, events that often involve catastrophic depletion of resources. All the kinds of resources identified in Hobfoll's conservation of resources model are affected.... Victims may lose their homes (object resources) and with them their sense of safety and security. Victims may lose their jobs (condition resources) and with them the sense of status and belongingness. Victims' self-esteem and sense of invulnerability (personal characteristic resources) are also potentially shattered. Victims may lose money and time (energies resources) and with them the chance for quick recovery.
>
> To cope with these losses, disaster victims need all the support they can get.... Unfortunately, natural disasters have the capacity to deplete social support. Although disasters tend to mobilize support immediately after the impact, it also appears that need soon exceeds the availability of those supports ... from an initial rush of spontaneous helping to a long-term depletion of supportive resources. (Kaniasty & Norris, 1993, p. 396)

Studying older flood victims involved in a major flood in Kentucky in 1981, Kaniasty and Norris examined the loss deterioration cycle prior to the flood and during an additional four interview occasions in the years that followed. As predicted, both personal loss and level of community destruction independently contributed to victims' depression. Also, initial social support decreased disaster stress and mitigated people's level of depression.

But at the same time, disaster stress caused a deterioration in social support, limiting the support that could be mobilized by victims. Personal loss's influence was more or less immediate, but community loss had a more delayed effect, suggesting that the community was unable to respond adequately to assist the older individuals' recovery. Both individual and community loss left victims with a sense of deterioration of the availability of social support, including help from kin and nonkin. Moreover, Kaniasty and Norris concluded that the older adults were particularly vulnerable because, as Baltes theorized (1987), older individuals are more reliant on cultural supports to buttress their personal strengths when loss occurs.

Norris and Kaniasty (1996) replicated this study on victims of two hurricanes. Hurricanes Hugo and Andrew struck Charleston, South Carolina in 1990 and southern Florida in August 1992. Both were major disasters that resulted in severe loss of homes and property, dislocation, and injury. In human terms, Andrew also was more devastating in that 55 related deaths were attributed to it. Again, these studies are exemplary in that they are among a select few that examined disasters longitudinally and replicate models across different disasters for different populations.

As illustrated in Figure 7.1, the scope of the disaster results in a simultaneous mobilization of received social support and a deterioration of perceived support. However, the mobilization of received support acts to bolster these lagging perceptions of support, which in turn mitigate the negative impact of the disaster. In other words, at the same time that circumstances are depleting perceptions of available support, the process of rallying of support is buttressing the support process from more rapid decline.

Their careful analysis also revealed an additional process predicted by COR theory. Specifically, as indicated in the FALL model outlined in Chapter 4, limitations in the use of resources were evidenced for lower status populations. Support should operate by the "rule of relative need," such that more support should be available to those who experience greater disaster-related loss. However, ethnic minority individuals and lower socioeconomic groups were noted as receiving less help than others who were comparably hit by the hurricanes. Because their resources were already strained prior to the disasters, the cycles of loss for these groups were more severe and long-lasting.

COMMUNAL SOCIAL RESOURCE DETERIORATION

The initial period of affiliation, heroism, self- and communal sacrifice, and sense of community that often follows disasters eventually gives way to

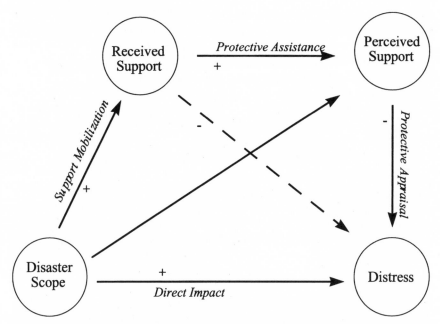

Figure 7.1. The social support deterioration deterrence model. *Source:* Adapted from Norris and Kaniasty (1996), copyright *Journal of Personality and Social Psychology* and reproduced with permission.

the harsh reality of the resource losses involved. After the media and govern-ment agencies migrate to new disasters, the community is left with its diminished resources and ongoing chronic stressors that follow in disaster's wake. As Pennebaker and Harber (1993) observed following the 1989 Loma Prieta earthquake in San Francisco, the pressure cooker effect translates to people becoming decreasingly tolerant of hearing others' disaster sagas, and perhaps due to underlying individualism, communal helping is difficult to sustain. The disaster brings people out into the schoolyard, courtyard, porch, and community center. Individualized culture returns them to their televisions, living rooms, and backyard patios.

Moreover, as Giel (1990) has observed even in more communal soci-eties, in-group versus out-group dichotomies within these cultures may similarly not only limit cross-group social support, but may stimulate dor-mant hostilities between haves and have-nots. Following the Peruvian earth-quake of 1970, an immense landslide entirely enveloped the village of 4,000 inhabitants in the provincial capital of Yungai. Early reactions were based on relative need, but soon middle- and upper-class survivors began to refer to the lower-class survivors as "nondeserving Indians." Indians were said to have had nothing and so deserved nothing of the resources distributed in the relief effort. In fact, the lower-class individuals were more in need of aid and were not even likely to be Indians, but these reactions mirrored underlying prejudices within the society. As Wallace (1957) theorized, human beings are

> organisms whose peculiarity it is to construct and modify slowly and laboriously, over centuries, very complicated sets of mazes for themselves and their posterity, with elaborate inter-connecting doors and pathways; and also to construct complex rules for interaction and even mutual aid in operating the maze, as "the way" to satisfy their multifarious wants. (Giel, 1990, p. 8)

Giel suggests that major physical disasters suddenly destroy the material resources, social cues, and pathways, rendering these complex mazes inoperative.

As early as 1812, these processes were outlined by Benjamin Rush, the father of American psychiatry. Referring to major, human-precipitated communal stressors, Rush wrote,

> Revolutions in governments which are often accompanied with injustice, cruelty, and the loss of property and friends; and where this is not the case, with an inroad upon ancient and deep-seated principles and habits, frequently multiply instances of insanity. Mr. Volney informed me, in his visit to this city in the year 1799, that there were three times as many cases of madness in Paris in the year 1795, as there were before the commencement of the French Revolution. It was induced, I shall say hereafter, [in the United States] in several instances, by the events of the American Revolution. (p. 71)

The nuclear disaster at Chernobyl on April 26, 1986, illustrates how social support deterioration is accelerated by a breakdown in the complex social fabric referred to here, where the traditional pathways and mazes are thoroughly interrupted. In discussing the disaster at Chernobyl, Bromet (1995) divides the episode into three highly stressful communal processes. First, came the radiation accident and release, followed by evacuation, and culminating in relocation. The nuclear episode was of enormous magnitude. An area of some 1,000 square kilometers, which included 98 villages, many farms, and a sizable populace was heavily contaminated and later declared unsuitable for continuing human habitation (Kidd, 1991). Technological disasters are particularly stressful, in part, because they challenge social trust if there is a perception that they could have been avoided or the affected population could have been handled more humanely and generously (Baum, Fleming, & Davidson, 1983; Green, 1995), and Chernobyl compounded this problem because of an underlying mistrust of government among the population.

The dispersal of the population resulted in a breakdown in social connections and natural and professional support patterns. Natural and formal resources that might have been brought to bear were fragmented, and official denials of the magnitude of the problem accelerated the sense of urgency and terror. This was felt in particular, Bromet writes, for parents who rightfully feared for their children's well-being. The truth about what did occur was held from the public for 2 years, and the health consequences were never openly divulged. Integration into their new communities was also problematic. Perhaps because their new neighbors accepted official versions of the minimalist nature of the disaster, they were unwelcoming to the refugees and jealous of their meager compensation packages. Children tend to be adaptive, but frequent sicknesses meant that children were often absent from school and had difficulty integrating into new school environments.

Overall, it is clear that initial resource losses were severe and that individual, group, and social resource reservoirs were already stretched before the disaster occurred. What resources were available were undermined by both the natural breakdown in support and resource chains, and official undermining in order to perpetuate the myth of little harm. Loss cycles were rapid, could not easily be curtailed, and had long tails, reaching far into families and children's lives. The negative lifetime effects on children are particularly upsetting and are a reflection in large part of the intertwined nature of children's resources with those of their parents, who are their major resource linkage (Pynoos, Goenjian, & Steinberg, 1995; Raphael, 1986).

Looking across these disasters, the social support deterioration model can clearly be generalized to other resources and illustrates that extreme stress diminishes a broad array of resources at the same time that these resources are in demand. Given the long-term nature of disaster's impact (Green, 1995; Solomon, 1995), we can expect these loss and gain cycles to extend many years following the original episode. Green (1995), McFarlane (1995) and Solomon (1995) all interpret existing research as showing that the degree of original threat and loss are good predictors of long-term sequelae. Breakdown of individual, family, and community resources accelerates and extends these negative spirals not for just weeks and months, but for years. Studying the victims of the Beaver Creek Flood after 14 years, Green and her colleagues (1990) noted significant overall improvement in mental health indicators among victims. However, 14 years after the flood, the affected population still showed significant impairment in the form of anxiety and depression.

It is notable that one of the major risk factors is degree of community dispersement. People who can rebuild their communities and refabricate prior resource and communal patterns have better long-term prognosis (deJong, 1995; deVries, 1995). Indigenous secular and clerical leaders are integral to this process and a reconstitution of the vague, but keystone, interweaving of families, institutions, and social practices must be reformulated (deJong, 1995). Being denied the possibility to rebuild the mazes and pathways of the community is a decidedly ominous indicator of future recovery.

Disaster may also disperse or destroy economic resources that underpin community integrity and are difficult to reconstitute. Palinkas and his colleagues noted that the Exxon Valdez oil spill disrupted fishing activities and the accompanying cultural patterns involved in maintaining traditional social structures in ways that made even long-term recovery of resource retrieval patterns difficult (Palinkas, Russell, Downs, & Petterson, 1992; Palinkas, Downs, Petterson, & Russell, 1993). Native Alaskans were particularly at risk, and the spill spiraled from economic problems to health problems and increases in drinking, drug abuse, and domestic violence. Perhaps because of fishing being more culturally embedded, Native Americans were not aided by family support in their recovery from the oil spill. This extends Kaniasty and Norris's support deterioration model in two ways. First, it is generalized to express and describe the process of resource deterioration and replenishment for a variety of resources, and second, it includes long-term influences whereby a rebuilding of resources is possible to the extent that communities can restrengthen their fabric and normalize the living process.

LOSS AND EXTREME STRESS: SUMMARY

Reviewing these complex stories and research on extreme stress, the principles and corollaries of COR theory seem to emerge with clearer focus in terms of their cycles and movements. As suggested by COR theory, those with greater resources were indeed less vulnerable to resource loss and more capable of orchestrating resource gain. Those with greater resources were less negatively affected by initial resource loss and were more likely to create gain cycles because they could borrow from resources that were not required for everyday functioning or reserve capacity. Conversely, those with fewer resources displayed greater vulnerability to resource loss and were less capable of achieving resource gain. Those with few resources were more deeply impacted by the initial onslaught of demand that accompanied extreme stress and less adequately addressed the chronic demands that ensued. Those particularly low in resources were especially disturbed by initial setbacks, resulting in immediate and rapid loss spirals that made recovery difficult if not impossible.

As COR theory proffers, those who lacked resources were not only more vulnerable to resource loss, but also their initial loss begat ancillary losses. Where individuals and social units relied on resources to counter losses, and because stress results from resource loss, at each iteration of the extreme stress cycle there were less resources available for mobilization or to invest in gain cycles that might have countered stress's negative influence. Thus resource reservoirs became depleted and were decreasingly capable of mobilizing to defend against ongoing demands. Moreover, the supposition that loss cycles have higher initial velocity for resource-poor individuals and groups was repeatedly revealed. Already vulnerable, they have limited capacity for protection of the self, family, or social system (see also Lepore, Wortman, Silver, & Wayment, 1996).

Individuals and communities who possessed strong backup resources were not only more capable of offsetting initial losses, but also were even able to optimize and compensate (Baltes, 1987) to parlay their resources to initiate resource gains that begat further gains. However, as suggested by COR theory, these gain cycles always appeared tenuous, and the cowboy or movie image of the invulnerable individual or combat unit is a gross romanticization, as even the finest units and individuals seem to teeter on the brink of demise with one false investment of resources or one demand from the environment at the moment when resource reserves are most challenged. Still, when initial gains are achieved, additional resources are produced or become liberated from other functions—enabling truly heroic efforts.

It was repeatedly made apparent that those who lack resources are likely to adopt a defensive posture to guard their resources. With few resources, the cost of resource investment for them outstrips demands and makes the individual or organization vulnerable. This leads to inaction, denial, avoidance, and seeking solace in drugs and alcohol. Care should be taken here, however, not to blame the victims, as it is also clear that if afforded more resources, they would be just as likely to be more effective copers. Moreover, those who seek defensive postures are often low-status populations that have been denied full access to the cornucopia of potential resources available in their greater society.

Finally, the concept of *fitting*, rather than fit of resources, becomes more obvious. Few individuals or groups have the exact resources required to answer the demands of disaster, war, and other extreme stress. Even trained troops, let alone civilians, confront unexpected circumstances and combinations of demands that were never anticipated and certainly carried no social metaphors that outlined functional alternatives. As the model of ecological congruence suggests, fitting of resources is an active process, where fundamental resources such as self-reliance, shared reliance, strong social ties, and a common sense of meaning and purpose seem to be the engine that fuels the operation of other resource elements and orchestrates their implementation. We saw clearly how resources were shaped, parlayed, traded, and sometimes corrupted in order to meet demands that themselves were constantly changing over time. Those who possessed richer resource reservoirs resisted the worst consequences of extreme stress of shaping and combining their resources to counteract challenges. Furthermore, they were at the same time capable of retaining adequate resource reserves for functioning, and even adequate resource stockpiles in case of emergencies.

STRESS AND BURNOUT:
CREEPING LOSS AND GAIN CYCLES

In the next section, I contrast these rapid cycles and spirals to the slow ebbing of resources that occurs in the process of burnout at work. If extreme stress may be compared to a typhoon, the stress burnout process is comparable to the movement of slowly creeping tides, almost unnoticed. Like the tide, however, burnout has a powerful effect and is one of the most critical areas of stress for modern, industrialized society because of the toll it takes on individuals, families, and business productivity (Shirom, 1989). By virtue of the stark contrast between extreme stress, on the one hand, and burnout, on the other hand, we can better understand how resource losses and gains operate on these two sides of the loss–gain cycle continuum. If we can identify common rules for extreme stress and for stress burnout, then it is likely that the kinds of stress that fall in between are governed by the same operations and properties. This is not to say that there are not major differences between traumatic stress events and the circumstances that contribute to burnout. The costs of traumatic stress on victims are more overwhelming, result in long-standing debilitation that is sometimes even beyond the realm of full recovery, and threaten much more deep-seated elements of the self, psyche, group, and society (Shalev, 1996). But this notwithstanding, inasmuch as there are common properties about the movement of resource cycles, we can learn important insights about the underlying process of stress in the full spectrum of the human drama.

> Look you, when life is brimful of success
> —Though the past hold no action foul—one feels
> A thousand self-disgusts, of which the sum
> Is not remorse, but a dim, vague unrest;
> And, as one mounts the steps of worldy fame,
> The Dukes; furred mantles trail within their folds
> A sound of dead illusions, vain regrets,
> A rustle—scarce a whisper,—like as when,
> Mounting the terrace steps, our mourning robe
> Sweeps in its train the dying autumn leaves. (Rostand, 1980)

The most widely cited definition of burnout comes from Maslach and Jackson (1986, p. 1): "Burnout is a syndrome of emotional exhaustion, depersonalization and reduced personal accomplishment that can occur among individuals who do 'people work' of some kind." Burnout has been extended by others to include other than those who perform "people work," but the three core elements remain, these being (1) emotional exhaustion, (2) depersonalization, and (3) reduced sense of personal accomplishment. By extension, organizations that are plagued by burnout among their workers will suffer from reduced accomplishment, absenteeism, avoidance of stressful aspects of the job, conflict between employees and between employees and management, and high rates of worker turnover. Kearns (1986) estimated that as much as 60% of work absence is the result of stress-related disorders. Although burnout is only part of this, its influence is likely to have major work costs (Hobfoll & Shirom, 1993).

A related phenomenon that I find is often confused with burnout is rustout. I have not seen any solid empirical work on rustout, but intermixed with the burnout literature are cases that seem to me to be better defined by rustout. By rustout, I mean work situations that fail to challenge individuals into using their resources. This can occur in the workplace and may be more common in institutional or bureaucratic settings, where individuals may be discouraged by a variety of forces from investing their resources and attempting to be productive.

By focusing on resource cycles, the differences between burnout and rustout become more striking. In burnout, individuals often have to draw on resources for long periods of time with little payoff, few rewards, and little sense of accomplishment. In rustout, resource cycles are stillborn, never allowed to be tried, invested, or challenged. These constitute very different kinds of cycles, with some overlapping consequences and many major differences in terms of processes and likely solutions. As we look at the burnout literature, we should be mindful of the fact that mixed in is the process of rustout.

COR Theory and Burnout

In developmental models of burnout, Shirom (1989) and Ezrahi (1985) suggest that during its early stages, individuals attempt to combat ongoing workplace stressors by a high level of resource investment directed toward coping. This stage may find individuals overaroused, anxious, and frustrated at the failure of their resources to impact the problem. Ezrahi (1985) noted that at this stage, people attempt problem-focused solutions expressed in terms of time investment, use of resources to address the problem, and seeking solutions. When and if these efforts fail, individuals switch to the more defensive posture suggested by COR theory. By behaving defensively, individuals garner what resources they can, reduce the indirect loss of resources that comes from continuing to invest in unrewarding solutions, and limit loss that comes from exposing themselves to the negative feedback they are receiving in the workplace. The price is paid instead in emotional exhaustion and a sense of depersonalization and failure, and concomitant negative emotions such as anxiety and depression.

The loss cycles involved in burnout are slow-paced, illusive, and even intentionally disguised by employers, unions, work rules, and people's own need to believe that their work is valued. A number of professionals are particularly vulnerable to burnout, including teachers, nurses, social workers, and service industry personnel who have frequent public contact (Burke & Richardsen, 1993). Teachers, for example, have one of the highest burnout rates of any profession (Schwab, Jackson, & Schuler, 1986). In many educational settings, teachers' hard work, initial zeal, idealism, and sense of accomplishment are continuously challenged. Factors such as large classroom size, children who are often unprepared to learn due to outside stressors of poverty, racism, violence, and family discord, lack of proper tools, and poor facilities combine to result in a long chain of microlosses. Isolation of teachers into single-teacher classrooms and frequent teacher–management labor unrest act to further exacerbate the situation.

Perhaps more than outright loss, the third kind of stressful circumstances identified by COR theory may play a damaging role. Specifically, *COR suggests that stress occurs when resources are invested without subsequent gain.* Teachers are commonly called upon to invest resources but may receive little resource gain for their efforts or investments. Gain might be expected in terms of seeing children learn new skills and advance, watching children mature, being thanked for a job well done, and parental involvement. Instead, teachers often receive little clear indication of children's advances, must concentrate efforts on a few children with severe discipline or learning problems, who seldom seem to benefit from teachers' investment in them, and hear the message from society that they are valued little for their frequent sacrifices. With poor funding in many settings, teachers must supplement supplies from their own budget and often travel into neighborhoods that are dangerous and where they are made to feel unwelcome. Rather than the perhaps idealized relationships they were expecting with children—grateful eyes, hunger for knowledge—they are more likely to confront disrespect, outright belligerence, violence, and apathy.

Whether more direct resource loss or failure to gain resources following significant resource investment characterizes their environment, the loss cycle undermines resource reserves in a process akin to a slow leak. Often unnoticed, resources become diminished, not in a rush, but bit by bit, with little opportunity for replenishment (Zohar, 1997). This results in loss of both personal and energy resources in particular. In this way, Pines, Aronson, and Kafry (1981) find burnout to be characterized by feelings of helplessness, hopelessness, entrapment, and a marked decrease in enthusiasm about work. Thus, resources of self-esteem, self-efficacy, hope, and a feeling of purpose are undermined, while on the physical level, exhaustion replaces earlier zeal.

Many other individuals are exposed to circumstances that encourage rustout. Again, there is little research on this, but I have frequently observed the process in my consulting with businesses. Many settings underutilize personnel. However, to reveal this would threaten too many individuals and sometimes the settings' very survival. Hence, a kind of conspiracy develops where workers agree to the myth that they are working hard. In unions, this has been termed *featherbedding*, the creation of work routines that appear to involve more work than they do. It is not merely a working-class phenomenon, however, as I have seen it in corporate headquarters and in academic departments as well. The price that is paid, however, is that those involved actually develop a sense that they do not have the resources or capabilities to do otherwise. The conspiracy of silence leaves resources untested, and untested resources disintegrate in disuse (Bandura, 1997). As in burnout, the failure to successfully utilize resources results in a slow trail of resource loss that is disguised by both its torpidity and the conspiracy of silence. At first, individuals are prevented from utilizing their resources, but eventually, they are left incapable of utilizing their resources, many of which become outdated, reduced, or obsolete.

COMMUNAL RESOURCE DETERIORATION

Just as in the case of extreme stress, it is notable that burnout has been frequently conceptualized in terms of a burnout not within the individual, but in the social connections between individuals (Maslach, 1993). The communal aspect of burnout is evidenced in the finding that environmental factors predict burnout better than individual factors (Cherniss, 1990). The processes that underlie burnout consist of cycles that fracture the interpersonal, relational roots that people have, or expect, at work. The supportive relationship resources between employees and their colleagues and supervisors, on one level, and the functional, competency-yielding ties between employees and their clients or students are interrupted and deteriorate.

Tying together the individual and organizational levels, Cherniss (1990) conceptualized burnout as more likely among individuals low in self-efficacy, but hinged this sense of efficacy on organizations' conditions that combine excessive workload with limited social support. Thus, the workplace as village fails to care for its citizens and leaves them isolated and lacking in supportive structures. Contrariwise, workplaces that encourage employee efficaciousness are structured in ways that Iscoe (1974) related to the competent community—allowing individuals to experience challenge, reasonable autonomy and control, accurate feedback on effort, rewards, and support from co-workers and supervisors (cf. Fisher, 1984). In their review of four separate burnout studies, Cutrona and Russell (1990) noted that settings that offered reassurance of self-worth and supervisor support were key in limiting burnout among teachers, nurses, and psychotherapists.

Glidewell (1987) noted the paradox here—that the very social structures that might be restorative were particularly weak within the existent social order. Studying teachers, he found that although teachers frequently communicated in the faculty lounge, they avoided discussion that might reflect their failure, inadequacy, or even problems in the classroom in ways that might indicate anything lacking on their own part. By so doing, they were expressing that such disclosure was a route to further resource loss, not to support and resource replenishment. Glidewell set his task to be the reversal of this natural, but unhealthy ecology, and to replace it with social standards that encouraged help seeking and help giving. By reversing the ecology to one that supported sharing and collaborative exploration of difficulties, he limited burnout and increased teachers' sense of effectiveness and of having a supportive base.

A similar approach was adopted by Freedy and Hobfoll (1994), when we intervened with hospital nurses in multiple hospital settings. In this work, led by my colleague, John Freedy, we attempted in a series of training sessions to increase nurses' sense of mastery by having them set winnable goals and work toward goal accomplishment. Simultaneously, we had nurses identify weaknesses in social support at work and at home, and taught them effective means of increasing social support. For example, they learned to ask more specifically for the kind of help they needed, to provide feedback to supporters about how their assistance aided them, and to make themselves available nonjudgmentally to their colleagues in offers of support. Only in groups where we addressed the cycles that result simultaneously in increased mastery and social support were we able to reverse burnout. When we intervened concerning mastery alone, we achieved little or no success. It was apparently important to alter both individual and collective patterns that created the shared and interwoven structure of the self-nested-in family-nested-in social organization that COR theory postulates.

Nor can it be said that burnout is a product of spoiled American workers who have become soft. It appears to be a cross-culturally valid proposition that people expect reasonable payback and effectiveness in response to their work-based efforts. Burnout phenomena occur worldwide and may be especially rampant in rapidly developing and economically underdeveloped countries (Golembiewski, Scherb, & Boudreau, 1993), perhaps because the expectation for a caring village, even at work, is even more expected in such cultures.

As I have emphasized in earlier chapters, people and their resources operate on a level that requires attachments and relationships from the individual to the dyad, family, organization, and tribe or village. In the historical village, family and work occurred in the same shared ecology. However, in the modern world, social relations at work are often geographically and socially disjointed from home and family. Yet, if we incorporate the workplace as part of the "village-extended," we see that many of the same rules apply as they do to the historical village. There exists an expectation of support, a need for supportive and friendship ties, and a perceived system of social understandings that reflect village, not corporate, expectations. The corporation may wish to segregate individuals from home and place impermeable borders between worklife and family life, but this neither seems possible nor ultimately successful. In America's vision of recreating Japanese success in the American workplace before the recent Asian crisis, there is the need to understand that these borders do not exist in Japan, where the company is traditionally local to workers and their families. This is not to say that Japanese firms have not asked for total dedication of their workers, even in ways that disrupt the family, but that they recognize and respect family and work obligations as inseparable (Fukuyama, 1995).

In the village, there is a high degree of certainty or predictability about how things occur and how people behave. Routines are somewhat repetitive and all the players are known entities, with more or less fixed social roles. In the modern workplace, there is often little certainty or ability to control outcomes. Buunk and his colleagues, studying Dutch nurses, found that uncertainty and social interactive patterns play a combined role in producing burnout (Buunk, Collins, Van Ypersen, Taylor, & Dakoff, 1990; Buunk, Schaufeli, & Ybema, 1990). First, consistent with COR theory, they found all three aspects of burnout—reduced sense of personal accomplishment, depersonalization, and emotional exhaustion—to be higher among nurses who invested more of their resources, but who received little gain in return. Moreover, as would be predicted by the thesis that the self is interwoven with the social–relational world, depersonalization was especially likely among nurses who lacked self-esteem.

Buunk and his colleagues also theorized that there is an expectation of exchange among people and that violations of these exchange principles contribute to burnout patterns. Those nurses who had these social expectations were more likely than others to experience depersonalization, in particular, as the lack of return from others made them feel isolated and cut off. Also of interest, Buunk and his colleagues (see also Van Ypersen, Buunk, & Schaufeli, 1992) found that nurses who were more communally oriented were able to resist feelings of depersonalization, because of their lower expectations of *quid pro quo*. The same was found for ideological communities such as Catholic religious orders, suggesting that it is not that they do not expect a return on their investment (Cherniss & Krantz, 1983), but rather than looking for immediate return on their investment, they see the return more long-term and derive satisfaction from knowing that they are contributing on some wider scale. These more communal individuals are also less likely to be socially isolated and may derive much strength from their particularly robust and committed collegial ties.

Buunk's work is particularly important in the way it illustrates the cycles of resource loss. The sequence is probably transactional, with many feedback loops, but it can be seen from his work that burnout is a product of lack of gain following resource investment. This results in losses that reverberate between the self in terms of loss of sense of control and lowered self-esteem and the social collective in terms of alienation, weakened ties, and feelings of being "cheated" in terms of failed payoffs for personal investments made. Those with a stronger sense of communal responsibility can invest more with fewer expectations for receipt of immediate payoff, but their cycles of investment and gain are more likely to be long-term than simply nonexistent. As Burke (1988) also noted, those with close, personal relationships at work are less vulnerable to burnout, further suggesting that it is not just a sense of attachment with others, but the presence of attachments that is critical in buffering the insidious effects of burnout's slow loss.

CONCLUSIONS: COMMON CYCLES AND PROCESSES

Although so very different in magnitude, speed, and impact, the processes of burnout and extreme stress combine to illustrate the pattern of cycles of resource loss and gain. Extreme stress causes a turbulent loss of resources that can virtually immediately outstrip all but the strongest resource reservoirs and in a short time devastate the individual and community. Burnout results in a slow ebbing of resources, slowly depleting resource reserves and making individuals and organizations incapable of successfully acting to counteract these cycles. Gain cycles can be instituted if the individual or group retains sufficient resources to begin the high demand necessary for halting losses and substituting slow, arduous processes that characterize gain cycles. Loss is rapid; gain is more painstakingly slow and stepwise.

Initial losses not only create stress and negative emotional sequelae, but also they deplete the very resource reservoirs that need to be called on to halt loss and seek solutions. At each turn of the cycle, emotional and physical health reactions increase in strength, and more resources are required to combat them. At each turn of the cycle, at the same time, less resources are available. Here lies the critical importance of communal ties. The group or collective is likely to be more capable than the individual to have pockets of sustained resources, even if the community is hit in some widespread manner with the circumstances that are the roots of the loss process. Family, friends, colleagues, professional sources, and religious and volunteer organizations may not be hit equally hard at all levels or for all members. Or they may have banked resources resulting in their being more resource rich, even after trauma or burnout has had time to operate. Thus, by sharing strengths, buttressing weak areas and mutual support efforts, loss cycles can be halted, reversed, or limited until individuals can regain their footing and themselves support the recovery process.

Even in the case of traumatic stress, the traumatized individual has great value to the group. A rape victim or victim of disaster becomes a cataloger of threat and a storyteller for others' recovery. Their deeply ingrained memory of the event, which for them is a terribly painful, intrusive legacy, is a reminder for others to be vigilant. Their survival tells a saga of how others may survive that is probably deeply rooted in human tribal nature. Seen in isolation, psychological and physical distress have little meaning. In collective, the value for group survival is striking and speaks to the intertwined nature of the individual, nested in family, nested in organization and village. Individuals borrow resources from others around them, and the collective relies on the individual in an interactive, repetitive, often turbulent manner.

Finally, on a cultural level, extreme stress and burnout share a tendency to create breakdown of the social fabric in ways that major and moderate stressors that lie in between do not. This may result from the nature of both extreme stress and burnout to threaten social contracts within cultures. Extreme stress threatens social contracts because it is out of the realm that culture has taught its members can occur. Consequently, social structures and regulatory systems have not instilled adequate coping metaphors. (Figley, 1978; Figley & Leventman, 1980). Burnout threatens social contracts because society inculcates the belief that work should be rewarding and that if you invest your resources, you will be rewarded. Stressors that are in between these two are more likely to be expected, to have established patterns of coping, and to be developmentally normalized. Death of a loved one is tragic, but if the death is at the appropriate time in the life span, it is usually accepted and can be grieved normally. Job loss, likewise, is common enough to be normalized, as reflected in unemployment insurance, work search agencies, and daily advertisements in newspapers for available employment. This translates to cycles with linked resources for midlevel to major stressors, but fragmented resource links for extreme stress and burnout. Because the culture does not produce appropriate supports, victims feel violated and isolated unless social support patterns are strong enough to rally in their defense and are not themselves deteriorated too extensively by the stress cycles that ensue.

8

Stress Crossover

The Commerce of Resources across the Borders That Divide and Unite People, Organizations, and Tribes

On the one hand, we rely on others for support and sustenance. Colleagues contribute critical resources for our work performance, loved ones are essential to well-being, and attachment to familial and tribal groups has been a constant feature of human social behavior since its earliest fossil record. Yet people's social relationships are also, and often, the bane of their existence. This chapter addresses how the stress process is influenced by the commerce and competition for resources across the borders that exist between individuals and between individuals and the social systems with which they interact—their families, their jobs, their places of worship, their neighborhoods, and their tribes.

SOCIAL INTERACTION AS CAUSE AND CURE OF MENTAL ILLNESS: EIGHTEENTH- AND NINETEENTH-CENTURY INSIGHTS

Although work on stress has only begun to examine the crossover of stress and stress resistance resources between individuals and between individuals and social systems, it has long been recognized that these resource transactions are paramount to mental and physical health.

The curative versus destructive properties of positive social interaction versus social conflict were first introduced in psychiatry by the French physician Pinel in the early nineteenth century and the English physicians,

Tuke and Conolly in the late eighteenth to mid-nineteenth centuries. Entering the madhouses of the time at Bedlam and the Bicĕtre, *maniacs* were treated by "copious and repeated blood-letting, water and shower baths, low diet, and a rigorous system of coercion" (Pinel, 1806, p. 101) at best, and more commonly "whipped out of their madness" and subjected to "terrible attendants, armed with whips, sometimes (in France) accompanied by savage dogs, and free to impose manacles, and chains, and stripes, at their own brutal will; uncleanliness, semi-starvation, the garotte, and unpunished murders" (Conolly, 1856, p. 5). Their insights are particularly remarkable when framed against the then-current debate as to whether mental illness was a product of physiological discord or moral turpitude. If mental derangement is a "change or lesion in some part of the head," wrote Pinel, "hence the popular prejudice that insanity is generally an incurable malady, and the custom very prevalent of secluding maniacs from society, and of refusing them that attention and assistance to which every infirmity is entitled" (p. 110).

Tuke and Pinel offered a radical variation on treatment. Although their innovations were quickly and quite unfortunately reversed for more "modern" biomedical cures (or more accurately the wait for such cures[1]), they laid the groundwork for the eventual recognition of the pathogenic properties of negative social interaction and the curative properties of positive social contact in a way that had never before been considered.

> The daily visits of the physician and his assistants ... should not be formal and hurried; but time should be given to each ward, and even to many individual patients.... The officers should dismiss all their own cares ... and be ready to hear with patience, to investigate with justice, and to remedy with kindness, all the little or great causes of dissatisfaction laid before them; so that the patients may be tranquillised, and, at the same time, the attendants not ruffled and discomposed, and left in an unfit state themselves to show kindness or exercise patience towards others through the rest of the hours of the day.
>
> ... When, later in the day, they see the chaplain come into the wards, and he converses with them gently and judiciously, their feelings are often evidently touched by a sympathy which, even from early childhood, they have been strangers.... When sitting down to comfortable dinners, they find that some of the officers still come to see that all is conducted properly, a conviction that they are carefully looked after necessarily arises in their thoughts.... The day soon becomes occupied by the men in the various workshops ... and by the women in the workrooms.... Wherever they go they meet kind people, and hear kind words; they are never passed without some recognition, and the face of every officer is the face of a friend.... Day after day these influences operate, and day by day mental irritation subsides, and suspicions die, and gloomy thoughts gradually disperse, and confidence grows and strengthens, and natural affections re-awake, and reason returns. (Conolly, 1856, pp. 56–57)

In this way, these champions of "morale treatment," as it was called, opened the cracks for later understanding that psychological distress and well-being were not the products of sin, and in many cases were not the outgrowth of biological roots, but instead recognized psychosocial causes as the common substrate, especially in what they saw as curable cases. They believed that by offering psychosocial, physical, and conditional resources to those left bereft of these was salutogenic and the best course of treatment. In the place of family discord, they offered ward harmony. In the place of censure, they offered understanding and an open ear. In the place of idleness and boredom, they offered productive work that encouraged self-confidence and reattachment to lost social roles. In the place of brutality, they offered respect and honor.

Coming on the eve of the American and French Revolutions, it is also clear that they were translating liberal, democratic principles to all citizens, even these most disenfranchised societal members. Hence, we again see the power of culture to infuse its ideals into the social sciences. Pinel, Conolly, and Tuke were not themselves inventing an alternative social construction. Rather, they were capable of reinterpreting what permeated the general cultural atmosphere in a manner that had previously not been considered, and the new social construction better fit their observations and empirical data (Erickson & Hyerstay, 1980). What followed was a period in which the "microbial revolution" overtook psychiatry, a social construction that actually had little evidence and shrouded the insane and the field of psychiatry under a long dark veil that resulted in a return to patient warehousing and lifelong incurability for the next 100 years (Erickson & Hyerstay, 1980).

SOCIAL ATTACHMENTS AND RESOURCES

A more modern psychosocial understanding of the role of social attachments in the sustenance of well-being can be attributed to Cooley (1909), who proposed the thesis that interpersonal contacts provided a roadmap for decoding the complexities of the world around us. He felt that interpersonal ties defined culture for us and what the individuals role was in that web of relationships.

Somewhat later, the Chicago School of Sociology, represented by Parkes, Burgess, and McKenzie (1926) in their classic book *The City*, proposed the novel thesis that health and well-being—versus deviancy and ill-health—were direct consequences of the extent that individuals were nested in social relationships in which they held a sanctioned social place and position. Their theory challenged the current *zeitgeist* that attributed deviancy to genetic or moral inadequacy, which indeed was the predominant psychological view of that time, held by such eminent scholars as Lewis Terman of Stanford and Robert Yerkes of Harvard, who argued that Jewish and other "brunette" immigrant groups were genetically inferior and should be prevented from immigrating (Kamin, 1974). In contrast, the

Chicago School held that individuals who did not have sanctioned place and position, such as immigrants, were vulnerable to deviancy and ill health. This concept of marginality became a keystone construct in sociology and is a principal explanatory mechanism offered by sociologists for mental health and social deviancy to this day. The concept implies that the social relations of the marginalized group are not only divided from the resources and rules of the majority society, but also that marginality fractures potential health-maintaining ties within the marginalized community and strains the ability of social relationships to aid the members of the marginalized group.

Psychology and sociology adopted these notions as work on stress evolved in the 1960s and 1970s. Cassel (1974) was a seminal theorist in this area, and reminiscent of the Chicago School of Sociology, looked to the complex urban environment for insights about the relationship between psychosocial processes and stress. Cassel, an epidemiologist, examined the influences of socioenvironmental conditions on infant mortality, tuberculosis, and mental illness. He concluded that social disorganization and negative social conditions were capable of undermining disease resistance on both psychological and physical planes. Consistent with the early work of Cooley and the Chicago School, Cassel reasoned that in such circumstances, people lacked or received insufficient informational cues from their environment to conduct their lives through the labyrinth of demands placed upon them. Moreover, Cassel identified that the strengths of primary social contacts, shared with the individual, could provide a protective, healthenhancing influence. Antonovsky (1979), building further on this concept, identified the nesting of individuals within social networks as general resistance resources. Social networks, he theorized, provided access to supportive ties and a sense of community. Antonovsky further underscored that many of these resources were tied to socioeconomic and ethnic minority status, and that the lack of resources in some groups was a product of classicism and racism, as well as differences that were related to other aspects of power differentials, cultural and subcultural factors, and finally familial and individual differences.

Another key pioneering investigation highlighted the importance of social ties in the maintenance of health and well-being. This study, perhaps more than any other, transformed what at the time was still considered more of a folk wisdom to an area of valid scientific inquiry. Berkman (1977) examined data collected on a random sample of adults in Alameda County, California. Of the original sample of almost 7,000 persons, Berkman identified the 682 persons who died during the following 9 years. Those individuals who were married, had close friends and relatives, church membership, and informal and formal group associations had the lowest mortality rates. The fact of attachment to social structures was a *primum mobile* upon which health turned. She concluded that social isolation and lack of social and community ties compromised people's disease resistance, and the presence of these attachments acted as a resistance resource.

Kanter (1968) identified three aspects of group attachment that are germane here. First, people must feel that it is worthwhile to be committed to the group. Second, they need emotional ties to the group that form the basis of social commitments. Last, they must be committed to the moral rightness or cultural validity of the group. Such commitments embody the resistance contribution of social attachments and their positive contribution to health and well-being.

The question becomes, how are these processes actually translated to aid individuals? That is, sociological theory and research noted the social structures that support health or that subvert it. But it is unclear as to what mechanisms translate these social structures from the setting to the individual or social group. In the nascent field of community psychology, S. Sarason (1974) deemed this transaction between the larger social network and the individual the *psychological sense of community*, and theorized that this sense of community was fundamental to well-being. Psychological sense of community emerges out of an ongoing positive attachment to a significant group that cares for the individual, makes him or her feel valued, and provides for his or her safety and protection, and access to society's resources. Sarason defined psychological sense of community as "the sense that one was part of a readily available, mutually supportive network of relationship upon which one could depend ... [which is] part of the structure of one's everyday living ... [and] available to one in a 'give and get' way," (pp. 1–2).

Iscoe (1974), another community psychologist, referred to this as the *competent community*—the kind of community that fostered healthy connections among people and catalyzed and nurtured their linkages to the fruits of the society, and protected individuals from potential harm, including harm that the community itself could deliver. Iscoe's and Sarason's perspective reflected a major transformation from more pessimistic views of society that had haunted the aftermath of both major post–world war periods. But Iscoe and Sarason made another critical point, that not all societies, nor all social commitments, are characterized by a sharing of the provisions necessary to preserve people's well-being. They deemed some communities competent and some incompetent, and even destructive, based on their relative ability to promote the self-worth and safety of the community's members through the provision of resources or the encouragement or fostering of resources already held by individuals.

The development of the competent community involves the provision and utilization of resources in a geographical or psychological community so that the members of the community may make reasoned decisions about issues confronting them, leading to the most competent coping with these problems. Coping is stressed rather than adjustment in keeping with a positive, activist point of view. Conceptually, the competent community is one that utilizes, develops, or otherwise obtains resources, including of course the fuller development of the resources of the human beings in the community itself. (Iscoe, 1974, p. 608)

Another important avenue of research emerged out of this more socio-cultural tradition. Specifically, the work of Cassel, Iscoe, Sarason, and Berkman began to be recast into the investigation of the protective, stress-buffering effects of social support. The study of social support individualized the work on social attachments and transformed it from its original epidemiological and sociological focus. Beginning with the work of the pioneering psychiatrist and social theorist, Gerald Caplan (1974), the area of social support has attracted literally thousands of studies. Gerald Caplan had come to Israel in the early days of independence and quickly found himself inundated with demands on his time. Paradoxically, Caplan was psychoanalytically oriented, with all the attendant emphases on intrapsychic processes and the professional approach that demands years of medical and postgraduate training. Yet, the realities of the fledgling State forced him to think in community rather than individual terms.

Caplan's community focus initially led him to develop the new field of psychiatric consultation, within which he championed the then-heretical idea that mental health professionals should provide professional support for non-mental-health professionals (untrained in psychiatric or medical terms). These non-mental-health professionals and paraprofessionals, in turn, would actually provide the direct services (1964). But this giving away of psychiatry, with its emphasis on professionals making more supportive connections, was only his first turn of the wheel. In the years to come, Caplan recognized that much of mental health lay in the natural commerce of social support between people, in particular, the provision of resources and aid in organizing, catalyzing, and implementing resources that individuals might possess but find constrained in some way. In this way, Caplan began to identify the nature of the process by which social relationships acted beyond their symbolic level and provided actual aid in the stress resistance process.

> The significant others help the individual mobilize his psychological resources and master his emotional burdens; they share his tasks; and supply him with extra supplies of money, materials, tools, skills, and cognitive guidance to improve his handling of his situation. (Caplan, 1974, p. 6)

Caplan felt that such support provision not only supplied and activated resources, but also enabled individuals experiencing stress to retain their sense of mastery, which Caplan thought was a paramount ingredient in mental health.[2] Social support research altered the focus to how individuals benefited from social support and social connections in times of stress, rather than how the stress process inevitably caused physical and psychological malady (Vaux, 1988).

FORGOTTEN SOCIAL CONFLICT

In the rush and excitement over social support and the curative value of positive social attachments, the negative aspects of social interactions were for a time forgotten in the stress literature (Rook, 1984). However, if social attachment is a necessary ingredient for health, social conflict is one of the most destructive to health and well-being. First, in the form of interpersonal violence and war, social conflict has direct impact on health and well-being. We live still in the shadow of the Holocaust, which saw the murder of 6 million Jews and probably an equal number of non-Jews in the German concentration camps. As I write this book, institutionalized murder in Rwanda and the former Yugoslavia has claimed millions of lives through starvation, slaughter, and forced migration, without any semblance of shelter or humanitarian respect for life. Although it is difficult to pinpoint accurately, as many as one in ten women in the United States is raped during her lifetime (Allison & Wrightsman, 1993). The prevalence of family violence is similarly difficult to estimate, as it occurs behind closed doors, but 10.7 percent of American parents admitted using "severe violent acts" against their children in one national survey (Straus & Gelles, 1986) and estimates of child abuse are estimated in the United States to be from 100,000 to 200,000 cases per year (Hayes & Emshoff, 1993).

Violence, however, is not the only means by which interpersonal conflict exacts its toll. On a less dramatic but more pervasive level, emotional conflict diminishes self-esteem and confidence, separates individuals from the very social ties that might protect them, and acts as a pathogenic agent. However, relationship research in the stress field emphasized the positive aspects of social attachments, and the negative influence of a lack of social attachments. Work by Rook (1984) was instrumental in reminding researchers and theorists that interpersonal relationships had simultaneous negative influences on health and well-being that operated through social conflict. Both sides of the coin are critical.

Culture, Malinowski (1944) wrote, provides a comprehensive range of answers as to how to address the demands that the world places upon us. On a psychological level, we learn these routines and incorporate them in our sense of self. On a structural level, institutions and laws are created that act as the mazes through which people are required to act. In societies, ancient and modern, these rules and paths are identified within religion, laws, traditions, and everyday cultural practices. However, whether we are speaking of modern, ancient, or future societies, cultural imperatives and interpersonal interaction within culturally prescribed norms are the structures that either enable health or create and exacerbate illness. What we need to explore is how the commerce of resource support, resource competition, and resource depletion processes operates between these structures.

THE COMMERCE OF RESOURCES ACROSS THE BORDERS THAT JOIN AND DIVIDE PEOPLE

In the prior chapter, I developed the concept of resource cycles and spirals. Implied in many of these cycles were the interpersonal processes and person-to-social-group processes that transfer, catalyze, actualize, impede, deny, or rob resources. Within the current *zeitgeist* of psychology and stress research, in particular, the emphasis is on self-reliance and self-efficacy (Bandura, 1997; Carver et al., 1989), and certainly individuals can do much to garner, develop, and advance their own resources. Nevertheless, as I have argued throughout this volume, many of the resources that we have at our disposal, however individually framed, are largely intertwined in complex social processes in terms of their development, possession, and implementation. What we must embark on at this point, then, is a disentanglement of these structures, mazes, and pathways across and through which resources are transferred, sometimes in aid of, and sometime injurious to, individuals-nested-in families-nested-in organization-nested-in villages and tribes.

Interestingly, the concept of stress and resource crossover was first proposed on an intraindividual level, as described by the concept of spillover. Spillover was defined as the process by which resources and demands spilled over from one aspect of the self to another. Discussed and researched widely in the literature on women's multiple roles, the idea was advanced that demands in one role, say, career, would spill over to other roles such as mother or homemaker, creating increased overall stress (Goode, 1974). In contrast, a spillover of resources was hypothesized by others, who argued that multiple roles exposed women to multiple opportunities to garner resources and that these resource gains would spill over across roles (Marks, 1977). Baruch and Barnett (1986) suggested that this process was more dependent on role quality within each role and that positive role quality led to resource enhancement, whereas negative role quality led to resource depreciation and increased stress. Thus, Stephens and Franks (1995) noted both positive and negative spillover among women who had primary caregiving responsibilities to an impaired parent, from their caregiver role to their parent and wife roles. These positive and negative spillover effects in turn had ameliorative and degenerative effects on psychological distress.

More recently, the spillover concept has been generalized to the process called crossover. Crossover, here, refers to the movement of demands and resources across borders between individuals (Westman & Etzion, 1995). The crossover of demands and resources raises a number of complex issues that may be key to understanding the interpersonal and person-nested-in family-nested-in social group nature of the stress process.

The simplest level of crossover is the dyadic process that transpires between two individuals, and I will begin with research that has addressed this level of analysis in couples. Although the diagrams and examples describe dyadic processes, many of the same principles can be applied to individual interactions with larger social units, such as the family, workplace, and tribe. These processes are schematically represented in Figure 8.1.

Hobfoll and London (1986) and Riley and Eckenrode (1986) suggested two processes that underlie stressful crossover. Hobfoll and London noted that many stressors made simultaneous demands on both individuals in the

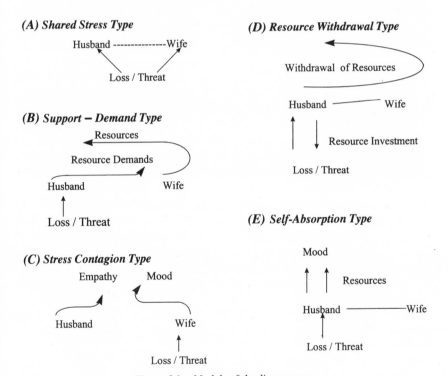

Figure 8.1. Models of dyadic crossover.

dyad and members of a larger group (e.g., family, co-workers; Figure 8.1a). Studying Israeli women whose male relatives and friends were recruited virtually overnight to serve in the Israel–Lebanon war, we noted that interpersonal transactions not surprisingly concentrated on the war and its real threat. This, in turn, led to a demand for resources from the stronger individuals, higher in mastery, to those lower in mastery through the process of social support, as illustrated in Figure 8.1b. This had two effects. Social support aided those lower in mastery, but depleted the resources of those higher in mastery (the wife in Figure 8.1b) at a time when they too needed all their stress resistance reserves. This intense sharing of multiple demands on all members of a common social grouping we called the *pressure cooker effect*, noting how effected individuals exacerbate their distress by their exposure to others of equal or worse need. Since no one in the system is free of threat, individuals who themselves have great need to depend on others must serve as supporters and lose precious resources that they themselves require at this time.

Riley and Eckenrode (1986), in their study of stress among inner-city women, also noted that the demand for resources caused a drain on others in the dyad or social group. They suggested that empathic processes, such that women felt "Your pain is my pain," further aggravated stress levels. They termed this process *stress contagion*, and it is depicted in Figure 8.1c. They underscore that two simultaneous processes need to be recognized here. First, there is the transaction of intimate support, whereby one individual or the social group share resources with those more needy. Second, those providing resources experience diminished resources both because they have shared their resources, and because they empathically experience the demands of the more needy individuals. With empathy acting as a conduit for stress, the greater their empathy, the more severe the stress contagion process.

In the occupational stress literature, still another stress crossover process is implied. This type of crossover is typically applied to the interactional style of men interfacing both work and home roles. The man, and increasingly true today for women, experiences demands or threats to his resources from work. In order to meet these resource demands, he withdraws resources that were reserved for the family (Figure 8.1d). This leaves his wife with an added burden, as she must meet family demands and her other demands. Hochschild (1989), in *Second Shift*, provides evidence that men are more likely to follow this script than women in dual career couples, placing much added burden on women in particular. This resource withdrawal includes time, energy, intimate support, and instrumental help with household labor and child care.

Finally, the need to meet internal demands that emerge from psychological distress may result in stress crossover, because resources that are intended for the dyad or family are dedicated to combat negative mood or physical dysfunction that emerges from stress. As illustrated in Figure 8.1e, when individuals are confronted with resource loss or threat of loss, they often experience psychological distress or physical health impairment. To counteract these threats to self, individuals must utilize their resources to reverse these negative spirals. Often, the resources that must be drawn upon had been banked for family or dyadic purposes. Individuals must apply their resources to limit the destructive sequelae that accompany depression, anxiety, exhaustion, and sickness. Hence, time, energy, self-esteem, and self-efficacy must be used to buttress the self, rather than for generative purposes. This again translates to a decreased availability of resources for the partner or family.

The complexity and richness of these crossover processes are exemplified in a study by Coyne and Smith (1991), who investigated the stress impact of myocardial infarction on men and their wives in a way that illuminates a number of the patterns that are outlined in Figure 8.1. They felt that dominant stress and coping models were narrowly focused on individual coping in isolation of others and that even social support research is generally reduced to mentalistic, cognitive models that dilute the complexity and real-world aspects of major stressful circumstances. Rather than seeing the heart attack as a stressor for the men alone, Coyne and Smith felt that "coping is best conceptualized as a thoroughly dyadic affair," where the "give and take, not just the perception of events" (pp. 404–405) determine how events unfold and reverberate in people's lives.

First, they found that husbands and wives were both at considerable risk for psychological distress 6 months postinfarct, indicating the direct effect of a shared stressor. Younger couples were also more distressed by the heart attack, and Coyne and Smith interpreted that this was a product of the greater degree of disturbance in resources that evolved from an early-life illness of this kind. It was further found that wives were less negatively affected if the couple's marital adjustment was better prior to the illness and suggested that positive relationship patterns limit stress crossover for both members of the couple. Most interestingly, patients' active communicating with their wives was related to wives' lower psychological distress, hinting at the beneficial effects of sharing resources. However, if patients tried to shelter their wives from their problems, women became more, not less, distressed. Particularly in marriages that had known more discord, this latter kind of coping acted to exacerbate stress's influence. Coyne and Smith speculated that for these troubled couples, what was superficially helpful may have had an underlying antagonistic message, "You are not able to help me."

COMPETITION FOR RESOURCES

The work of Coyne and Smith (1991) and Rook (1984) hints at a second set of processes that co-occur with the provision of social support and interactive coping. Specifically, as detailed in Chapter 3, shared systems also compete for resources. Resource competition can be antagonistic or cooperative and often are simultaneously cooperative and competitive. What is efficacious in reducing one's own distress or supporting one's own social role may be negatively related to what the relationship or partner needs at one point in time, and positively related to joint well-being at another time.

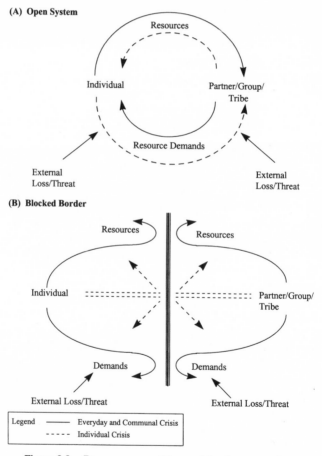

Figure 8.2. Resource competition and border transaction.

Individuals must not only protect themselves for selfish reasons, but also for their value to the family, social group, or tribe. Psychology has often imagined that resources are endless and that people should just cope in the most effective ways, but because resources are usually finite, their investment needs to be more carefully economized.

The system of competition and sharing of resources can be conceptualized in a way that aids understanding if we imagine that the borders between individuals and between individuals and social units, such as family or organization, may be more or less porous and may be unidirectional or bidirectional; that is, resources flow more easily across open borders, and borders may be more open or more blocked in one direction than another. These border diagrams are presented in Figure 8.2 and their significance is only beginning to be appreciated. The work of Duck (1990) is particularly

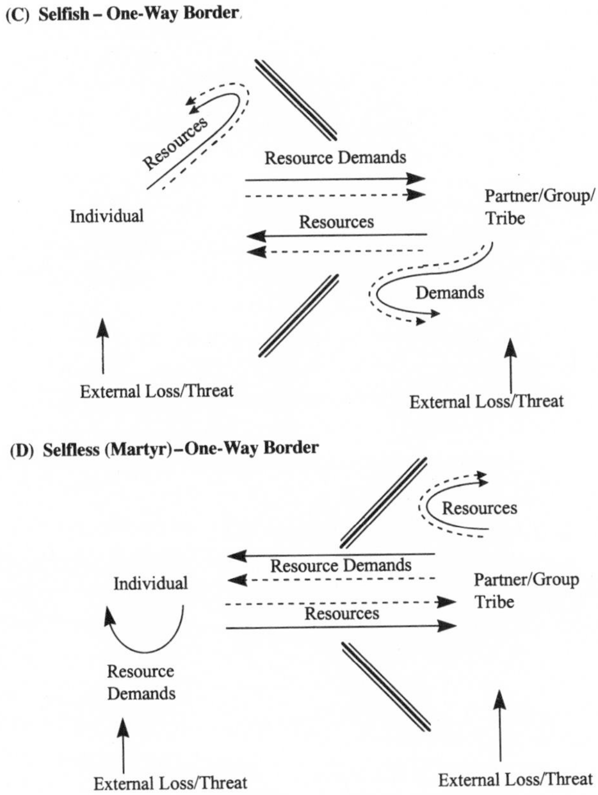

(C) Selfish – One-Way Border

Resources
Resource Demands
Individual
Resources
Partner/Group/Tribe
Demands
External Loss/Threat
External Loss/Threat

(D) Selfless (Martyr) – One-Way Border

Resources
Resource Demands
Individual
Resources
Partner/Group Tribe
Resource Demands
External Loss/Threat
External Loss/Threat

Figure 8.2. (*Continued*).

instructive on this point, as he emphasizes that social support should not be considered outside of the ecology of the relationship. Because stress research has tended to ignore relationship quality, there has been a tendency to decontextualize the transfer of resources between people as if it transpires under the same rules and regulations for all kinds of relationships (see also Pierce, Sarason, & Sarason, 1996).

The concept of borders is a particularly good metaphor here, because just as nations have rules, regulations, and histories that influence how they exact commerce across their borders, so do people in their various attachments. In fact, Argyle and Henderson (1984) demonstrated through rather creative investigations of social interactions that most social relationships are strictly governed by socially sanctioned patterns with little deviation. As outlined by COR theory, Argyle and Henderson find that these rules mainly address the exchange of rewards and intimate contact that is the give and take of material and social resources.

Coyne and Smith (1991) imply that the couple should be viewed as an open system, as denoted in Figure 8.2a. In an open system, demands on resources and offering of resources are conducted across a borderless space. External demands that act outside the system act equally on all members of the system. During everyday life, resources are both shared and built up for later need. During high-stress periods, exchange occurs actively, openly, and successfully, because a bank of resources has been created by positive social interaction prior to the hour of need. The open system is the least competitive for resources, as that which aids one member of the system aids all. However, the idealized nature of this state should be recognized. Further, even in this idealized system, it might benefit all members of the system to enrich the resources of some members more than others, if they were most needy at that time (the weakest members) or could support the neediness of others (the strongest members). Most social support research has assumed an open system, as if borders do not exist between members of the system, but this assumption is easily challenged in real-world relationships (Rook, 1984).

We can contrast the open system to one in which the border is fully blocked (see Figure 8.2b). In such a system, external demands act on each individual independently, and there is no rallying of resources across the blocked border. This model is reflected in insecure relationships that are isolationist and withdrawn (Roberts, Gotlib, & Kassel, 1996). Often, in such relationships, there is either a very poor relationship history, the presence of deep-seated psychological disturbance, or both. These circumstances differ significantly from instances where the individuals in the social system are not in some way tied to one another, so the blocked border should not be confused with the situation where no relationship exists (i.e., no common border). Because most cultures impart a sense and expectation of social obligations among members of social groupings (Argyle & Henderson, 1985), be they a couple, a family, or colleagues at work, there is resentment added to the prior history and an even further reduced chance of further helping in the future. Hence, because we expect not only help when we need it, but also to be asked for assistance when those with whom we have close relationships need it, a disturbance occurs when requests for help and the mobilization of resources do not transpire.

A selfish, one-way border is the next kind to consider. As illustrated in Figure 8.2c, in relationships described by the selfish, one-way border, demands can move in one direction only, and resources only in the opposite direction. In this manner, one individual (or one group) receives benefits from others, makes demands on others, but does not answer the demands of others or share his or her resources. The individual in such a system is exploitive of the group and is highly competitive in resource acquisition, fostering, and promotion. By almost exclusively studying social support on an individual basis, much of this research may inadvertently have been promoting the virtues of this exploitive kind of support seeking. Since virtually all social support studies only ask individuals what support they received, persons who report receiving much support are seen in isolation of the support they, in turn, may have provided (Vaux, 1988).

Hence, one may receive much support from others but be an albatross on those relationships (the helpless victim), or worse, may be actually seeking to drain the resources of others in order to gain some advantage (aggressive, antisocial). Those who are demanding in this way on their social attachments may be able to sustain relationships in a variety of ways. A woman may be "required" to have a husband or be dependent on his limited provision of material resources alone. Some relationships are sustained by violence, where mutual support provision would no longer sustain the tie. Many of these types of relationships are socially demanded, such that society does not provide for dissolution of the relationship once entered (e.g., parenthood, some work relationships, slavery, immigrant labor, etc.).

The next kind of border type is the selfless, one-way border. In such relationships, demands flow onto the individual, and the individual is responsible to provide resources, but he or she may not make demands for resources. In a way, this is simply the opposite border region of the selfish partner. However, what I imply here is that this kind of martyred sacrifice is voluntary in many cases. So, in the selfish, one-way border, the members opposite their selfish, demanding counterpart are forced to provide resources and cannot make demands. In contrast, the self*less*, one-way border is created by an individual (or social group) who sacrifices him- or herself and will not ask for help. Selfless persons choose both to answer the demands of others and make demands only on themselves. If support were offered them, they do not accept it. Women may be socialized to behave in this manner, especially in traditional cultures. In such cultures, women come to demand this of themselves as well, wishing always to be a helpmate, never a burden (Wethington, McLeod, & Kessler, 1987).

In our own research, we found the selfless profile actually to be quite common among men and women. Individuals would much prefer to offer support, then ask for it, and tend to feel uncomfortable seeking aid. Fisher et al., (1982) suggest that this may also stem from discomfort at showing vulnerability in need, as asking for help in many cultures implies weakness. This also may reflect a competitive ecology or culture, because in a more supportive system, a call for aid could be made comfortably with the expectation of help without any negative judgments. But again, this may be an ideal that is not attainable in either an individualistic society, because in it needing help from others denotes dependency, or in a communal society, where one is expected to give more than to receive.

Although I have outlined these borders as types, they actually represent continua. Few border are fully open, fully closed, or conduct the commerce in resource exchange unidirectionally. Moreover, relationships are typically compartmentalized as to task, such that a border may be open for exchange of instrumental help on tasks, one-way on emotional aid, and blocked fully on financial and material resources. This means that in many cases we should not speak of the relationship as having a type of border as much as the border being a concept that helps us understand the transport of different kinds of resources across it. Returning to the metaphor of the borders that separate nations, two nations may have different treaties as to the commerce of some goods and not others. Likewise, people have different understandings as to what is allowed to be transmitted between them.

Because most systems have multiple relationships, these kinds of borders also exist in different combinations for different members of the system. Priests seldom confess to their parishioners. Romantic relationships are allowed to transport resources that are contraband in other relationships. Parents may share some emotional material with their children, but other areas would be unhealthy to share and would burden a child. Hence, as we consider relations within a family, between families that are related, and between such social units as families and the workplace, there must be understood to be a complex system of connections. These connections allow different resources to be requested and offered, depending on the type of relationship, their relational history, and the cultural traditions that govern acceptable interactions at different levels (Argyle & Henderson, 1985).

Moreover, the transport of resources across borders often diminishes under conditions of sustained stress as resource pools are depleted. Even significant others may withdraw support as they themselves become emotionally drained or must gear their resources toward other directions after time. Bolger, Vinokur, Foster, and Ng (1996) found, for example, that significant others provided support to women with breast cancer in response to their physical impairment, but withdrew support in response to women's ongoing emotional distress. These processes, then, are dynamic and change over time and conditions.

What is critical also to remember is that borders are unequal in their sharing, distribution, and transfer of resources. The open system that psychology often suggests is more accurately a complex system that differentially favors some members of the social group over others. From the outset, the position of resources is in part a function of social position and social status (Aneshensel, 1992; Ross & Mirowsky, 1989). This means that resource depletion will be faster for some than others, expectations of replenishment more realistic for some members than others, and that which appears positive for one member of the group may come at a heavy price to other members (Kessler, McLeod, & Wethington, 1985).

UNDERMINING: DIRECT CHALLENGE TO RESOURCE EXCHANGE

In stress crossover, I examined how stress may impact members of a shared social group, be they family, coworkers, or community residents. In discussing borders, I outlined how resources may cross or fail to cross interpersonal bridges that people share. Undermining is still another key facet of resource exchange. Undermining does not merely designate the absence of or withdrawal of resources. Undermining can be defined as "behaviors directed toward [a person] ... that display (a) negative affect (anger, dislike); (b) negative evaluation of the person in terms of his or her attributes, actions, and efforts (criticism); and (c) behaviors that hinder the attainment of instrumental goals" (Vinokur, Price, & Caplan, 1996, p. 167). In these ways, undermining can be construed as actions that directly or indirectly diminish the value of resources, create obstacles for resource investment, or create further stress that requires the investment of resources for managing relationship problems rather than other external threats. If there are mazes and pathways for investing resources toward goal attainment, undermining acts to divert those resources, mine the bridges, and blockade the pathways that might otherwise lead to problem resolution or stress resistance. As I have throughout this chapter, I would underscore that undermining may also occur between larger social groups, such as family and workplace.

Individuals and social groups, according to COR theory, act to mobilize their resources to combat or prevent loss or, in some circumstances, to embark on gain. If I am correct in arguing, as I have throughout this volume, that most individuals and social systems are doing what they can just to keep up with ongoing resource demands and are usually stretched in times of crisis, then imagine the toll taken by undermining. Just at the time that resources are being instituted and plans made, likely under crisis conditions, people's energy, emotions, and attention are sabotaged from their purpose and subverted to deal with undermining by members of their social network. If this were emanating from people's sworn enemies, then so be it, but more typically, the undermining that has been studied and that plagues us is proffered by the very individuals and social groups that we had expected to rely on for support. Indeed, a large portion of stress crossover is a by-product of undermining itself (Westman & Vinokur, 1995). Moreover, stressful circumstances, by impinging on the members of a family, couple, or workplace as a group, may elicit undermining as one unfortunate spin-off of the stress process.

Bolger, DeLongis, Kessler, and Wethington (1990), in a very careful microanalysis of how stressful events unfold and impinge on interpersonal processes, found that interpersonal conflicts are the fuel that fires daily stress. Major stressors, in this way, often lead to microstressors in the form of conflict among the individuals people need for succor. They found that 80 percent of the variability in people's daily mood was an outgrowth of negative conflict. This may help explain why microstressors or hassles can be so stressful. If they become the means by which major stressful events are interpreted within the family, in the form of everyday multiple, minor irritations and flare-ups, they would negatively color life as a reflection of the greater stress events unfolding. Social undermining increases depression (Coyne & Downey, 1991; Krause, Liang, & Yatomi, 1989), and depression, in turn, tends to foster an environment characterized by social undermining (Nelson & Beach, 1990; Gotlib & Whiffen, 1989). In this way, those with fewer resources, or those more drained of resources by ongoing stress, are more vulnerable, as not only external events contribute to undermining, but they do so more intensively and more likely in relationships where one or more members are in a weakened resource state.

A number of possible combinations of social support and social undermining can coexist, and low social support does not necessarily indicate high undermining and vice versa (Vinokur et al., 1996; Vinokur & van Ryn, 1993). As an ideal, a relationship between individuals, between individuals and social groups (e.g., family, workplace) and between social groups (e.g., family to family, or family to work) would be denoted by the presence of high social support and low undermining (Vinokur & van Ryn, 1993). In such relationships, social support exists at a maximum and undermining at a minimum. Abusive relationships, in contrast, would combine low levels of social support and high levels of social undermining (Vinokur & van Ryn, 1993). These relationships are particularly destructive and would be likely to end in dissolution if they are not kept intact by some other powerful force, such as severe psychopathology or external pressures.

Clinically, I have witnessed many relationships that are sustained by a seductive combination of high social support and high undermining. Such relationships can be mystifying, as one aspect of the relationship camouflages the other. When confronted, the spouses who are sending both these contradictory messages appeal with the many examples of their good will, love, and nurturance. The transfer of resources through the support process disguises the undermining of resources that co-occurs. The high support–high undermining relationship may be sustained by the need for the support that is provided, by the difficulty in clearly identifying the undermining, and by social sanctions on dissolving many relationships (e.g., marriage) if there is a modicum of good. For example, friends and family may point to the good things the spouse is providing and overlook or be unaware of the undermining. Gotlib and Whiffen (1989) suggest that the undermining may be subtle, and, although partly observable, parts may only be interpretable from inside the relationship or by those who intimately know the relational history.

Still other relationships are best described as low on both social support and social undermining. These relationships might be described as apathetic or neglectful relationships. The individuals exist in a cold peace, offering each other little in terms of interactions that are other than lukewarm. Such relationships, however, may also exist as outgrowths of chronic or severe crisis, where members of the social group's resources have been exhausted (Ensel and Lin, 1991). At this state, they have nothing more to give and must rely on the earlier period of hopefully positive resource interaction to sustain the relationship through this period (Kaniasty & Norris, 1993; Norris & Kaniasty, 1996).

In one of the most well-designed studies of this type to date, Vinokur et al. (1996) followed a large sample of unemployed job seekers and their spouses or partners over a six-month period. This investigation is particularly valuable in the way it illuminated the dynamic rather than static nature of these processes. They noted that with the ongoing strain of unemployment, depressive symptoms increased in both partners. As depressive symptoms increased, partners tended to both withdraw support and increase their undermining. With reduced support and increased undermining, in turn, depression and relationship discord further increased. This process clearly supports COR theory's supposition that stress causes cycles of resource loss. Moreover, Vinokur et al. noted that those who had greater initial financial resources were better able to withstand the potential threat of unemployment on depression, supporting another important stanchion of COR theory, that the presence of resource reserves forestalls loss cycles.

Vinokur and his colleagues also highlight the cultural theme that is suggested by the COR principle that threats occur to individuals that occupy a certain culture at a certain historical moment (see Chapters 2–4, this volume, and Baltes, 1987). Comparing rural to urban settings, Vinokur et al. (1996) theorized that threats to resources are more impactful in domains that are identified by the culture with that gender. Hence, in cultures where men hold the primary breadwinner role and women are more centrally identified within the family support and leadership role, economic downturns threaten men more than women (see Conger, Lorenz, Elder, Simons, & Ge, 1993). Vinokur et al. interpreted their lack of gender differences in economic impact to recent changes in women's roles, especially in urban settings (cf. Barnet, Marshall, Raudenbush, & Brennan, 1993), such that men and women are more equally responsible for and committed to work, employment, and financial domains.

RESOURCE QUALITY AND INTERPRETATION

The preceding discussion implies that the resources and stressors that are experienced are somehow uniform. In fact, resources differ in quality, but research to date has barely begun to consider this important factor. For example, virtually all research on social support examines amount of support. Hence, they look at amount of emotional support, amount of advice, or amount of help on instrumental tasks. How good that support was, that is, its quality, is only recently being considered (Pierce et al., 1996). Pierce et al. make the important point that we have probably indirectly assessed support quality, but have mainly examined the amount of resources that are offered and received, not whether they were the right ones or good ones. Likewise, individuals might share their self-efficacy, in order to tackle a joint problem. Research has considered how much self-efficacy persons think they have, but not the quality of that strength. A false bravado would be unlikely to have the influence that a deeply-seated sense of self-worth and competence, backed by actual competence, would have.

In our research on kibbutz couples, we examined social support quality by a number of means (Johnson, Hobfoll, & Zalcberg-Linetzy, 1993). In order to test the cross-cultural strength of our ideas, we looked at support transactions on two kibbutzim, where about half the members were Israeli born and about half were born in Europe and South America. First, we developed a test of social support knowledge, knowledge being one measure of quality. Those who knew more about social support would at least have a head start on how to offer support when it was required. Second, we had spouses report on each other's support behavior using careful descriptions of helpful and unhelpful kinds of interactions as assessed by external judges familiar with the area of social support. For example, spouses rated the extent to which their partner "Listens when they have something to say," "Asks questions that do not close the discussion or the expression of emotion," and "Encourages you to express emotions, even painful feelings" (positive support) versus "Gives a philosophical reason for the situation," "Reverses the conversation to talk about him- or herself," or "Tells you to simply get over what has happened" (negative support). By tapping both interactions that are typically positively received and those that are typically negatively received, we again were able to assess an aspect of support quality (see Wortman & Lehman, 1985).

We then examined the question of whether those with greater support knowledge and who supported their spouse with better quality support behavior had more intimate relationships and whether their support was received by their partner with greater satisfaction. This model tests the theoretical treatise of Reis and Shaver (1988), which proposed that the commerce of quality social support was an important underpinning of sense of intimacy in relationships. Our findings were quite clear. Those who were more knowledgeable about support were viewed by their spouses as offering better quality support during stressful circumstances. Moreover, both support knowledge and support behavior contributed significantly to greater relationship intimacy for men and women. Those who offered support of poor quality reduced the intimacy felt by their partner. Support satisfaction, in turn, was to a great extent a by-product of that intimacy. Hence, we can see how the quality, not amount, of support that is transferred during stressful periods is the critical variable. The commerce of poor-quality goods and supplies has little value.

It is also necessary to remember that the commerce of social support transpires within a framework that is screened by perceptions (Lazarus & Folkman, 1984). Perceptions, if I am not overstretching the border metaphor, are the customs agents that decide the value of commodities crossing the border. Kelley (1979) suggests that these perceptions of interpersonal transactions are influenced by relationship history, setting factors, and individual biases and motivations. If individuals do not wish to have a close relationship with another, they will be prone to ignore or discredit the resources they receive.

In a recent study, we found that when men underestimated the stress in their partners' lives, women's stress reactions were much more severe (Chapman et al., 1997). It would be easy to interpret the differences between partners' views of stress as an outgrowth of differential perception of the proverbial parts of the elephant, and this is how individual differences in appraisals are usually explained. However, it is more difficult to explain why men were underestimating the stress that was going on for the women. It is possible that men were seeing the stress, but ignoring it. It is possible that the stress was experienced by the women outside of the men's purview and that women had not communicated their concerns. It is possible that women communicated their concerns, but were not heard because either they or their partners are poor tellers or listeners, respectively. We still know very little about how resources and stress are shared between people and why and where the potentially open system breaks down or is interrupted.

If people desire a close relationship, they will be prone to positively evaluate help and to interpret it in the best possible light (Clark, 1983). Hence, support may receive a booster effect when there is the hope of a sustained close tie, and undermining may be ignored to the extent possible, so that the relationship can proceed on course. Those who are particularly neurotic may be less capable of correctly interpreting interpersonal interactions, but even here, there is reason to believe that they may be causing poor interactions more than they are misinterpreting truly positive interactions as negative (Coyne, 1976). Nevertheless, because we often are not privy to people's relational history, their perceptions will provide insights both as to the actual nature of their interactions and their interpretative biases.

ECOLOGY, CLIMATE, AND CULTURE OF RESOURCE INTERACTIONS

Community Principles and Ecological Notions

I have been traversing between individual–interpersonal and systems levels of interactions. James Kelly (1966), in thinking about the commerce of resources on a more systems level, speaks of four ecological principles that are helpful in understanding how we might bridge from an individual to a more systems' level of analysis and understanding of the processes of crossover of stress and resources. His insights, I believe, hold equally for micro- (e.g., couple, family) and mesolevel social systems (e.g., workplace, village) and may help the reader understand the ecological nature or backdrop rules that govern resource transactions.

First, he suggests that members of a social system should always be viewed as *interdependent*. Changes at any point in the system alter the entire system in some fashion. This concept reminds us that it is dangerous to break apart the system into its component parts, because in so doing, we lose the meaning of resource transactions. When a resource loss occurs at one level of the system or to one individual, it in some way involves all other parts of the system. When multiple players in the system gain resources, it is likely to reverberate broadly along all connections. When a woman gains employment with greatly increased salary and responsibility, this will exact a multitude of changes throughout the ecosystems of both family and workplace.

Kelly's (1966) second principle is that systems naturally *cycle* resources. This means that as long as a resource remains in the system, it is often reused at different levels. Hence, when resources are transferred, they may very well not be lost to those who gave them up, but instead may be again available to them later, if perhaps in a different form. Many resources may in fact be shared and used by more than one party simultaneously, and even be fostered and advanced in the process. Many abstract resources that embody close relationships, such as love, caring, and trust, can only truly be enlarged if shared. On the other hand, this also means that when resources are lost, the stress will deplete the resource reserves that might have been called on later in resource cycling. Hence, if the Hispanic community of a city loses its leadership because educated members move from the *bario*, these resources are lost to the potential future cycles that might need to call on those strengths.

Kelly's third principle is *adaptation*; that is, people are not entirely free to act. Traditions, rules, and relationship histories constrain some behaviors and facilitate others. Moreover, as resources are made available to the social system or taken away, the system adapts, offering new opportunities through the creation of new niches and making new constaints through the loss or significant alteration of other niches. Hence, a community might think it cannot survive without electricity and water, but may learn to do so quite well during times of disaster. Human systems are adaptive systems. In the Spielberg movie *Schindler's List*, a wealthy family that has lost its home huddles in a single room in the new ghetto created by the occupying Nazis. The husband asks how things could possibly be worse, when in walks two or three more families to now share the single room. And yet, the ghetto adapted with orchestras, theater, and schools for children. The greatly reduced level of resources was met quickly, even if painfully, with rapid adaptation to new resource cycles and commerce. The resource exchange patterns adapted to the resources and constraints available in the new, revised circumstances of the ecology.

Kelly's last principle is *succession*. Environments are constantly changing, because systems lie within systems and have a natural progression through maturation and outside influences of history. For example, immigrant groups in Chicago at the turn of the century were at first at the bottom of the economic and social ladder. Over time, two things transpired. One, the immigrant group acclimated by learning new skills in terms of language, work, and cultural fluency. Second, history evolved such that new immigrant groups would enter, making the prior immigrant group the veterans of the system and tending to push it up the social ladder economically and educationally (Park et al., 1926). Urban dwellings that were in poor repair have been revitalized by the gentrification of many American cities during the past 20 years. This makes new housing available for middle- and upper-middle classes and revitalizes cities, greatly broadening their economic base and attracting new business and taxes. At the same time, it limits the inexpensive housing available for the urban poor and may increase homelessness. This transfer of resources is constant and influenced by many factors, most of which are beyond the scope of this volume. However, we must recognize that these successions occur, and, as they do, the ecological landscape is transformed and reshaped (Trickett, 1995).

Resource commerce takes place through a combination, then, of the influences of interdependence, resource cycling, adaptation, and succession. Many of these systems are too complex to predict precisely. But by acknowledging this level of systems movement, we are able to outline various configurations and background characteristics that meaningfully impact the stress process. The changes are multidetermined enough to be chaotic, but at any given point, they can be identified, described, and understood (Bronfenbrenner, 1977). This is illustrated, for example, in the work of Siegrist (1996), who illustrates that resource investment of workers becomes increasingly stressful when their workplace does not provide rewards consummate with their resource investment. This imbalance translates over time to heart disease, and can be expected to lead on another level to increased labor unrest and alienation from work. We can also, as the work of Siegrist shows, probably project forward to the next few iterations of the cycle, but not further. Systems level changes on the global economic level translate to investment–reward imbalance on the individual level, and an unhealthy workforce, in turn, at the level of production. This, then, cycles to potential labor unrest, demands for higher pay, inflation, and further tightening of the job market. As Kelly reminds us, for long-term changes, we need mainly just be aware that unanticipated spinoffs will occur and be cognizant of their inevitability when trying to understand the process of resource loss and gain and whenever we move to intervene to help others or influence systems.

Communal versus Exchange Principles and Crossover: The Influence of the Culture and Climate of Relationships on Resource Commerce

I have been discussing borders and commerce of resources between people as if one culture or climate exists. In this way, I have been speaking as if there is no background set of traditions and rules that influences these processes, and that they are only dictated by the nature of the relationships (i.e., the structures) between persons and social groups. I would suggest that such an assumption is grossly inaccurate. The culture of a society and the climate (the small culture of traditions within social settings) have an enormous impact on how we see calls for assistance, the offering of assistance, and the commerce of resources (Argyle & Henderson, 1984, 1985; Bronfenbrenner, 1977). Luckily, there is already excellent theoretical work that has been done that can aid the translation of greater sociocultural processes to exchange transactions between individuals and between groups that are nested within cultures. For this, I look next to tie the work of Kelley (1979) and Clark and Mills (1979) on exchange versus communal relationships to the greater cultural models of individualistic versus communal cultures. In so doing, I hope to illustrate that the continuum from exchange to communal relationships is not only a product of relationships as these authors presented, but also can be applied to greater cultural traditions.

I offer an anecdote to introduce this critical point and perhaps underscore the entire cultural theme of this book. As a young man, I lived for a period on an Israeli kibbutz. Kibbutz Sarid was a member of the left-wing kibbutz movement, and at the time, socialist ideals were strongly held by its members. I was assigned to the dairy, the kibbutz's most profitable wing, and one that demanded intensive labor, and hence, where young men and women who were willing to work hard chose to be placed and where I was unwittingly assigned. As a volunteer, not a member, I was on the lowest rung of the kibbutz hierarchy, and being from Chicago, I knew nothing about farm work. The manager of the dairy was a young man named Yehuda, only 4 years my senior. Yehuda was the first on the scene in the morning and labored tirelessly. When he finished his long day, he would come find me, usually assigned to some physically demanding task at which I was usually behind. At first, I would have fully expected him to admonish me or, at best, point out how I could do better. Instead, he would grab a pitchfork, or jump up on the back of my tractor and simply take the lead. He would pitch more silage and load more feed than I and only occasionally suggest I watch how to do some task better. He would lead by example, occasionally talk about his American girlfriend, Lorel, and always stay until the task was complete. At times, when there was more work for the two of us, others from the dairy would find us and lend a hand. There was never an admonishment, even when I had made a mistake that added extra hours. Cheerful, positive, they would never go to lunch (after having worked 8 hours already) or finish the day without me.

The kibbutz rules of help and relationships are built on a culture of unit and communal ties. There was an expectation in the dairy that I work hard, and seeing that I worked hard, even if inadequately, they were there to work with me. I intentionally should avoid the word *help*, because that implies they were doing it for me. They were pitching in for the fact that it was our joint obligation and as a weak link in the chain, I needed support. As I grew stronger and more capable, I learned never to leave my job when my own task was done, but when our joint work was completed. Yehuda Rosenfeld, a war hero in the 1967 Six Day War at the age of 20, fell in the Yom Kippur war in a tank battle somewhere in the Sinai engagement. He epitomized the kibbutz spirit that was adopted as a model by the Israeli army, "After me, with me, by my example."

Exchange Codes within Cultures

How individuals and groups respond to calls for help, and if they call for help, is dictated by the ecology of exchange principles on the kibbutz as elsewhere. These rules are known by individuals through social scripts that are learned by watching others, and in the lifetime of learning that occurs through being a member of a family, village, and culture (Cantor, 1990; Markus & Nurius, 1986). On a broad level, they are depicted by the background cultural pathways that govern resource transactions as exemplified at their extremes by two models: (1) individualistic exchange codes versus (2) the more communal sharing principles of collectivist climates and cultures (Triandis, 1994).

Individualistic exchange codes and climate are exemplified in the work of Harold Kelley (1979) and Kelley and Thibaut (1978). In this model, relationships are defined by patterns of reciprocity. Kelley describes two essential types of reciprocity. The first is positive reciprocity, where people give in order to take later, and take with the expectation that they will later be expected to give. The second, competitive interaction type is the eye for an eye. Here, one undermines with the expectation that there will be probable retribution and avoids undermining in order to avoid such retribution.

The accounting in this system, although later revised by Kelley, was originally described in a very much tit-for-tat manner. People, according to this system, keep a careful accounting of the resources and actions that transpire in the relationship. There may be some banking of resources, such that reciprocity does not require immediate reaction, but Kelley largely described a system wherein fairly close tabs were kept on the account books. These accounts could be calculated in a number of manners. For example, the matching of a dyad's behavior could be considered to the extent to which partners match the specific behavior of their spouses. Hence, we would expect a jibe to be matched by a jibe, and help at a task to be matched by help at a task. Alternatively, reciprocity could be viewed on the basis that one partner's behavior will increase the likelihood of subsequent behaviors of similar kind in the second partner. Gottman (1979) found, for example, that spouses from clinical mental health samples and nonclinical samples both tended to reciprocate negative interactions, but that spouses from clinic samples were more likely to reciprocate negative affect. This further suggests that there is a spiraling of interactions, such that reciprocity is cast in the shadow of past interactions.

Kelley emphasizes that relationships are governed by rules, and this is true of relationships in all cultures. But he assumed that reciprocal interaction was the basic rule upon which other rules (i.e., how much reciprocity is normal or expected) were based. Kelley's thinking accurately describes many informal relationships or ones that are not close, but he also meant his theory to apply to close personal ties. The application to closer or more formalized relationships may depend more than Kelley suggested on dominant cultural and subcultural patterns. Kelley may also have been describing a particular cultural pattern at a particular historical time: Northern European and North American, rather than more Mediterranean, Latin, African American, or Eastern.

As discussed many years earlier by Max Weber (1946, 1978), Northern European and American models of individualism demand a more rule-based ecology, in which the give and take of transactions is suspect. This stems, quite clearly, from individualistic competition for resources, such that survival of the fittest means that some will survive and others will not. If individuals let others gain an advantage on them, then they are likely not to thrive. Hence, individuals and groups must conform to a rather immediate, piecemeal accounting of resource give and take.

Margaret Clark (1983) and Clark and Mills (1979) depicted the kinds of relationships that Kelley outlined as *exchange relationships* and contrasted these to what she called *communal relationships*. She was speaking of relationships, and not communal cultures, and there are both similarities and differences in the concepts on the interpersonal and cultural plane.

> In communal relationships, members have a specific obligation to be responsive to one another's needs, whereas in exchange relationships they do not.... In communal relationships a norm exists to give benefits when the other has a need for them. Benefits are also appropriately given when something can be provided that would be particularly pleasing to the other.... People with whom we have communal relationships expect such benefits ... [but the] general obligation that members of communal relationships have to benefit one another when needs arise is not altered by receipt of a specific benefit.... When one member of a communal relationship provides another with aid, the two people's obligations to be responsive to one another's needs are not altered.
>
> In exchange relationships, benefits are given when one person owes the other for a benefit received from that other in the past, or they are given with the expectation of receiving a benefit of comparable value in return. In other words, recipients of benefits

expect to repay the other for a specific benefit, and know that the other expects to be repaid as well. (Clark, 1983, pp. 283–284)

Clark suggests that relationships become communal when those involved see themselves as a unit. Because they are part of a collective, the notion of self loses dominance. Instead, benefits that are derived and resources that are lost are experienced equally by all members of the collective. On the kibbutz collective, this is formalized in that everyone receives the same benefits, and even those members who work outside the kibbutz contribute their paycheck directly to the kibbutz, whether they work as physician, professor, or building contractor. Likewise, many families place all funds in a common pool and seek to share the families' resources with members on the basis of need.

Clark makes an additional point that is critical to understanding the nature of communal ties. In communal ties, the benefits and losses are perceived by the group as defining of the relationship; that is, a close friendship is defined by mutual helping and sharing. In families, likewise, the helping, sharing, and commonly experienced consequences are what defines the concept of family for members. In extended families, common historically among African Americans, many "aunts" and "uncles" were counted as family, even if not related by blood. What made them extended family was their contribution to the family unit, often caring for children, helping in work, and lending support in times of sorrow (Dressler, 1985). Similarly, a kibbutz is defined as a setting in which resources are shared and needs met by common benefit to the group.

In exchange relationships, the relationship will be ongoing to the extent that the rules of exchange are met. In communal relationships, direct exchange may actually undermine the communal nature of the tie. Parties of the collective believe that this careful accounting specifically does not occur, and their safety lies in this belief. If it was the case instead that they must be repaid in any immediate and direct way for providing resources to another, then they would have to expect the same when the tables were turned. This means that if they were unable at times to repay a debt, then the relationship would be quickly jeopardized. In times of sickness, unemployment, disaster, or some victimization, individuals may be debilitated for prolonged periods. Exchange relationships would be expected to evaporate due to the inability to provide *quid pro quo*, but communal ties should be sustainable over long periods.

Exchange Patterns and Resource Transactions

Applying these two relationship constructs to these detailed patterns of crossover, borders, and undermining, it can be seen that the commerce of resources will depend on whether the relationships are exchange or communal in nature. Exchange ties will be more competitive, less likely to sustain aid, more short term if resource exchange is not reciprocal, and less given to trust. Communal ties, in contrast, are likely to work more toward mutual benefit, to sustain unequal benefit for prolonged periods, to be more long term, and may be quite unbalanced in terms of reciprocity.

However, just being a close relationship does not make the relationship communal. Nor does social distance necessarily mean that exchange principles will guide relational transactions. This will depend on relationship history, the social climate of the setting, and sociocultural traditions of the broader society. In the kibbutz, even distant relationships are communal in nature. Unity includes all members of the kibbutz. Old-timers may have not said hello for 50 years, because such greetings were seen as bourgeois, despite passing one another daily. However, they remain tied to work for their collective benefit. Couples married 50 years may interact daily, but work to undermine each other the moment an imbalance in mutual benefits occurs. Hence, the exchange and communal nature of that particular relationship and the ecology in which that relationship exists must both be considered. The rules of resource commerce will vary meaningfully in reflection of these differences.

> The likeness of those who expend their wealth in the way of God is as the likeness of a grain of corn that sprouts seven ears, in every ear a hundred grains. So God multiplies unto whom He will; God is All-embracing, All-knowing. Those who expend their wealth in the way of God then follow not up what they have expended with reproach and injury, their wage is with their Lord, and no fear shall be on them, neither shall they sorrow.
> (*The Koran*, II, The Cow)

CONCLUSIONS

Throughout this chapter, I have concentrated on the relational space between people. Although many of the examples concern individual interactions, the same general principles apply for individual to group and group to group interactions. Integrating this chapter with the prior one on resource spirals, it is clear that when communities respond to disasters, or when business drains people's resources, stress and resource transfers occur along similar lines. Indeed, as I have considered these resource transactions, I have grown increasingly comfortable with seeing people's behavior in groups as tribal in nature. What I mean by that is that people seek these affiliations, want strongly to identify with them, and take cues from those in their group as to how they should behave. I think these patterns form what we might call tribal behaviors. Thus, from the individual to the village level, the reason that a similar set of principles may hold is that we look to the tribe to learn how to behave and carry these traditions, routes, and mazes to our interpersonal interaction. It is not the tribe that reflects the family, but the family that translates communal values and practices to the individual.

Finally, I am aware that the use of terms such as *commerce, borders, goods,* and *supplies* may appear too materialistic and mechanistic. It might pertain to the transfer of monies or materials between people or help with instrumental tasks, but does it relate to love and caring? Obviously, I believe that it does. Even when moving from exchange to the close, loving relationships to which Clark refers, the principles of commerce in the way I have been using them seem to apply. When Coyne and Smith (1991) examined the caring and support that transpires between spouses following a heart attack, they were referring to an experience that for many is the darkest hour of their lives. Although research is always in danger of making the meaningful into something so abstract that it appears meaningless, I hope that through my choosing examples of real threats occurring to people in all kinds of settings, from all kinds of backgrounds, this makes for a good test of the transportability of these concepts to real-world concerns.

I would also turn to a very informal kind of study that I have conducted over the years. Readers can also judge by their own standards, especially non-English speakers. When I meet people from different cultures, who speak different languages, I ask them two questions. What is the language used in your culture to explain why and when close, loving relationships go well? What is the language used in your culture to explain why and when close, loving relationships dissolve? I have done this in over 30 languages, and the answer has uniformly been the same. Relationships that thrive do so because people "*give* it their all," "*invest* in their relationship," "are there for the other person in times of need." Relationships do poorly when "people *withdraw* from the other," "*spend* their time elsewhere," "*dedicate* themselves to work," and other similar statements. People talk about "*giving* the best years of their lives," "*giving* their all," "all that was mine was his," and "I *gave,* and *gave,* and *gave,* but never got back." In Turkish, when a woman does not receive positive regard for her efforts she says, "And I swept their floor with my hair," and in Arabic, when a relationship does not give back despite resource investment, people say, "I gave him/her my skin." In each of these cases, people are expecting a return on their investment, even if they will wait until their beauty (metaphorically hair) is gone and their skin is flayed. This spontaneous language of love speaks in similar ways to the commerce of support that this chapter and this volume has presented.

On the other hand, I would not use the same language I use in the volume when working with patients or couples in therapy. What serves an academic and philosophical level of understanding must be put in lay terms to be appreciated in clinical work. When my wife and I translated COR theory to a self-help book for dual-career couples, we were able to find lay terms for all these concepts, I think, precisely because people quickly resonate to the resource analogies, because they reflect how they have often thought and felt (Hobfoll & Hobfoll, 1994). In the next and last chapter, I present clinical principles that follow from COR theory. I address issues of prevention and intervention, and do so on individual, family, organizational, and community levels. If COR theory and the individual-nested-in family-nested-in neighborhood or tribe framework is robust, it should not only translate to a better understanding of stress and stress resistance, but also be helpful for stress interventions in real-world settings and for real-world problems.

NOTES

1. More accurately, psychiatry was medicalized at this juncture, but with little data to support this period of biologicalization of mental illness and even less in the way of cures. For over 100 years, patients were again mostly warehoused and often subjected to many of the same horrors about which Tuke and Pinel wrote. It would wait until the 1960s, when humanistic psychology, the advent of psychotropic drugs, and the expense of the megainstitutions on the state combined to return to the practices advanced by Tuke and Pinel, and then more often leading to mere revolving-door therapy as chronic patients were shuffled in and out of hospitals and many more were released to homelessness and nursing home care (Shadish, 1984).

2. Although I could cite Caplan and Antonovsky as providing insights and research that supports COR theory, this would be deceptive scholarship. Their work supports COR theory because COR theory emerged quite directly from their work. Although I had not realized it at the time, my work under Antonovsky's tutelage at Ben Gurion University in Beersheva, Israel, and in frequent discussions at Hadassah Hospital in Jerusalem with Caplan in the early years of my career, acted to shape my thinking and the formulation of the theory that this book attempts to illuminate.

9

Aiding Resource Acquisition and Protection in Ecological Context

I have focused throughout this volume on the natural processes by which resources are obtained, retained, protected, and fostered in order to preserve the individual-nested-in family-nested-in tribe. When this process is threatened or interrupted, stress ensues. Not only do individuals seek to safeguard resources and the rituals, traditions, and paths meant to foster resources as individuals-nested-in families, nested-in tribe, but they create their families, institutions, and societies for this purpose. Because of the fragility of many of these systems, and of the human body itself, people are also biologically, socially, and psychologically loss sensitive. A gain may be postponed, but a loss of resources or circumstances that makes individuals vulnerable to loss cues an immediate vigilance and reaction to circumvent that loss or minimize its impact and aftermath (see Chapters 2 and 3).

In this final chapter, I address how Conservation of Resources (COR) theory and a resource perspective in general can guide intervention. Because resources are products of individuals' interactions with social systems, any comprehensive intervention strategy must include individual, family, organizational, and social policy levels. This will take us far from the intervention offered through traditional avenues in schools, clinics, and workplaces. Indeed, I argue that if we continue to individualize the intervention process, we do little more than repair the wounded for rewounding and worse. Rather, a resource perspective is guided by an alternative blueprint. Individuals do not so much need to change their mind or biology as to alter their acquisition of resources and ability to use their resources (Baltes, 1987; Iscoe, 1974). They and we must endeavor to reshape their social ecologies to foster their resource acquisition and retention (see Albee, 1980; Antonovsky, 1979; Baltes, 1987; Brandstädter & Wentura, 1995; Bronfenbrenner, 1977). As many systems are shaped in ways that either unintentionally or intentionally diminish, deplete, and reject people's resources, changing individuals alone will serve to mystify them into believing that their failure is indeed their own (Laing, 1969).

This resource perspective does not reject individual interventions, as they are necessary and often effective paths. My thesis here is that if they are all that is in interventionists' armamentaria, intervention will often fail and continue to be part of the problem. Moreover, there are, of course, some percentage of mental health professionals who already adopt a resource-in-systems perspective and visit their patients' and clients' schools and workplaces and endeavor to alter these settings, aid their entering schools and training programs, help them seek shelter and employment, and intervene on their behalf in the courts. But mental health professionals are seldom taught these skills building, environment shaping strategies or techniques in their training programs, and they will generally not find them in the mainstream literature of their professions. They acquire these skills and perspectives, if at all, because of the limitations they experience when they intervene by traditional means alone. And again, they need not abandon their traditional methods and models, but they must radically alter them by entwining them with amore resource-attentive, adaptation-based strategies.[1]

CULTURE AND INTERVENTION

Culture and Individual Intervention

The individualistic, mentalistic focus of psychology and psychiatry offers one possible model of health and wellness. Its principal advantages are the identification of individual needs, establishment of the biological correlates of psychopathology, and an understanding of the complexity of individual differences. It might be helpful at this juncture to step back and analyze the individualistic model of psychology and psychiatry in terms of its possible cultural origins as well. As I have argued earlier (see Chapters 1–3), the psychology of the individual grew out of a historical period in which society was experienced as dangerous and personal liberty as an ideal (see Baumeister, 1987). This might be seen as a particularly American archetype, but the two world wars of this century did much in Europe and even in Japan to undermine confidence in nation, nationalism, and society. During World War I, French soldiers went on strike and refused to attack enemy trenches— they would only defend (Elting, 1963), and Russian soldiers left the battlefield to overthrow the government that sent them to slaughter (Golovine, 1931). In post–World War II Japan, the connection between social obligation and obedience to the state became unhinged (Fukuyama, 1995). More recently, the post-Vietnam generation in the United States refused or avoided service and reawakened these sentiments, challenging any blind societal litany. It is not then coincidental that a decontextualized, individually based perspective gained favor in the post-Vietnam era, where once again society was seen as suspect and even dangerous. The self in such a climate became a safe harbor. If the world was the cause of our stress, the self, and close personal ties, held the route to stress resistance.

The independent self, and mental health professionals' goal of supporting a healthy independent self, can also be seen as outgrowths of another revolution that was founded in the "beat generation" of Alan Ginsberg and Jack Kerouac of the 1950s. The beat generation, too, was germinated during the post–World War II era and the mind-numbing lack of consciousness that seemed to comprise the 1950s. Rather than following society's goals and wishes, the beat generation donned black garb and embraced abstract modern art forms such as the Pop Art of Andy Warhol that rejected a society that expected social conservatism and sameness (Nathanson, 1976). The beat generation and the later Hippie Movement of the 1960s and early 1970s may be said to have marched under the banner of "Do your *own* thing." Their catchphrase was "Tune in, turn on, drop out," expressing the rejection of social norms and promoting a personally defined sense of self. Psychology reflected these social cross currents and in fact cross-pollinated with them, as noted by two of the defining figures of the Hippie generation, Timothy Leary and Baba Ram Das, who were both Harvard faculty in psychology prior to their own dropping out. The language of Fritz Perls's gestalt therapy (1969), Carl Rogers's client-centered therapy (1951, 1961), and the later cognitive-behavioral therapies of Meichenbaum (1977) and Ellis (Ellis & Greiger, 1977) all can be seen as focusing on the need of the individual: to "thine own self be true." Rather than doing what they were supposed to do, individuals were encouraged to find their own path, develop their self-esteem, and seek genuine personal expression.

The distrust of society, which seeded and fed individualism, also helps explain the social meanings of the often-unintentional offshoots of such a philosophy. Although one might as well disparage apple pie and the flag as criticize self-esteem and self-expression, there is a negative side to these very healthy goals. In rejecting social norms and standards in the service of the self, or at least making them suspect, it is a model that risks placing individuals in isolation and competition. The goal is for self-identity, self-esteem, and attainment of individual goals. In so doing, it construes the borders between people and between people and institutions as circumscribed and solidly demarcated (Baumeister, 1987; Sampson, 1988). These borders imply separateness. Indeed, individualism, and even more so, the mentalism that accompany the cognitive revolution and the psychodynamic schools of therapy, argue for an intervention that meets the individual on a mentalistic level in kind. If individuals must find their own best path, intervention must make the patient's or client's needs primary. As such, intervention preserves and promotes individual mental health, even if it sacrifices the family, social traditions, and others' welfare. Therapy does not embark with these goals, but if we serve one master, we cannot serve another. If individual well-being is paramount, social well-being is secondary at best.

With the current emphasis in the United States on the importance of the family, my argument that we champion the individual over the social group must seem misplaced. However, one only need compare this Western sense of family with Japanese or Chinese construals of family to appreciate my meaning. In Chinese culture, for example, it would be unacceptable to assert that the self even has needs that are inconsistent with the family (Lee, 1953). In Japan, the individual and the family serve the welfare of the greater social milieu (Fukuyama, 1995). In religious Jewish homes, even today, in the United States, a Rabbi intervenes in the case of marital problems not by helping the individual find his or her own path, but by constructing a *Shalom Byeet*, a plan for a peaceful household. Psychotherapy itself may not have a place in such cultures insomuch as it inherently seeks to solve conflicts between individual and social needs with an individualistic bias; its patron is the welfare of the individual.

If the individual was to be independent of the society, psychology and psychiatry also needed to become decontextualized in other ways. Freud, Adler, and Erickson each saw their views of personality as linked to societal norms, values, and structures. Likewise, the American personality theorist, Gordon Allport (1937, 1961), whose ideas of personal traits were to underpin the early thinking about stress and anxiety, conceptualized personality as intrinsically linked with social values and social behavior. The healthy self was a self as citizen and good Samaritan, the self as linked to family, the self as linked to religion and morality. By separating the self from society and construing that behavior was a function of personal appraisal, broader social structures and linkages evaporated by atrophy. When applied to the study of stress, this risks reducing people's stress as something in their minds, and therefore something that can be changed by changing their minds. Although Lazarus and Folkman (1984) included real-life circumstances and how people address these challenges and threats in their model, their emphasis was clearly on the appraisal portion of their field-dominating model. As Sampson (1988) concluded, individualism seldom focuses on the environment or the connections between people as more than background.

Appraisal goes further and seldom considers the environment and social connections as more than cognitions, or mental models. The environment remains out of focus in stress intervention, as dull backwash that can hardly be honestly called background, let alone a defining context that influences behavior (Trickett, 1995).

Culture, Resources, and Contextualized Intervention

We also need ask what cultural phenomena are being reflected in the rise of interest in resources, a renewed focus on the environment, and a wellspring of attention to non-Western, nonmale views of psychology and psychological processes as they apply to stress. This is a more difficult process, because these changes are new enough that it is difficult to acquire the necessary distance to decipher social trends—the wheels of change are still in spin.

As this is this volume's final chapter, however, I take one more chance. I would argue that those who created the current *zeitgeist* naturally mirrored their own culture. Specifically, the focus on the self in psychology and in stress theory and research evolved at a time when those creating this focus in universities and medical settings, principally white, American men, were fairly safe. They were economically safe, they were socially safe, they were safe from war (others went to Vietnam), and opportunity was on the horizon in the post–World War II years of the 1960s through the 1980s. In 1960, only 36 percent of U.S. women were in the paid workforce, whereas today, 57 percent of women are employed (U.S. Census Bureau, 1997). From 1967 to 1994, enrollment rates in college for whites compared to blacks changed from almost 2 to 1, to only 1.25 to 1, still favoring whites, but with a rapidly closing gap (Snyder & Hoffman, 1995). Notwithstanding continued racial, ethnic, and gender biases, there has been a rapid alteration of who constitutes the defining members of society. Critical to my argument, this shake-up has meant a redistribution of object, condition, personal, and energy resources (see Chapter 3).

The computer and modern transportation technologies have also changed home markets to global markets. Here, too, the defining standards have become global and multicultural. America may be a world leader, but its competitors are everywhere and on ever more equal footing worldwide. If "money talks," then new social perspectives and worldviews gain the bully pulpit (Moran & Riesenberger, 1994)

These enormous and fundamental changes translate to a rearrangement of the allocation of resources that has, in turn, led to a shake-up of an expectation of stability (Siegrist, 1996). Hence, resources have again become of paramount importance because the rules pertaining to their creation and protection are in transition. Who has the resources, who will acquire them, and who will maintain them was always at issue, but there were few who expected major changes. The Berlin Wall, American economic supremacy, and the nuclear family were seen as permanent edifices. Today, changes are everywhere and no one appears quite sure where they will be in the resource hierarchy tomorrow. The expectation of working for one company from graduation to retirement is over, even in Japan. Part-time work is substituting for full-time employment, and high-paying manufacturing jobs are being exported from the richest nations to poorer nations and being replaced by lower paying service opportunities (Moran & Riesenberger, 1994; Nollen, Eddy, & Martin, 1978). Indeed, the militant white, male militia movements have been interpreted as a backlash against just these changes, as white males sense their supremacy ending (Abanes, 1996).

Accompanying this upheaval, a white, Western, male-dominant view of the world encapsulated by rugged individualism becomes contested by other idealogies. Individualism is faced with the challenge of collectivism as East meets West. Competition as a defining model is faced with the alternative of cooperation as less male-dominant, less Western viewpoints gain attention. Even within the borders of Western nations, and particularly the United States, the voices of various nonwhite ethnic groups are being heard. They demand attention to their cultures and reject the ideal that they must acculturate to the white, Western norm. It would be wrong to amalgamate these disparate cultures into any one, uniform image, but compared to Western, white culture, they tend to be more familial, more collectivist, more spiritual, and less individualistic (Triandis, 1995a,b). They may also be more xenophobic, more in-group versus out-group oriented, and no less prejudiced and biased in many of their own ways.

Social changes are and will always be reflected in the makeup of the social and behavioral sciences and psychiatry, even if social-behavioral scientists and mental health professionals themselves are not aware of the sociocultural roots of their own work (Baumeister, 1989; Foucault, 1965; Sarason, 1977). These most current trends may be too dynamic to name exactly or categorize at this time, but I believe that the evolving resource perspectives and the attention to culture, context, and collectivism are reflections of these newly evolving social tides. For intervention, this translates to a need for mental health professionals to aid individuals' acquisition, retention, and protection of resources. This means working on individual, familial, organizational, and social policy levels. Women may come to therapy not to seek self-actualization at the expense of family, nor to sacrifice themselves for the good of family, but to find balance between both roles—a more collectivist ideal. Women experiencing bias at work may expect assistance in breaking corporations' glass ceiling (Powell, 1988). Parham (1989), a leading African American psychotherapist, envisions a psychology that incorporates promoting the welfare of the individual as inseparable from social change and a strong African American community. As mental health professionals, we are suddenly expected to become "culturally competent," which entails ability to work with people from different cultural perspectives, even before we know how to train cultural competence and prior to having any scientific evidence that we can transform current psychological interventions in culturally effective ways across all cultures. These social and economic changes will cause social and behavioral interventionists naturally to think in new ways and force them to address a very new world order.

PSYCHOPATHOLOGY: DEFECT VERSUS ENVIRONMENTAL EXPLANATIONS

In the early chapters of this volume, I discussed the seductiveness of convenient paradigms, paradigms that we would like to adopt because they would make our lives as researchers easier (Kuhn, 1962). Individualistic models of psychology are particularly seductive paradigms because they fit investigators' needs to conduct research with relatively simple methodologies and without the need to leave the walls of the university and the ease of paper-and-pencil tests. If reality is not what matters, but only interpretation, then undergraduate student samples are as reasonable as research targets as factory workers, soldiers, refugees, parents, or the elderly. If reality is not what matters, then ethnicity and the associated racism or preferential treatment of certain groups is a matter of perception. If reality is not what matters, then the laboratory is as acceptable a setting for study as the inner city, or the homes of families with serious health problems. If reality is not what matters, women's higher depression lies in some problem within them, some greater vulnerability, and not environmental inequalities that must be addressed. Even investigating coping with major illness, for example, individualization treats the extent or severity of illness as a control variable, focusing on individual differences rather than the differences generated by the external causes of stress as reflected in illness severity.

If researchers are seduced by the ease of the paradigm, the more so for clinicians. Since the time of Freud, no major innovation in treatment has been seriously considered and incorporated within psychiatry or psychology that forces clinicians to leave their clinics, offices, and hospitals. Indeed, virtually all talk therapies involve the same 50-minute hour. Cognitive individualism further encourages the therapist to work through talk therapy alone, one mind with another, and without family members or co-workers present (although they may be present, it is a less preferred option). Biological individualism goes further and allows the clinician to merely prescribe a drug with perhaps a 5-minute contact, and perhaps through an intermediary altogether. No need to see the family, visit the workplace, take social action, or act to change an environment.

The movement toward prevention-oriented, skills-building, community-based mental health centers created by the 1963 Mental Health Act has been all but totally eradicated. Community mental health centers have been turned into traditional treatment centers largely dedicated to medicating the chronically mentally ill (Rochefort, 1989). Mental health professionals, when in work settings, answer calls for psychological problems using short-term counseling or referring callers back to colleagues' guarded offices in so-called employee assistance programs (EAPs). Employee assistance does not consider that the assistance that employees need may be that workplace changes are due. The mentalist, biological, individualistic paradigm sanctions this approach, and once the paradigm is accepted, there is little incentive to do otherwise. The background of the environment is taken as a given.

By turning to individuals as the source of problems, inherent in clinical models is the concept of sickness, defect, or illness as the primary explanation of disturbed behavior (Albee, 1977). Once again, because illness or defect is envisioned as a trait of individuals, their minds, and their biologies, there is little impetus to examine either aspects of the social environment or even competencies of the individuals.[2]

COR theory challenges this paradigm, even for those rich in resources, for whom resource loss is less critical an issue, because COR theory envisions resources as the keystone in the activation and exacerbation of stress and its consequences. For those lacking in resources, COR theory contests the individualistic paradigm even more forcefully because individualistic treatment offers them still less of what they need from their resource-depleted and therefore vulnerable station (Dohrenwend & Dohrenwend, 1974).

Since COR theory depicts certain cardinal resources as cognitively based, such as self-esteem or self-efficacy, and other fundamental resources as physical, such as stamina and a state of physical healthy functioning, I have no agenda to dismiss talk therapy or use of medications. The problem with the individualistic, mental, and biological paradigms is that they circumscribe treatment within this confining perimeter. They reduce the stress of the real world to the neuroticism (i.e., defect) of individuals' minds and biologies, and sanction clinicians disengaging from environmental concerns, social action, social policy or, for that matter, ever leaving their offices (Albee, 1977; Caplan, 1964; Dohrenwend & Dohrenwend, 1974; Laing, 1969; Rappaport, 1977). COR theory spans between individualistic and collectivist notions because it conceives resources as intertwined between individuals, their thoughts, their actions, their social relations, and their biology (see Chapters 1–3). Indeed, I would even fear that when we move on from the cognitive revolution that we will dismiss its gains, as we did with the psychodynamic revolution for the most part. Rather, we need to incorporate intervention aimed at bolstering cognitive resources and changing cognitive biases that are self- or socially destructive (Ellis & Greiger, 1977; Meichenbaum, 1977; Meichenbaum & Cameron, 1983), with a greater awareness of other resources and the place of environments as the fountainhead and battleground for resource acquisition, retention, and protection.

A few professionals notwithstanding, psychology and psychiatry, and even social work, with its more community-based foundation, risk failing people by conceptualizing intervention on the individual level void of context, and this is precisely what they are trained to do. In our schools and workplaces, if the individual fails, it is a matter of individual failure, not the system that is seen as at fault (Albee, 1977; Goffman, 1963; Rappaport, 1977). Sociology may focus on this systems level, but again, mental health professionals are hardly influenced by sociological theory or research. Their work is not read in medical schools or departments of psychology, and even such important sociological classics as Goffman's *Stigma* do not appear on reading lists. In the prevailing intervention ideologies and sciences, health, well-being, illness, and dysfunction are all defined within the parameters of the sphere of individual biochemistry, thought, emotions, and action. Most resources that exist outside of the self, if addressed at all, are seen as the purview of social work, and social workers have been seduced into practicing individual psychotherapy rather than intervening to aid people's resources as well. To the extent that psychiatry, psychology, or social work address how people interact with systems, it is for the sake of diagnosis. Specifically, dysfunction in any of these realms is seen in diagnostic manuals DSM-I through DSM-IV (1952, 1968, 1980, 1994) as indications of individual psychopathology.

ALTERNATIVE VISIONS

Paradigms are so pervasive and overpowering that it is even difficult to imagine how another paradigm would look. I will touch on three individual-nested-in systems approaches that have already been applied and proven successful, hoping that their elucidation may help frame the nature of a clinical world that would include greater linkage between depressions, their families, their workplaces, and their communities. I use examples that, however imperfect, have already been well developed to illustrate that the intervention recommendations that follow from COR theory are not fanciful and that they have already been practiced. If nothing else, I mean to illustrate that the traditional individualized treatment model is only one alternative and that it is far from the only possibility. Moreover, I hope to show by way of these examples that they and the individualized, cognitive, psychodynamic, biological, and behavioral models reflect sociopolitical choices with major implications for how we conceptualize intervention and where we lay the responsibility for action and change. They are not, as they claim, apolitical.

Hull House as a Model, Ideology, and Setting

The first approach I would offer as a model was developed at the beginning of this century by Jane Addams and her famous Hull House (McCree Bryan & Davis, 1990). Hull House is important as an illustration because it is both a place and a philosophy, and both aspects are fundamental to a paradigm whose primary underpinning is that people exist with others in settings, not alone, and not in isolation of their environment. The Hull House model personifies Sampson's (1988) ensembled individualism, characterized by fluid interaction with others, lack of clear self–other boundaries, and sharing of control between the self, others, and the environment.

Hull House developed in Chicago during the fastest period of U.S. immigration at the turn of the twentieth century. The ideology of Hull House was to foster the process of acculturation and independence of immigrants and the poor. Hull House became a center where immigrants learned competencies that fit the demands of their new country, and where the poor found an advocate for change. Language competencies, work competencies, and social competencies were objects of concern and focus.

Hull House was also a place for advocacy. The diversity of Hull House's programs defies imagination. This meant working on housing conditions, workplace opportunities and fairness, and, at times, ethnic and union organizing. The very concept of a public playground, that children should have a safe, fun place to play, was introduced to Chicago by Hull House. Hull House was instrumental in the passage of the landmark Illinois Factory Act of 1893 that provided for the inspection of factories and tenement lofts, and prohibited the employment of children under the age of 14 years for more than an 8-hour day, and still found time to fight for academic freedom in American universities during a period of rising outcries for censorship. Hull House ran an arts program, a lecture series, a number of small industries, sports clubs, a competitive women's basketball team, day care, summer camps, naturalization classes, dances, and worked to create the first juvenile court in the nation.

A primary goal of Jane Addams was promoting personal and group efficacy and control, and Addams encouraged use of her center for political organizing as well. Indeed, her willingness to allow Greek Americans to use Hull House for their own ends almost cost her the Nobel Prize. The award was held off for years, because although herself an ardent pacifist, she allowed them to conduct military training that was organized in order to prepare troops to fight Turkey. Workers at Hull House could not simply see clients in their offices, but had to become involved as catalyzers and advocates of change, and as shown by the example of its Greek constituents, chose to allow the community self-determination rather than expert-directed control. The attempt to break down expert–client barriers was also demonstrated by the fact that Jane Addams, many of her staff, and researchers from local universities, such as the University of Chicago, also lived at Hull House. They did not return to their comfortable suburban homes at night.

The Hull House philosophy is reflected in the later writings of George Albee (1977, 1980). Albee suggested that psychological and physical well-being are functions of a combination of organic causes (e.g., genetics, communicable diseases) and stress. This first point would not differentiate Albee's model from traditional psychiatric and psychological treatises on mental and physical illness. However, Albee further theorized that many of these disease- and dysfunction-producing factors, in turn, were by-products of ethnic and economic discrimination of minorities and the poor within a society that demands their resource contribution but offers them little return on their investment. Albee also theorized a health-driving dimension of his model, specifically, that the deleterious effects of organic causes of disease and stress were potentially offset by competencies, coping skills, self-esteem, and supportive social ties. Albee presented his model in terms of the following equation:

$$\text{Health/Illness} = \frac{\text{Organic Causes + Stress}}{\text{Self-Esteem + Resources + Supportive Ties}}$$

Linking this model to intervention, Albee asserted a need to focus on both lowering the causes of illness and infirmity and bolstering people's resources. Furthermore, consistent with the earlier Hull House model, Albee depicted environmental conditions as largely responsible both for generating illness and for limiting people's abilities to develop the competencies and social ties that might combat the causes and consequences of those negative environmental conditions. Hence, his two-prong approach involves social action to change environmental conditions and enhance resources to improve people's accommodation with a demanding world. Wrote Albee (1980):

> When did we switch from an *evil-is-in-the-system* social reform philosophy to the more conservative *evil-is-inside-the-person* individual-treatment philosophy? Probably sometime in the decade of the 1920's. Psychiatry and social work focused on individual need, on psychic determinism, and on the one-to-one intervention method. The early involvement of social workers in social action—storming the citadels of the establishment, organizing the poor, working with the unions, leading and encouraging tenant strikes, gave way to the ascendant psychiatric notion that evil is inside the person, and that if we can get the person across a desk from us, we can somehow patch up the problem. Our training programs all teach this model.... If evil is inside the person, then we do not need to change anything except the person, and the damaging status quo is left intact.... The fundamental question is whether we *represent the client* or whether we *represent the agency*, institution, and society that pays the salary. (p. 100; emphasis in original)

Occupational Medicine: Combining Individual and Systems Intervention

Another potentially exciting model is presented by the medical sub-discipline of occupational medicine. Although I am afraid to say that I often find that its ideals are corrupted in practice, it offers a challenging vision for psychology and medicine. I would even argue that its apparent weaknesses are instructive if we wish to adapt it and improve upon it, because the same obstacles would await a systems-oriented mental health approach.

Occupational medicine sees itself as nested within the nexus that ties worker, work setting, management, and employment policy. Occupational medicine addresses treatment, prevention, work conditions, and lifestyle issues simultaneously. Unlike most areas of medicine that focus on treatment of disease, occupational medicine addresses the span from wellness to illness and the natural history of health–disease continuum. In the natural history of health–disease continuum, wellness is not only considered, but also fostered through preventive interventions.

Environmental factors as causes of disease and promoters of wellness are integral to occupational medicine's approach. Hence, the clinician must be knowledgeable in acute-care medicine, public health intervention, and public policy. There is no parallel to this among mental health professionals. Clinical psychology and psychiatry have often turned to the argument that they acknowledge environmental conditions as a cause of health problems, but that the explosion of information in their professions prohibits their learning about intervention outside of individual and family treatment. The areas covered by occupational medicine are no less broad, however; yet because they adopt a different model, they feel it is incumbent upon them to gain expertise in individual and systems intervention, even if no one practitioner is expected necessarily to work at all these levels.

Although I admire occupational medicine's model, its U.S. reality, in particular, tends to favor the employer over the worker. This, however, is not endemic to the model and is not as representative of the European interpretation of the discipline. In the United States, as the workplace is typically the employer of the occupational physician, they risk becoming conspiratorially related to the business rather than the worker, in a climate that has relatively few laws regarding work conditions (see Lurie, 1994). Indeed, occupational medicine has often been found to be ineffective because of the disincentives American businesses place on occupational physicians even to report occupational disease or danger (Lurie, 1996). In Europe, in stark contrast, recent pan-European legislation has demanded that all countries that wish to join the European Union must adhere to a comprehensive set of principles for worker well-being. This legislation goes well beyond workplace safety issues, and addresses such areas as limiting the degree of boredom on a job and the need to maximize worker involvement in decision making.

With a backdrop that simultaneously values employees' rights and needs, and the requirement for a productive workplace within a market economy, a model of what occupational medicine and occupational health psychology could offer emerges. Maes, a health psychologist in the Netherlands, and his colleagues (Maes, Kittel, Scholten, & Verhoeven, 1996) have been instrumental in developing model programs that comprehensively alter the worker–workplace interaction in a way that places quality of work life and productivity as mutual, noncompeting goals. Again, Dutch law and social traditions in Europe that are historically worker friendly make this approach more palatable to business. Maes's programs include providing incentives for self-help (e.g., stopping smoking, exercise), making work conditions conducive to health and well-being, including workers in decision making, and integrating work routines to support worker well-being. For Maes, the structure of work must be conducive to health and psychological well-being if we are to limit such diverse workplace problems as alcoholism, heart disease, burnout, and frequent sick days. Here too, the words of Albee (1977) come to mind.

> My thesis is that industrialization requires the dehumanization of work.... We are merely dealing with a small part of the problem when we try to build competencies into children who are destined to take their places as workers in endlessly boring and routine jobs in manufacturing, sales, service, and agribusiness. (p. 79)

The promise and problem of occupational medicine as a model for psychosocial intervention is illustrated in the coal mining, lead, asbestos

(Bayer, 1988), and dairy industries (Corbett, 1982). The promise is that occupational medicine would work to preserve the health of workers as its foremost obligation and to help workplaces to shape their settings to promote worker health. Instead,

> physicians and scientists avoided blaming the asbestos industry for workers' illnesses. They set acceptable levels of exposure to lead so as to define this an engineering rather than a medical problem, and attributed black lung disease of miners to silica rather than coal particles.... [In another instance] polybrominated biphenyls (PBBs) were inadvertently mixed with feed for dairy cows, contaminating feed of other animals, with deleterious consequences for the public. Major health effects were ignored because both the responsible industry and state public health department were unwilling to risk economic losses by acknowledging the diagnosis by a dairy farmer ... until public outrage led to litigation. (Lurie, 1994, p. 1370)

Even public health officials, who are charged to work for the public good, are prone to this same deception. In the famous case of the toxic-waste-polluted Love Canal in New York, health physicians and scientists consistently argued in favor of governmental and industry leanings, and against citizen rights (Levine & Perkins, 1987). They ardently claimed they saw no convincing connection between the pollution left by industry and the high rates of disease and congenital disformity among residents or, at least, no connection that would justify compensating families and allowing them to evacuate the toxic waste's immediate site. A carefully conducted survey by local families of the pattern of homes where illnesses were occurring was dismissed by health officials as the work of "housewives," that is until "housewives" took two U.S. Environmental Protection Agency officials hostage, and took their case to national television, forcing President Carter's hand in an election year. Carter himself, in the end, came to the area to announce that all residents would be compensated so they could relocate. Here again, the problem of who employs the occupational and public health professionals is paramount, and the weakness as well as the potential of this area of intervention expertise is underscored.

Thus, although occupational medicine and public health science hold a promising model, they again point to the problem that paradigms become bent toward the power of the purse strings. This is not to say that occupational physicians or public health scientists are unethical; rather, they are forced to work within a certain power structure and must endeavor to do the "most good" for patients considering the constraints placed upon them as employees or contractees of industry. Moreover, working for one entity, they are naturally influenced by the interpretations and climate fostered in those corridors. Further, if they are seen in today's business climate as worker advocates, they will not be hired or contracted by industry and so can do little good. They are placed in the dilemma that if they do too little, they wrong workers and the public, and if they do too much, they are removed from positions where they can intervene on people's behalf whatsoever (Lurie, 1994).

Community Psychology

The one area of psychology that has promoted a person-nested-in environments approach with an attendant emphasis on people's needs and rights has been community psychology.[3] Indeed, the recognition of the multidisciplinary nature of such an intervention ideology has resulted in the professional society representing this field to change its name to the Society for Community Research and Action, formally leaving the structure of any one discipline. It is also noteworthy that the key concept around which community psychology has almost entirely constructed its interventions is empowerment (Rappaport, 1981). Inherent in this ideology is a focus on simultaneously enhancing people's competencies and changing social systems so that they can utilize these competencies in a productive fashion that is meaningful to their lives. Such an approach underscores the need to avail individuals and groups to resources and allow them to develop within their culturally defined pathways both in acquiring and utilizing resources. The interventionist in community psychology may be viewed as a kind of organizational consultant who identifies person-nested-in settings problems. Once problems are identified, community psychologists develop an intervention plan by mobilizing professional, community, and individual resources to alter the persons or setting. This also means that community psychologists may not themselves have the intervention "technique" required to solve the problem, insomuch as they recognize that they must call on lay and professional resources in the way a building contractor calls on carpenters, plumbers, and bricklayers.

Community psychology has from its onset been deeply ecologically minded (Kelly, 1966). Its hallmark has been a devotion to an understanding that the context surrounding people is what is critical in promoting or frustrating their healthy functioning. There is a basic belief here that given a healthy environment, people will find healthy means to accomplish their goals. Contrariwise, psychopathology and poor functioning are depicted as the inevitable consequences of environments that form obstacles to people's basic capacity toward healthy, productive functioning. This has led community psychology to look closely at the various "isms"—racism, sexism, ageism—and to see broad social and political processes as fundamental to any successful intervention (Levine & Perkins, 1997). It has also led community psychology to challenge expert–client models and to promote advocacy and partnership models where professionals lend their expertise to communities and as partners owe a debt to the communities with which they work. This means that their involvement, like in the Hull House model, does not begin and end with some research project, but must be looked at as an ongoing relationship.

Community psychology's strength has been in providing both an ideology and model programs in such diverse settings as schools, industry, and community (Cowen, 1983; Felner, Ginter, & Primavera, 1982; Jason & Bogat, 1983; Sandler et al., 1992; Trickett, 1978). The failure of community psychology has been an inability to secure a stable funding base. Who will pay for the prevention of dysfunction, the building of competencies, and the advocacy of individuals against the often prevailing winds of social institutions, industry, and government? This problem of payment and the general decline of social activism since its heyday in the 1960s and early 1970s has led to a decline of community psychology programs. However, with the increased pressure being created by women and ethnic minority groups for society to conform to them, and not just for them to conform to society, community psychology has an enormous potential contribution. By emphasizing a systems perspective, community psychology is well situated to provide leadership in many areas of prevention, resource enhancement, and altering systems to meet people's needs and respect their rights (Levine & Perkins, 1997).

Having some potential models to serve our understanding with Hull House, occupational medicine, and community psychology, the question arises as to what special blueprint COR theory offers to an intervention discipline that might emerge from psychology and other mental- and physical-health-promoting disciplines. It is this I turn to next, with the caveat that COR theory does not offer a complete plan of action and will be weak in the areas in which traditional psychology is strong, in particular where individuals' problems are more a function of psychopathology (e.g., severe neurosis and psychosis) than problems with resources, competencies, and settings. Nevertheless, even in areas where psychopathology must be attended to by traditional intervention methods, COR theory offers suggestions for intervention that would addend traditional treatment and improve quality of life.

COR PRINCIPLES OF INTERVENTION

COR theory lends itself directly to intervention guidelines on the individual, group, and systems levels. In fact, inherent in COR theory as I have presented it throughout this volume is that the individual-nested-in family-nested-in tribe is an indivisible unit. We may, at times, focus on one level of the unit, but as an interactive system, our intervention will automatically reverberate to other levels (Bronfenbrenner, 1977; Kelly, 1966, 1988). We may choose to ignore these ecological interactions at different trophic levels of the ecology, but that does not change the fact that they will react. In part, they will react with the intended result. However, they will also react to resist change in order to preserve the system intact, they will incorporate the change as a part of the natural process of succession, and they will reshape the intervention by placing constraints on the very source of intervention (Kelly, 1966, 1988).

Following the principles introduced throughout this volume and the research that supports a Conservation of Resources position, I can now outline a number of principles for intervention.

First, act to prevent or limit loss. Because resource loss is potentially so devastating, intervention must first act to prevent resource loss through individual and systems strategies. This step may be volitional on the part of the target person or population when they are capable of moving out of harm's way. This may be the case in many family, work, and school settings. For example, adolescents may be helped to extricate themselves from a problem situation. Family members with a major conflict may choose to limit their contact, and some behavior that is producing the conditions of loss may be discontinued or postponed. At other times, it requires nonvolitional steps such as evacuation, finding shelter, police intervention, or acting to alter the aspects of a setting that are harmful, such as a harassing supervisor. These types of interventions require linkages with other professionals, managers, police, and the courts, and can even be made by private clinicians who recognize the importance of such professional relationships. Because mental health professionals are not taught to think in a systems manner, they may move immediately to therapy that involves individual change, and therefore requires weeks or months, and not attend to the crisis conditions. Indeed, rugged individualism would decry attempts to escape from bad conditions, as we are taught to "face our problems."

Because resource loss cycles are more rapid than resource gain cycles, acting to limit or interrupt loss cycles must be quick. If momentum is allowed to build, the amount of damage will be great and the resources necessary to halt the loss spirals and their spinoffs may be beyond the means of the interventionist and social institutions charged with this intervention responsibility (e.g., clinics, hospitals, social services). Although this, of course, should not be done haphazardly, a slow response can prove devastating.

Second, begin initiation of gain-focused interventions. Because resource gain is secondary to loss, intervention should next act to create new resources and to facilitate their implementation. Because gain cycles are slower acting and take time to evolve, intervention aimed at fostering gain cycles can be designed and implemented more methodically, as it will require greater acquisition time and must be placed in ecological context. Time should be taken to consider primary and secondary ramifications of such programs and their fit to the overall ecology in the individuals' life space, for that family's style, and for community regularities (deVries, 1995; deJong, 1995).

In devising gain strategies or loss deterrents, one also need not necessarily look to change the individual or group. Rather, if loss cycles have not been too devastating, systems level changes can alter the ecology such that loss spirals will be halted and gain cycles more easily engaged. If the individuals or organizations have adequate resource reserves and a favorable ecology to utilize those reserves, negative trends can be reversed and healthy trends initiated. Examples of such intervention include alternative classroom environments for more active children, promotion of policies that effectively eliminate racist and sexist practices in the workplace, flexplace policies (e.g., allowing individuals to do some work at home), and elder care leave.

Intervention must consider the resource strengths and weaknesses of the target. Both traditional diagnosis and intervention seldom consider the resource strengths or weaknesses of the target, but focus instead on specific pathologies (e.g., heart disease, depression). If individuals, families, groups, or communities have weak resource reservoirs, they will need major investment of resources from external sources because they will have few resources to themselves invest to aid and support the intervention scheme. For example, mental health professionals make little effort in facilitating people's making it to therapy or what they do once they leave the therapist's office. Failure to enjoin therapy is simply attributed to lack of patients' motivation: "They weren't ready for therapy."

COR theory, in contrast, suggests that enjoining an offered intervention requires considerable resources, and targets of intervention are often in such a resource-depleted state that they lack resources to engage the intervention. They may lack the self-esteem, social support, transportation, money, insurance, time, or energy necessary to form a partnership with the interventionist. Individuals and systems that are extremely lacking in resources will, in fact, resist intervention, because enjoining the intervention demands a resource investment that threatens their "final defense" position (cf. Schönpflug, 1985). They will instead act to conserve their limited resources and cannot afford to do otherwise (cf. Aspinwall & Taylor, 1997).

If individuals or systems (e.g., families, communities) have moderate to strong resource systems, these can and should be utilized in intervention strategies. This will both increase the amount of resources available for intervention, thus increasing the likelihood of success, and provide the target individuals or organization a sense of ownership in their recovery. As

Iscoe (1974) suggested, many communities already possess certain competencies, and by calling on and enriching these, we show respect and acknowledge the natural strengths of the community, and not only its failings or difficulties.

Target resources, not illness. The target of intervention is not only the symptom, but also perhaps more the resources and conditions that facilitate healthy functioning. Such a strategy will simultaneously influence traditional health and mental health outcomes (e.g., blood pressure, heart disease, depression, anxiety), and will also enrich resources that may be incorporated in people's resource armamentarium. These stronger resource reserves can, in turn, be utilized to offset future resource threats and loss, and to enhance resource gain cycles. Interventions aimed at limiting resource loss and facilitating gain will create positive, resource-generating spirals that should be anticipated and further fostered. The original intervention can begin a positive process, and shepherding that process will create resource bridges between the intervention and the target population that can be called upon to continue the recovery process and adapted in the defense against other threats already present or evolving. This bridge operates in two directions (see Chapter 8) and the strengthened recipient of resources becomes an ally with enriched resources for future stress interventions that will be required elsewhere in the overall system. Such partnerships challenge traditional expert–client and doctor–patient models because they imply that the patient or client is an ally (read equal).

Focus on key resources. Certain resources will be key to resource loss and resource gain chains. This will be determined by the nature of person–environment interactions in settings and cultures (Bronfenbrenner, 1977). Self-efficacy may be so strong a focus in Western psychology (Bandura, 1997) because of its fit with the emphasis on individual achievement and the expectation that individuals are often isolated from others within North American culture and the settings created within this culture. A study of culture and settings, and an appreciation of multiculturalism in many societies will aid in the identification of key resources.

For example, understanding the process of divorce and its influence on children within a given culture allows for development of an ecologically valid intervention strategy based on the natural strengths, weakness, and pathways represented in that system as represented in the ecologically rich and methodologically advanced prevention efforts of Sandler et al. (1992). On a community level, this has been illustrated in the disaster work of Giel (1990), who advises that intervention must consider the natural mazes and pathways of the stricken culture and community. Acquiring these management resources will assist in overall adjustment and adaptation (Aneshensel, 1992; Thoits, 1994).

Target multiple resources. Because resources are linked, and because multiple resources are often needed for any stress challenge, it is advantageous to target multiple resources for intervention. In our work helping nurses find better coping strategies to prevent burnout in hospital settings, we found that if we targeted a single resource, such as mastery or social support, that the intervention had minimal impact (Freedy & Hobfoll, 1994). However, when we target both personal and social resources, participating nurses gained meaningfully from the program. Their resource acquisition was greater, and their stress resistance was enhanced. Multiple resource interventions (Jason, McMahon, Salina, & Hedeker, 1995; Sandler et al., 1992) capture the more real-world nature of people's problems. Most stressful circumstances influence people on multiple levels (e.g., socially and emotionally) and so require multiple resistance resources to offset negative sequelae. It may also be the case that different members of the target populations are more capable of changing in one resource area first, and they can then use this to bootstrap to other strengths because resource gains create more fertile ground for further resource acquisition.

Targeting multiple resources is illustrated also in the linkage of resources in stress resistance, even if treatment focuses on a key resource. Ozer and Bandura (1990) taught women who had been raped an aggressive means of self-defense. The course was taught in groups and included acquisition of aggressive fighting skills. The intervention also taught verbal persuasion techniques, how to display a confident tone and demeanor, how to issue aggressive verbal warning, how effectively to yell at an attacker, and decision making when under attack. Although their goal was to increase *perceived* self-efficacy, Ozer and Bandura emphasized that the underpinnings of such appraisals are actual behavioral efficacy and successful utilization of acquired resources.

> The most effective vehicle for developing a resilient sense of efficacy is through mastery experience. Performance successes build a sense of personal efficacy....
>
> Mastery modeling served as the principle vehicle for instilling dependable self-protective skills and a strong sense of personal efficacy to execute them as well. It combines the power of performance mastery experiences, modeling of effective coping strategies for variable circumstances, physiological indicants of capacity, and repeated verification of personal coping capability. (p. 473)

The work of Ozer and Bandura and our own investigations (Freedy & Hobfoll, 1994) suggest further that the targeted resources should be pieces of naturally existing resource chains linked to stress resistance. This enables a multiple defensive strategy by tying together the reservoir of acquired resources in a problem-focused manner. A single resource defense risks being overwhelmed and may not be the principal resource required at that time in the history of the problem. It follows from this that one must clearly understand the ecology of the circumstances in which target individuals or groups find themselves, so that an optimal set of resources can be marked.

Adaptation and change have definite and sometimes overwhelming costs. Because coping, adaptation, and attempts at resource gain demand resources, these processes deplete already jeopardized resource reservoirs (Schönpflug, 1985). Intervention must prepare and respond to this, because these intervention-generated losses will exacerbate and accelerate the very loss cycles that are the targets of intervention. This, in turn, undermines intervention success and creates new problems that will draw individuals' and organizations' attention and resources away from the original focal problem. Family therapy may entail ill-afforded financial costs, time, and loss of work. Likewise when an organization addresses a problem area, it may need to borrow resources necessary for competitive production. If resources must be drawn away from production, this may imperil the company economically or force it to cut costs elsewhere. Interventionists must plan for these costs and incorporate a response within the intervention.

Because of the costs of coping and adaptation, individuals, organizations, and communities that have depleted resources will respond in odd and unanticipated ways. What is often described as dysfunctional may be a creative application of a set of resources that has poor fit with *ideal* adaptational needs. What must be kept in mind is that, however maladaptive, it may still be the best fit that the individuals involved can mobilize given their available resources and the heavy demands they are facing (see Chapter 4). Given that one only has a hammer, it will be the tool both used and misused, when other tools are not available. Rather than depicting this as a weakness, as traditional models would have it, these solutions should be used to aid more effective adaptation by building on them as a foundation. Inner-city gangs may thus be seen as a response to social isolation, physical threat, and a lack of educational opportunities and employment. The tendency to associate in groups may be built upon, as it represents an attempt to address massive threats to loss and substantial resource loss. Building alternative pathways does not necessarily need to use these gangs (as their leadership may well resist this), but the path of social affiliation in strong groups provides an insight for potentially successful response.

Look to alter systems–individual resource fit. Individuals and groups often do possess the resources they require. Stress may still be encountered because their settings are rejecting their resource investment or blocking the way resources and the rules by which resources are used might benefit them (Bronfenbrenner, 1977; Felner, Ginter, & Primavera, 1982; see also Chapter 4). This means that intervention should in many situations direct itself at altering social systems, not individuals or group targets. This is especially germane for people who have little power or exist in prejudiced systems. Women, the elderly, African Americans, Hispanics, children, and refugees may have many resources to invest, but may find their potential blocked. Interventionists should be aware that some of this is unintentional, but that it may well be an intentional process aimed at preserving the resources of those in power. Political naivete, either in the larger political sense or in the sense of office politics of an organization or family politics, will result in sabotage of intervention efforts.

Jason has been a pioneer in this area and his work promoting health has been innovative and instructive. In one model program, Jason, Anes, and Birkhead (1991) noted that the ecology of certain communities promoted adolescent smoking by ignoring laws forbidding sale of cigarettes to minors. This, in turn, made tobacco products easily accessible to young people. Rather than targeting the youth with antismoking campaigns, Jason joined with local law enforcement officials to increase the vigilance of fining merchants who sold cigarettes to minors and made sure this change was well-publicized. This effectively reduced smoking rates in local teenagers by greater levels than could be expected from programs that target the teenagers directly.

In another model program, Winett, Neale, and Williams (1982) examined the use of flextime scheduling for government employees. By allowing workers to arrive at work earlier or stay later, families were able to use their resources to spend more family time together and increase their leisure time. Clearly, workers and their families already had the necessary resources to make these changes but were thwarted due to a lack of time resources. With flextime, they gained time resources in two distinct ways. First, they gained in terms of reduced commuting time, because they could now avoid peak traffic periods. They also gained time by now having the particular hours in the day they needed to meet their task demands. It is also of interest that most workers chose to commute to work earlier and leave earlier. This suggests that work schedules may be generally based on the needs of single breadwinner, two-parent families that constituted most of the workforce when schedules were first instituted. This group then becomes a preferred class, and others such as dual-career and single-parent families have to fit their resources to meet the demands of an ecology with which their resources have less good fit.

Watch for spinoff effects. Because resources are linked, and because loss and gain spirals are likely to follow unpredictable courses, it is necessary to be vigilant about probable spinoffs (Kelly, 1966). Some spinoffs will be positive, such as where those gaining resources enter more robust gain cycles. However, spinoffs of programs that are otherwise effective may nevertheless have deleterious effects. DeVries (1995) and deJong (1995), working with disaster, refugee, and famine victims in nonindustrialized nations, speak of the need to attempt minimodel programs within an overall intervention and to use the natural environment as a laboratory to test these preliminary trials. In their work, they often enter disaster-stricken areas and work with indigenous groups on codeveloping interventions. This may include distribution of medical care, policing temporary refugee camps, developing educational programs, and planning and implementing means to enhance future economic viability. This multistep approach allows interventionists to watch for intended and unintended effects, and to shape the program as they evolve. Desirable spinoffs can be further fostered, or at least not interrupted. Undesirable spinoffs can be approached as interventionists learn from the ecology and may be remedied at their source or down the road. A major negative spinoff may require a rethinking of the entire program effort, but a minor spinoff may be addressed with some follow-up service.

Traumatic resource loss leads to lifelong loss vulnerability and vigilance. According to COR theory, people are prone to be sensitive to resource loss and vigilant against loss, especially when loss-producing circumstances are cued by environmental conditions. However, those who experience severe resource loss in early life may have even more exaggerated loss sensitivity (Janoff-Bulman, 1992). Their natural response to protect against losses will have been mobilized at a time when it was either too immature or simply unable to meet the challenge it confronted. Parental or sibling death, loss of basic trust following abuse, periods of hunger, lack of shelter, and social instability not only have direct profound effects, but also they shatter the fundamental belief that the social fabric of society in the form of parents, elders, and the community, will provide protection. Lomranz (1995), studying child and young adult Holocaust survivors into late adulthood, speaks of the long-term sequelae of such events. The pattern of loss vulnerability remains throughout their lifetime, and they endow it to their own children through parent–child interactions. Psychologists similarly have become aware of similar, long-term effects on children that were individually traumatized through sexual and physical abuse (Janoff-Bulman, 1992; Herman, 1981).

If my thesis is correct that we have a biological drive to create resource-generative and -protective linkages with others, and self-sustaining, protective behavioral repertoires, then severe loss experiences should be particularly destructive from midchildhood through adolescence. During these periods, adaptive capabilities (i.e., learning to live in the world) are rapidly formed and would be vulnerable to the most serious impairments. This does not suggest that earlier life trauma would be less devastating, but it might not interfere as deeply with the learning of adaptational mechanisms. Of course, earlier life trauma may result in other forms of psychopathology, but not necessarily the inability to resist stressful conditions, although the two are likely to be connected.

Translating this principle to intervention, individuals and groups with early life severe trauma and later life chronic, severe trauma will develop oversensitized loss vigilance. On the individual level, this will often require the need for both individual and social interventions aimed at restoring basic trust (Bowlby, 1980). Individuals will need to develop self-understanding of what in most cases will mean deep-seated fears and frequent bouts of depression, anger, and other loss-generated emotions. They will also have difficulty creating the very close interpersonal relationships that are necessary to meet life's challenges. On the community level, such historical events as the Great Depression, the Holocaust, and the turmoil now going on in the Balkan States will produce a generation of such individuals. As the Israeli experience teaches, these individuals will not all be devastated by the experience, and some will thrive. However, they will be imprinted with a lifelong sensitivity to loss that will appear exaggerated if one is not familiar with historical context (Lomranz, 1995).

Obstacles to Intervention

Stress research in sociology has often focused on the social status of target populations, because a basic premise of sociology is that resources are competed for and social power often influences the causes of stress and the process of stress resistance (Aneshensel, 1992; Brown & Harris, 1979, 1989; Pearlin & Schooler, 1978; Kaplan, 1983). Community psychology may be the one subdiscipline in psychology that similarly acknowledges these broader social and political processes (Albee, 1977; Sarason, 1977), but community psychology has been in general retreat since its heyday in the 1960s and 1970s. Once these systems level processes are understood, they must be incorporated in intervention efforts. COR theory (see Chapter 4, FALLS model) posits that the environment often contains obstacles to adaptation and impediments to the process of fitting resources to demands. A number of intervention principles follow from this understanding as to expected obstacles to intervention (Hobfoll, Briggs, & Wells, 1995).

Communities are nested within communities. The first principle regarding expected obstacles to intervention, which follows from an understanding of the competition that exists for resources, is that communities exist within communities. These subcommunities will vie for access to the resources being offered. Even if intervention only intends to halt loss cycles, such action may oppose existing power structures and their agendas. Offers to aid the Hispanic community in the inner city may produce jealousies in the growing African American political hierarchy, which sees its role as garnering these resources for its own constituents. Offering assistance to women in the workplace may threaten men that share this ecology and they are likely to resist and even undermine intervention if they feel threatened. Moreover, if the losses, however fortuitous, enhance one community over another, they may contribute to agendas already operating. In family therapy, this is a long-known process, and the veteran family therapists know that as they act to strengthen the identified patient, they will likely meet resistance from other family members, however much they claim to have the patient's interests alone at heart.

Pressure cooker effects. Because resources are finite, their maintenance is often fragile, and because resources are shared by people within social ecologies, intervention may produce pressure cooker effects. Intervention in individual and family therapy, worksite intervention, and communities often call on the strong, more resource-endowed individuals to offer their resources. It also involves them in the problem. This produces pressure cooker effects (Hobfoll & London, 1986) and stress contagion (Riley & Eckenrode, 1986) wherein stress is placed on all those who share a system that is in crisis or under chonic stressful demands.

The stronger individuals and systems will resist having their resources depleted by the shared stressors of the pressure cooker phenomenon. Such defensiveness is not necessarily selfish either. A mother may resist helping one needy child if it means the abandonment of her time, energy, and other resources for other children. A school that has limited resources may resist helping children with special needs if it means that other children they can help will be at risk or encounter failure.

This means that resources must be supplied to aid the strong as well as the resource weak. It means that individuals must see that the overall strategy will not weaken them or the entire system in some way that will be difficult or impossible to reverse. Like a general on the battlefield, asking one's best troops to sacrifice themselves for an entrapped and surrounded unit may be counterproductive not only to them, but also to the overall objective.

Intervention is a political process. Psychology and psychiatry have traditionally attempted to avoid political processes as outside of their milieu, and social work has backed away from this earlier tradition. A resouce perspective challenges the possibility and feasibility of this apolitical stance. Communities and organizations are by their very nature political. This means that they have a leadership and an agenda. Intervention must consider that leadership and agenda, and incorporate it in intervention. Leaders will, on the one hand, have a knowledge of their communities and be able to facilitate intervention. However, this may only be the case when the intervention matches their own designs and plans. A competent, sound leadership will act in its constituencies best interest. But not all leadership is competent or sound. Many leaders will look out for their own best interests.

Also, given multiple communities within communities, there will be a competition for resources that already exist or that are being offered or altered. In schools, teachers and administrators make up this leadership. In organizations, the elected or appointed managers occupy positions of resource control. In families, parents, or one particular parent, may hold the reins. For communities, there will be a secular and a religious leadership. Interventionists must learn about and study the power structure and engage it in any intervention strategy.

Motivation encourages short-term solutions. Competition for resources means that after initial needs are met, individuals, organizations, and communities may on one hand lose their motivation to address long-term needs, and on the other hand, be cut off from resources in the long-term, because after initial setbacks are countered, there will be a tendency to move on to fresh needs of others. In the case of communities hit by natural disasters, the news media and federal agencies may bring resources and interest to bear in the short term, and communities themselves may foster altruistic interaction. However, this honeymoon of heroic responding will be quickly dissipated (Norris & Kaniasty, 1996).

This means that the interventionist must often be the advocate for long-term change. Rather than passively waiting for victims, patients, or clients to come to their office or exit early from intervention, they must develop strategies for long-term follow-up. On an individual level, this might include educating those who come for therapy from the outset that change is necessarily long term. Managed care insurance will resist payment for such efforts, so on the individual level, therapists may need to develop strategies through other than individual, face-to-face mechanisms. Educational literature, videotapes, follow-up with support groups, and occasional home visits are examples of alternate strategies that, if practiced at all, are not taught or implemented regularly.

On a community or institutional level, interventionists need to make their case for the wisdom of long-term approaches through solid evaluation research that illustrates the ultimate benefit of such practices and unveils the risks of short-term intervention. If part of the intervention is strengthening the target group and the host setting, intervention may often be turned over to the individuals, organizations, and communities involved (deVries, 1995). Indeed, this should be a fundamental goal wherever feasible.

The Place of Cognitive Processes in Resource Interventions

One last principle of intervention deserves special attention, because it is both a complex axiom and it is fundamental to change. This principle is that *attempts to alter appraisals must follow and be consistent with social norms and will be more effective if they dovetail attempts first to optimize resources–demand fit and compensate for lacking resources.* People will resist attempts to make appraisals that are counterindicated by reality or that attempt to substitute for problem-focused change if this is feasible. It is interesting and instructive that some of the most innovative theories on balancing resource-based and cognitive models emerge from recent work with the elderly. I have wondered about this since being presented with these models, and I have come to some conclusions that I would like to share as I near the end of this volume.

Why should work with the elderly lead to special insights? I think one reason is that psychological and sociological models have both failed in predicting what would occur for the elderly, not completely, but enough to raise important new questions that have widespread importance for all psychosocial intervention. Psychological and sociological models would each predict major difficulties of functioning and psychological well-being for the elderly. Psychologically, the elderly should become more helpless and therefore more psychologically frail (Abramson, Seligman, & Teasdale, 1978; Seligman, 1975). Sociologically, with culture being tuned to the young, and with little respect or social position for the aged, the elderly should fall victim to the same consequences as other disadvantaged groups. They do not (Blazer, 1989; Brandstädter & Greve, 1994; Stock, Okun, Haring, & Witter, 1983). Instead, the elderly tend to remain vital, psychologically well, and active until severe health problems emerge, and this, on average, is an outcome with later and later onset (Brandstädter & Wentura, 1995).

A second reason that examination of the adaptive capabilities of the elderly may lead to special insights is that health advances have led for the first time to a whole older generation exploring the territory of a new culture. What I mean by this is that until recently, the number of years after retirement was so limited that there was a relatively short period of renewed adjustment between retirement at age 65 and average death within less than 10 years. Significant leaps in the average life span in many Western nations at least means that the models of adaptation are tested on a new frontier. Whenever a new frontier is explored, there is much to learn.

The third reason that work with the elderly offers special insights is that on average, the elderly are average; that is, the elderly represent a normal distribution of the population that is simply older. With later and later onset of dementia, this means that problems that the elderly encounter cannot be conveniently blamed on them. Given the economic and political power of many elderly, they also will not allow themselves to be made the whipping boy for their own problems.

One obvious place to turn for answers concerning problems that are confronting the elderly is the fitting of resources with new demands within a culture that was not designed to support them. Following the work of Baltes (1987) and Brandstädter (Brandstädter, 1989; Brandstädter & Greve, 1994), we see emerge a resource-based perspective that also comfortably incorporates the role of cognitions. According to their models, individuals will adapt to the extent their resources can be applied to meet situational demands. Consistent with COR theory, they do not suggest that fit is static, but rather that individuals attempt to optimize their resources and the settings they select to maximize benefit (see also Chapter 4). Because they have worked with the elderly with an assumption that, on the average, the elderly were and are effective copers, they do not so quickly move into a victim-blaming explanation when this fit begins to break down. Rather, they assume that the emerging lack of fit for the elderly is a joint process of inevitable functional losses experienced by the elderly and the lack of a supportive culture for the aged.

Baltes's first step in reaction to this widening gap between resources and demand is optimization (see Chapter 4). Individuals optimize by selecting from demands those conditions that best suit their resources. Hence, they might choose a desk job over one that demands a great deal of travel, or choose a walking regimen over jogging. Similarly, they might choose a first-floor apartment or a smaller home. Intervention would thus act to facilitate this optimization, not forgetting that culture and organizations can change as well. Returning to the example of the Israeli kibbutz, the elderly are allowed to switch professions and work more limited hours as they age, and the society endeavors to offer work that is consistent with their changing resources.

When developmental losses become great enough, or cultural supports grow so weak as to cause major problems in resource fit, individuals move to attempts to compensate for these resource–demand gaps, as optimization interventions may no longer be adequate. Compensation involves retraining and use of technical aids, as two examples. Although a 70-year-old individual may no longer be fit enough to work in construction, he may be able to learn supervision skills. Sight may be failing, but computers are capable of larger print. Baltes suggests that people have a natural tendency to compensate when they cannot optimize, and intervention can facilitate this process by providing normative solutions that have worked for others and helping work and other settings implement them.

With decreasing resource reserves, Brandstädter suggests that compensation efforts are subject to the principle of "decreasing marginal utility." As argued in COR theory, adaptation demands costs and these costs begin to outweigh benefits. At this juncture, Brandstädter provides evidence from both life settings and the laboratory for the role of more cognitive kinds of coping, which he terms *accommodative coping*. Because resources and societal demands are often ambiguous, individuals may accommodate by downgrading past goals or adjusting their aspirations. In this way, individuals may choose new goals, let old battles rest, and realign their comparison set to other elderly rather than younger individuals.

However, Brandstädter is also insightful of the pitfalls of any such intervention aimed at reframing reality. He argues that *these cognitive changes must be consistent with pervasive social models for the elderly,* and that individuals will not make appraisals that fly in the face of widely accepted beliefs. He argues that it will be difficult to induce artificially such changes because people's worldviews are reality-based and not given to easy cognitive rearrangement. He further theorizes that where the loss is in the realm of a principal aspect of identity, cognitive reframing will be resisted. As the stress that truly matters concerns losses that are central to people's values (see also Kaplan, 1983), this means that cognitive reframing is a tenuous process. He stresses that cognitive immunization efforts are best played in ambiguous circumstances, where realities are more of a fuzzy set than rock hard. He also never loses sight of the role of culture in this self-defining process.

Some efforts at cognitive reframing may be enhanced, notes Brandstädter, by the fact that already, in everyday language, concepts related to many important areas of adaptation, such as health, physical functioning, or psychosocial competencies, are often used in an "age-relativized" way. So, social norms already allow for individuals to reframe success as different at age 70 than 35, and what it means to be healthy is different for the young and the old. As I have noted elsewhere in this volume, cognitive reframing is most advantageous when the environment is ambiguous and the ambiguity can be used to create favorable personal meanings.

Borrowing from this work, we can apply the concepts of optimization, compensation, altering of settings, and cognitive reframing, as long as they are restricted within socially accepted norms to any target population and are adopted as blueprints for interventions. Because these concepts were generated by work on normal populations, they tend to be free of gender, ethnic, or pathology-conceived biases, which does much from the outset to avoid the pitfalls of defect-derived pathology models (Albee, 1977). They also illustrate the relative place of resource change at individual and systems levels, and how cognitive interventions can operate if balanced within a more culturally sensitive, reality-based conceptual system. Recalling the model of ecological congruence (see Figure 4.1), resources may fit, be fitted to, or not fit stress demands dependent on individual, social, historical, and maturational factors. This translates to interventionists thinking in cultural, historical, and maturational terms in applying their intervention that help people optimize their position or compensate for areas where they lack the necessary resources. It also places the role of the interventionist in the mode of a resource facilitator, and places more shared responsibility for change with the target population. It implies that people will naturally seek a healthy path if offered healthy alternatives and given the means of traversing inevitable obstacles toward meeting their goals. It also strongly asserts the premise that goals are tied to broad social processes of persons within settings, where we must know both about the persons and the settings.

The model of ecological congruence, along with the work of both Baltes and Brandstädter, illustrates that resources may act to aid adaptation to the extent they complement task, emotional, and biological demands placed on the individual or group. This resource suitability, we must remind ourselves when intervening, is always dependent on the individual, familial, group, and cultural value system. Intervention that borrows from these conceptualizations would follow a more resource-nested-in systems mode, and mental health professionals would have to increase their knowledge base regarding the ecology of resources in various settings. Values dictate whether resources are appropriate for application, the acceptability and social ramifications of adopting a certain adaptational posture, and the sanctions that may be imposed that prevent or demand certain response courses. Because values emanate from culture, interventionists must truly be culturally competent. However, since no interventionist can know all cultures, this also means that interventionists must utilize indigenous experts and involve them in therapeutic processes.

CONCLUSIONS

In writing this book, I have probably taken on an impossible task. However, for years, I have been frustrated by a psychology that is increasingly devoid of context, by psychological science that has claimed to be apolitical while it uses political processes, and in so doing becomes ever more conservative, and that has come to depict behavior as a by-product of thought, personality, and biology, ignoring the environment. Had I not worked in the area of stress, these characteristics of psychology, psychiatry, and even sociology, to some extent, would have not been so obviously problematic. But in a world where individuals and social systems are wanting solutions to stressful conditions, I have become less sanguine with attempts to explain away real-world problems with such decontextualized solutions.

This, in turn, took me to the study of history, culture, and philosophy. If the reader feels that I was ill-equipped for these tasks, I can only serve as the first voice of my own guilt. However, as I searched for answers along avenues of scholarship in psychology, and particularly in the stress literature, for which I was well equipped, I came away wanting. Few others, perhaps with good reason, have attempted to integrate the study of any major psychological phenomenon within its sociopolitical, historical, and philosophical context. Philosophers of science may attempt to do so from their own discipline, as in the case of Kuhn (1962), Popper (1959), and especially Foucault (1965), but while they offer important insights, they know little about psychology and less about the study of stress. Hence, I found that they failed in ways that I might succeed, just as I have surely come up lacking in ways in which their work excels.

In the face of rapid changes occurring today in the social order, the instability of resources, and the demand of different worldviews to gain voice, it is increasingly difficult to seek a pure science and absurd to seek a pure social and behavioral science. The social and behavioral sciences are steeped in a complex interweaving of culture, environmental context, biology, and political issues. Their successful application depends on their being directed at all the populations in need, and the most needy may demand a science in context most of all, because their problems largely emerge from a society in which they have a marginal foothold for the acquisition, protection, fostering, and maintenance of resources necessary to preserve the individual-nested-in family-nested-in tribe.

The endemic, human saga of vying for resources must overcome the dilemma of the "tragedy of the commons" (Lloyd, 1833; Hardin, 1968). As rational beings, according to the tragedy of the commons, each herdsman alone wants to maximize his gains. Adding an additional animal to his herd means a clear gain if he is relying on a commonly shared pasture because there is no cost to graze on common land. The potential loss is less clear, because as long as the commons is not overcrowded, overgrazing will not occur and the herd will multiply—the commons are large. The tragedy occurs because if all seek this gain, then there will not be enough for all animals to graze and substantial loss will at some point become the dominating theme for all herdsman. At this point, conflict over the rights to the commons develops and a competitive hierarchy of ownership and rights of use evolves. In England, this very problem was solved by canceling ancient rights of commoners over the commons and allotting them to the liege lord—let others starve.

> The rational herdsman concludes that the only sensible course for him to pursue is to add another animal to his herd. And another; and another.... But this is the conclusion reached by each and every rational herdsman sharing a commons. Therein is the tragedy. Each man is locked into a system that compels him to increase his herd without limit—in a world that is limited. Ruin is the destination toward which all men rush, each pursuing his own best interest in a society that believes in the freedom of the commons. Freedom in a commons brings ruin to all. (Hardin, 1968, p. 1244)

In a world where threat to resources and resource loss are inevitable, and where tenuous resource gain may be the only protection for the individual-nested-in family-nested-in tribe, it is incumbent on us to find mutually benefical means of action in the commons. Resources are finite and must be shared. Finding a balance between individual and collective good will be a major agenda for political and social processes as we enter the twenty-first century. The question remains as to whether insights from stress research will be able to provide answers to these real-world problems and challenges. Resource loss, and protecting against it, defines the human drama, just as described in the biblical Book of Job, and we are entering an era where these issues will loom larger than in recent decades. If stress is principally in the mind, then we must only manage people's stress individually, as it occurs. If stress is in the competition for resources and the need to sustain an adequate resource reservoir, we have much to learn about stress in context and must concern ourselves with aiding peoples acquisition, protection, fostering, and maintenance of resources that they share as a part of the social fabric of membership in families, organizations, and villages. With national borders breaking down, this process will be increasingly global, and communities worldwide, with their varying worldviews, must find relevance in our work.

The resources, goals, and consequences of action are tied among the individual, the family, the village, the nation, and, as communication shrinks distances, the world.

> If there be righteousness in the heart,
> there will be beauty in character.
> If there be beauty in character,
> there will be harmony in the home.
> If there be harmony in the home,
> there will be order in the nation.
> If there be order in the nation,
> there will be peace in the world.
> CONFUCIUS

NOTES

1. I am speaking here principally of clinical and counseling psychology and psychiatry. However, even in such areas that originated with a systems perspective, such as school psychology and social work, social systems and social action interventions tend to be taught more historically, and current trends tend to be individualized and seldom are structured to change the system. This is not to say that all of these professions do not learn something about the influence of television violence, overcrowded schools, and economically depressed neighborhoods. However, they are taught to respond to the consequences of these problems by treating the individuals, not changing the systems that engendered them.

2. I refer mainly to cognitive models of therapy, but the same generally holds for psychodynamic models. I treat the latter in less detail, as there is relatively less work on stress from the psychodynamic perspective. Likewise, radical behaviorism (i.e., behavior modification that does not even accept a role for cognitions) tends to be individually administered and, outside of the work on token economies with children, has not tended to consider stress solutions that go beyond the individual.

3. Organizational psychology might be used as another example, but because organizational psychologists are almost exclusively hired or contracted by business, they could serve no different an example than occupational physicians. Moreover, because they do not identify themselves as necessarily concerned with workers' needs, rights, or health (although they sometimes are), they cannot even necessarily be held to the same standards as occupational physicians, who have an ethical obligation to preserve workers' health.

References

Abanes, R. (1996). *Rebellion, racism and religion: American militias.* Downers Grove, IL: Intervarsity Press.

Abrahams, R. (1975). Negotiating respect: Patterns of presentation among black women. In C. R. Farrer (Ed.), *Women and folklore.* Austin: University of Texas Press.

Abramson, L. Y., Seligman, M. E. P., & Teasdale, J. D. (1978). Learned helplessness in humans: Critique and reformulation. *Journal of Abnormal Psychology, 87,* 49–74.

Acitelli, L. K., & Antonucci, T. C. (1994). Gender differences in the link between marital support and satisfaction in older couples. *Journal of Personality and Social Psychology, 67,* 688–698.

Adelman, J., & Enguidanos, G. (Eds.). (1995). *Racism in the lives of women: Testimony, theory, and guides to antiracist practice.* New York: Harrington Park Press.

Adler, A. (1927). *The practice and theory of individual psychology.* New York: Harcourt Brace.

Adler, A. (1933). Advantages and disadvantages of the inferiority feeling. In H. L. Ansbacher & R. R. Ansbacher (Eds.), *Alfred Adler: Superiority and social interest.* Evanston, IL: Northwestern University Press.

Ainsworth, M. D. S. (1979). Infant–mother attachment. *American Psychologist, 34,* 932–937.

Ainsworth, M. D. S. (1989). Attachments beyond infancy. *American Psychologist, 44,* 709–716.

Albee, G. W. (1977). Problems in living are not sicknesses. *Clinical Psychologist, 30,* 5–6.

Albee, G. W. (1980). Competency model must replace the defect model. In L. A. Bond & J. C. Rosen (Eds.), *Competence and coping during adulthood.* Hanover, NH: Published for the Vermont Conference on the Primary Prevention of Psychopathology by the University Press of New England.

Aldwin, C. M. (1994). *Stress, coping, and development: An integrative perspective.* New York: Guilford.

Allen, L. R., & Britt, D. W. (1983). *Social class, mental health, and mental illness: The impact of resources and feedback in preventative psychology: Theory, research and practice.* New York: Pergamon Press.

Allison, J. A., & Wrightsman, L. S. (1993). *Rape: The misunderstood crime.* Newbury Park, CA: Sage.

Allport, G. W. (1937). *Personality: A psychological interpretation.* New York: Holt, Rinehart & Winston.

Allport, G. W. (1961). *Pattern and growth in personality.* New York: Holt, Rinehart & Winston.

American Psychiatric Association. (1952). *Diagnostic and statistical manual of mental disorders.* Washington, DC: Author.

American Psychiatric Association. (1968). *Diagnostic and statistical manual of mental disorders* (2nd ed.). Washington, DC: Author.

American Psychiatric Association. (1980). *Diagnostic and statistical manual of mental disorders* (3rd ed.). Washington, DC: Author.

American Psychiatric Association. (1994). *Diagnostic and statistical manual of mental disorders* (4th ed.). Washington, DC: Author.

American National Red Cross. (1931). *Relief work in the drought of 1930–1931: Official report of operations of the American National Red Cross.* Washington, DC: Author.

Amirkhian, J. H. (1990). A factor analytically derived measure of coping: The coping strategy indicator. *Journal of Personality and Social Psychology, 59,* 1066–1074.

Aneshensel, C. S. (1992). Social stress: Theory and research. In J. Blake & J. Hagan (Eds.), *Annual review of sociology* (pp. 15–38). Palo Alto, CA: Annual Reviews.

Antonovsky, A. (1979). *Health, stress, and coping.* San Francisco: Jossey-Bass.

Aponte, J. F., Rivers, R. Y., & Wohl, J. (1995). *Psychological interventions and cultural diversity.* Boston: Allyn & Bacon.

Arberry, A. J. (Trans.). (1955). *The Koran Interpreted.* New York: Simon & Schuster.

Argyle, M., & Henderson, M. (1984). The rules of friendship. *Journal of Social and Personal Relationships, 1,* 211–237.

Argyle, M., & Henderson, M. (1985). *The anatomy of relationships.* London: Heinemann.

Aspinwall, L. G., & Taylor, S. E. (1992). Modeling cognitive adaption: A longitudinal investigation of the impact of individual differences and coping on college adjustment and performance. *Journal of Personality and Social Psychology, 63,* 989–1003.

Aspinwall, L. G., & Taylor, S. E. (1997). A stitch in time: Self regulation and proactive coping. *Psychological Bulletin, 121,* 417–436.

Aspy, D., & Roebuck, F. (1974). From human ideas to humane technology and back again, many times. *Education, 95,* 163–171.

Atherton, H. M., (1961). *The cattle kings.* Bloomington: Indiana University Press.

Atherton, H. M., & Barlow, J. J. (1991). *The Bill of rights and beyond.* Washington, DC: Commission on the Bicentennial of the United States Constitution.

Baltes, P. B. (1987). Theoretical propositions of life-span developmental psychology: On the dynamics between growth and decline. *Developmental Psychology, 23,* 611–626.

Baltes, P. B. (1991). The many faces of human aging: Toward a psychological culture of old age. *Psychological Medicine, 21,* 837–854.

Baltes, P. B. (1994). *On the overall landscape of human development.* Invited address at the 102nd annual convention of the American Psychological Association, Los Angeles.

Baltes, P. B. (1997). On the incomplete architecture of human ontogeny: Selection, optimization, and compensation as foundation of developmental theory. *American Psychologist, 52,* 366–380.

Baltes, M. M., & Baltes, P. B. (1982). Microanalytic research on environmental factors and plasticity in psychological aging. In T. M. Field, A. Huston, H. C. Quay, C. Troll, & G. E. Finley (Eds.), *Review of human development* (pp. 524–539). New York: Wiley.

Baltes, M. M., & Baltes, P. B. (1990). Psychological perspectives on successful aging: The model of selective optimization with compensation. In P. B. Baltes, & M. M. Baltes (Eds.), *Successful aging: Perspectives from the behavioral sciences* (pp. 1–34). New York: Cambridge University Press.

Bandura, A. (1982). Self-efficacy mechanism in human agency. *American Psychologist, 37,* 122–147.

Bandura, A. (1996). Reflections on human agency. In H. Georgas, M. Manthouli, E. Bessevegis, & A. Kokkevi (Eds.), *Contemporary psychology in Europe: Theory, research and applications.* Seattle, WA: Hogrefe & Huber.

Bandura, A. (1997). *Self efficacy: The exercise of control.* New York: W. H. Freeman.

Banfield, E. C. (1958). *The moral basis of a backward society.* Glencoe, IL: Free Press.

Barnett, R. C., Marshall, N. L., Raudenbush, S. W., & Brennan, R. T. (1993). Gender and the relationship between job experiences and psychological distress: A study of dual earner couples. *Journal of Personality and Social Psychology, 64,* 794–806.

Barrera, M. (1986). Distinctions between social support concepts, measures, and models. *American Journal of Community Psychology, 14,* 413–445.

Baruch, G. K., & Barnett, R. C. (1986). Role quality, multiple role involvement, and psychological well-being in midlife women. *Journal of Personality and Social Psychology, 51,* 578–585.

Baum, A., Fleming, R., & Davidson, L. (1983). Natural disaster and technological catastrophe. *Environment and Behavior, 15,* 333–354.

Baumeister, R. F. (1987). How the self became a problem: A psychological review of historical research. *Journal of Personality and Social Psychology, 52,* 163–176.

Baumeister, R. F. (1989). The optimal margin of illusion [Special issue: Self illusions: When are they adaptive?]. *Journal of Social and Clinical Psychology, 8,* 176–189.

Baumeister, R. F., Heatherton, T. F., & Tice, D. M. (1993). When ego threats lead to self-regulation failure: Negative consequences of high self-esteem. *Journal of Personality and Social Psychology, 64,* 141–156.

Bayer, R. (1988). *The health and safety of workers: Case studies in the politics of professional responsibility.* New York: Oxford University Press.

Beck, A. T., Ward, C. H., Mendelson, M., Mock, J., & Erbaug, J. (1961). An inventory for measuring depression. *Archives of General Psychiatry, 12,* 63–70.

Beehr, T. A., Johnson, L. B., & Nieva, R. (1995). Occupational stress: Coping of police and their spouses. *Journal of Organizational Behavior, 16,* 3–25.

Beresford, M. (1967). *New towns of the middle ages.* New York: Praeger.

Bergin, A., & Garfield, S. (Eds.). (1971). *Handbook of psychotherapy and behavior change: An empirical analysis.* New York: Wiley.

Berkman, L. F. (1977). *Social networks, host resistance and mortality: A follow-up study of Alameda county residents.* Unpublished doctoral dissertation, University of California, Berkeley.

Bettleheim, B. (1960). *The informed heart.* New York: Free Press.

Bhatnagar, D. (1988). Professional women in organizations: New paradigms for research and action. *Sex Roles, 18,* 221–227.

Billings, A. G., & Moos, R. H. (1984). Coping, stress and social resources among adults with unipolar depression. *Journal of Personality and Social Psychology, 46,* 877–891.

Binswanger, L. (1963). *Being-in-the-world: Selected papers of Ludwig Binswanger.* New York: Basic Books.

Blazer, D. (1989). Depression in late life: An update. *Annual Review of Gerontology and Geriatrics, 9,* 197–215.

Bledin, K., MacCarthy, B., Kuipers, L., & Woods, R. T. (1990). Daughters of people with dementia: Expressed emotion, strain and coping. *British Journal of Psychiatry, 157,* 221–227.

Blumberg, R. L. (Ed.). (1991). *Gender, family, and economy: The triple overlap.* Newbury Park, CA: Sage.

Bolger, N. (1990). Coping as a personality process: A prospective study. *Journal of Personality and Social Psychology, 59,* 525–537.

Bolger, N., DeLongis, A., Kessler, R. C., & Wethington, E. (1990). The microstructure of daily role-related stress in married couples. In J. Eckenrode & S. Gore (Eds.), *Stress between work and family: The Plenum series on stress and coping.* New York: Plenum Press.

Bolger, N., Vinokur, A., Foster, M., & Ng, R. (1996). Close relationships and adjustment to a life crisis: The case of breast cancer. *Journal of Personality and Social Psychology, 70,* 283–294.

Bowlby, J. (1980). Attachment and loss: Vol. 3. *Loss.* New York: Basic Books.

Brandt, D. E. (1993). Social distress and the police. *Journal of Social Distress and the Homeless, 2,* 305–313.

Brandtstädter, J. (1989). Personal self-regulation of development: Cross-sequential analyses of development-related control beliefs and emotions. *Developmental Psychology, 25,* 96–108.

Brandtstädter, J., & Greve, W. (1994). The aging self: Stabilizing and protective processes. *Developmental Review, 14,* 52–80.

Brandtstädter, J., & Wentura, D. (1995). Adjustment to shifting possibility frontiers in later life: Complementary adaptive modes. In R. A. Dixon & L. Backman (Eds.), *Compensating for psychological deficits and declines: Managing losses and promoting gains.* Hillsdale, NJ: Erlbaum.

Breznitz, S. (1983). Anticipatory stress reactions. In S. Breznitz (Ed.), *The denial of stress* (pp. 225–255). New York: International Universities Press.

Brody, E. M. (1990). *Women in the middle: their parent-care years.* New York: Springer.

Bromet, E. J. (1995). Methodological issues in designing research on community-wide disasters with special reference to Chernobyl. In S. E. Hobfoll & M. W. deVries (Eds.), *Extreme stress and communities: Impact and intervention.* Dordrecht, The Netherlands: Kluwer Academic Publishers.

Bronfenbrenner, U. (1977). Toward an experimental ecology of human development. *American Psychologist, 32,* 513–532.

Broverman, I. K., Broverman, D. M., Clarkson, F. E., Rosenkrantz, P. S., & Vogel, S. R. (1970). Sex role stereotypes and clinical judgments of mental health. *Journal of Consulting and Clinical Psychology, 34,* 1–7.

Brown, C. (1994). The impact of divorce on families. *Family and Conciliation Courts Review, 32,* 149–167.

Brown, G. W., & Harris, T. O. (1979). *The Bedford college life-events and difficulty schedule: Directory of severity for long-term difficulties.* London: Bedford College, University of London.

Brown, G. W., & Harris, T. O. (1989). *Life events and illness.* New York: Guilford.

Burke, R. J. (1988). Sources of managerial and professional stress in large organizations. In C. L. Cooper & R. Payne (Eds.), *Causes, coping and consequences of stress at work.* New York: Wiley.

Burke, R. J., & Richardsen, A. M. (1993). Psychological burnout in organizations. In R. T. Golembiewski (Ed.), *Handbook of organizational behavior.* New York: Marcel Dekker.

Burton, R. (1624). *Anatomy of melancholy,* London: Democritus Minor.

Buunk, B. P., Collins, R., Van Yperen, N. W., Taylor, S. E., & Dakoff, G. (1990). Upward and downward comparisons: Either direction has its ups and downs. *Journal of Personality and Social Psychology, 59,* 1238–1249.

Buunk, B. P., Schaufeli, W. B., & Ybema, J. F. (1990). *Occupational burnout: A social comparison perspective.* Paper presented at the ENOP Conference on Professional Burnout, Krakow, Poland.

Cannon, W. B. (1932). *The wisdom of the body.* New York: Norton.

Cantor, N. (1990). From thought to behavior: "Having" and "doing" in the study of personality and cognition. *American Psychologist, 45,* 735–750.

Caplan, G. (1964). *Principles of preventative psychiatry.* New York: Basic Books.

Caplan, G. (1974). *Support systems and community mental health.* New York: Behavioral Publications.

Carroll, L. (1866). *Alice's adventures in wonderland.* London: Macmillan & Company.

Carver, C. S. (1993). *Coping with Hurricane Andrew.* Paper presented at the 15th International Conference of the Stress and Anxiety Research Society, Madrid, Spain.

Carver, C. S., Scheier, M. F., & Weintraub, J. K. (1989). Assessing coping strategies: A theoretically-based approach. *Journal of Personality and Social Psychology, 56,* 267–283.

Cassel, J. (1974). An epidemiological perspective on psychosocial factors in disease etiology. *American Journal of Public Health, 64,* 1040–1043.

Caughey, J. (1948). *The California gold rush.* Berkeley: University of California Press.

Chapman, H. A., Hobfoll, S. E., & Ritter, C. (1997). Partner's stress underestimations lead to women's distress: A study of pregnant inner-city women. *Journal of Personality and Social Psychology, 73,* 418–425.

Cherniss, C. (1990). *Organizational negotiation skill and the prevention of burnout: Lessons of a long-term follow-up study.* Paper presented at the 98th Annual Convention of the American Psychological Association, Boston.

Cherniss, C., & Krantz, D. L. (1983). The ideological community as an antidote to burnout in the human services. In B. Farber (Ed.), *Stress and burnout in the human service professions* (pp. 198–212). New York: Pergamon Press.

Choi, S. (1994). *Shimjung psychology: The indigenous Korean perspective.* Paper presented at the Workshop on Asian Psychologies: Indigenous, social and cultural perspectives. Chung-Ang University, Seoul, Korea.

Claassen, H. (1960). *Ronald encyclopedia of football.* New York: Ronald Press.

Clark, M. S. (1983). Reactions to aid in communal and exchange relationships. In J. D. Fisher, A. Nadler, & B. M. DePaulo (Eds.), *New directions in helping* (Vol. 1). New York: Academic Press.

Clark, M. S., & Mills, J. (1979). Interpersonal attraction in exchange and communal relationships. *Journal of Personality and Social Psychology, 37,* 12–24.

Clark, M. S., Mills, J., & Powell, M. C. (1986). Keeping track of needs in communal and exchange relationships. *Journal of Personality and Social Psychology, 51,* 333–338.

Cohen, S., & Hoberman, H. M. (1983). Positive events and social supports as buffers of life change stress. *Journal of Applied Social Psychology, 13,* 99–125.

Cohen, S., & Wills, T. A. (1985). Stress, social support, and the buffering hypothesis. *Psychological Bulletin, 98,* 310–357.

Collins, L., & Lapeirre, D. (1972). *O'Jerusalem!.* New York: Simon & Schuster.

Colvin, C. R., & Block, J. (1994). Do positive illusions foster mental health. An examination of the Taylor and Brown formulation. *Psychological Bulletin, 116,* 3–20.

Colvin, C. R., Block, J., & Funder, D. (1995). Overly positive self-evaluations and reality: Negative implications for mental health. *Journal of Personality and Social Psychology, 68,* 1152–1162.

Compas, B. E., Forsythe, C. J., & Wagner, B. M. (1988). Consistency and variability in causal attributions and coping with stress. *Cognitive Therapy and Research, 12,* 305–320.

Conger, R. D., Lorenz, R. O., Elder, G. H., Simons, R. L., & Ge, X. (1993). Husband and wife differences in response to undesirable life events. *Journal of Health and Social Behavior, 34,* 71–88.

Conolly, J. (1856). *The treatment of the insane without mechanical restraints.* London: Smith, Elder.

Cooley, C. H. (1909). *Social organization: A study of the larger mind.* New York: C. Scribner's Sons.

Corbett, T. (1982). Ethics and environmental health. In J. Lee & W. Rom (Eds.), *Legal and ethical dilemmas in occupational health.* Ann Arbor, MI: Ann Arbor Science.

Costa, P. T., & McCrae, R. R. (1990). Personality: Another "hidden factor" in stress research. *Psychological Inquiry, 1,* 22–24.

Cowen, E. L. (1983). Primary prevention in mental health: Past, present and future. In R. D. Felner, L. A. Jason, J. N. Moritsugu, & S. S. Farber (Eds.), *Preventive psychology: Theory, research and practice.* New York: Pergamon Press.

Coyne, J. C. (1976). Toward an interactional description of depression. *Psychiatry, 39,* 28–40.

Coyne, J. C., & Downey, G. (1991). Social factors and psychopathology: Stress, social support, and coping processes. *Annual Review of Psychology, 42,* 401–425.

Coyne, J. C., & Smith, D. A. F. (1991). Couples coping with a myocardial infarction: A contextual perspective on wives' distress. *Journal of Personality and Social Psychology, 61,* 404–412.

Cozzarelli, C. (1993). Personality and self-efficacy as predictors of coping with abortion. *Journal of Personality and Social Psychology, 65,* 124–126.

Cronkite, R. C., & Moos, R. H. (1984). The role of predisposing and moderating factors in the stress–illness relationship. *Journal of Health and Social Behavior, 25,* 372–393.

Cutrona, C. (1990). Stress and social support: In search of optimal matching. *Journal of Social and Clinical Psychology, 9,* 3–14.

Cutrona, C., & Russell, D. (1990). Type of social support and specific stress: Toward a theory of optimal matching. In B. Sarason, I. Sarason, & G. Pierce (Eds.), *Social support: An interactional view.* New York: Wiley.

Darwin, C. (1845). *The voyage of the beagle.* Danbury, CT: Grolier. (Reprinted in 1988)

Darwin, C. (1859). *The origin of species: By means of natural selection or the preservation of favoured races in the struggle for life.* New York: New American Library.

deJong, J. (1995). Prevention of the consequences of man-made or natural disaster at the (inter) national, the community, the family, and the individual level. In S. E. Hobfoll & M. W. deVries (Eds.), *Extreme stress and communities: Impact and intervention* (pp. 207–228). Dordrecht, The Netherlands: Kluwer Academic Publishers.

DeLeon, D. (1978). *The American as anarchist: Reflections on indigenous radicalism.* Baltimore: Johns Hopkins University Press.

Depue, R. A., & Monroe, S. M. (1986). Conceptualization and measurement of human disorders in life stress research: The problem of chronic disturbance. *Psychological Bulletin, 1,* 36–51.

DeSilva, P. (1993). Buddhist psychology: A therapeutic perspective. In U. Kim & J. Berry (Eds.), *Indigenous psychologies: Research and experience in cultural context* (Vol. 17). Newbury Park, CA: Sage.

deVries, M. W. (1995). Culture, community and catastrophe: Issues in understanding communities under difficult conditions. In S. E. Hobfoll & M. W. deVries (Eds.), *Extreme stress and communities: Impact and intervention.* Dordrecht, The Netherlands: Kluwer Academic Publishers.

Diener, E. (1994). Assessing subjective well-being: Progress and opportunities. *Social Indicators Research, 28,* 35–89.

Diener, E., Diener, M., & Diener, C. (1995). Factors predicting the subjective well-being of nations. *Journal of Personality and Social Psychology, 69,* 851–864.

Diener, E., & Fujita, F. (1995). Resources, personal strivings, and subjective well-being: A nomothetic and idiographic approach. *Journal of Personality and Social Psychology, 68,* 926–935.

Dohrenwend, B. S., and Dohrenwend, B. P. (1974). A brief historical introduction to research on stressful life events. In B. S. Dohrenwend & B. P. Dohrenwend (Eds.), *Stressful life events: Their nature and effects.* New York: Wiley.

Dohrenwend, B. S., Dohrenwend, B. P., Dodson, M., & Shrout, P. E. (1984). Symptoms, hassles, social support, and life events: Problem of confounded measures. *Journal of Abnormal Psychology, 93,* 222–230.

Dohrenwend, B. B., Raphael, K. G., Schwartz, S., Stueve, A., & Skodol, A. (1993). The structured event probe and narrative rating method for measuring stressful life events. In L. Goldberger & S. Breznitz (Eds.), *Handbook of stress: Theoretical and clinical aspects* (2nd ed., pp. 174–199). New York: Free Press.

Downs, R. F. (Ed.). (1970). *Japan yesterday and today.* New York: Praeger.

Dressler, W. W. (1985). Extended family relationships, social support, and mental health in a southern black community. *Journal of Health and Social Behavior, 26,* 39–48.

Duck, S. (Ed.). (1990). *Personal relationships and social support.* Newbury Park, CA: Sage.

Dunahoo, C. L., C. L., Geller, P., & Hobfoll, S. E. (1996). Women's coping: Communal versus individualistic orientation. In M. J. Schabracq, J. A. M. Winnubst, & C. L. Cooper (Eds.), *Handbook of work and health psychology.* Chichester, UK: Wiley.

Dunahoo, C. L., Hobfoll, S. E., Monnier, J., Hulsizer, M. R., & Johnson, R. (1998). Even the Lone Ranger had Tonto: There's more than rugged individualism in coping. *Anxiety, Stress, and Coping, 11,* 137–165.

Dunkel-Schetter, C., Folkman, S., & Lazarus, R. S. (1987). Correlates of social support receipt. *Journal of Personality and Social Psychology, 53,* 71–80.

Durkheim, E. (1952). *Le suicide: Suicide, a study in sociology.* Glencoe, IL: Free Press. (Original published 1897)

Dylan, B. (1964). Lonesome death of Hattie Carroll. On *Bob Dylan: Times they are a-changin'* [cassette]. Los Angeles: Warner Chapel Music.

Eagly, A. H. (1987). *Sex differences in social behavior: A social-role interpretation.* Hillsdale, NJ: Erlbaum.

Eagly, A. H. (1995). The science and politics of comparing women and men. *American Psychologist, 50,* 145–158.

Eckenrode, J. (Ed.). (1991). *The social context of coping.* New York: Plenum Press.

Eckenrode, J., & Gore, S. (1981). Stressful events and social supports: The significance of context. In B. Gottlieb (Ed.), *Social networks and social support.* Beverly Hills, CA: Sage.

Eckenrode, J., & Wethington, E. (1990). The process and outcome of mobilizing social support. In S. Duck (Ed.), *Personal relationships and social support.* Beverly Hills: Sage.

Edwards, J. R., Baglioni, A. J., & Cooper, C. L. (1990). Stress, type-A, coping and psychological and physical symptoms: A multi-sample test of alternative models. *Human Relations, 43,* 919–956.

Eliot, C. W. (Ed.). (1980). *The sayings of Confucius: Sacred writings: Confucian, Hebrew, Christian, Part I.* Danbury, CT: Grolier.

Eliot, C. W. (1989). Essays: *English and American.* Danbury, CT: Grolier.

Ellis, A., & Greiger, R. (1977). *Handbook of rational emotive therapy.* New York: Julian Press.

Elting, J. (1963). *Dare call it treason.* New York: Simon & Schuster.

Emerson, R. W. (1841). *Essays and English traits.* Danbury, CT: Grolier.

Endler, N., & Parker, J. D. A. (1990). Multidimensional assessment of coping: A critical evaluation. *Journal of Personality and Social Psychology, 58,* 844–854.

Ensel, M. W., & Lin, N. (1991). The life stress paradigm and psychological distress. *Journal of Health and Social Behavior, 32,* 321–341.

Erikson, E. H. (1968). *Identify youth and crisis.* New York: Norton.

Erikson, R. C., & Hyerstay, B. J. (1980). Historical perspectives on treatment of the mentally ill. In M. S. Gibbs, J. R. Lachenmeyer & J. Sigal (Eds.), *Community psychology: Theoretical and empirical approaches.* New York: Gardner.

Etzioni, A. (1994). *The spirit of community: The reinvention of American society.* New York: Touchstone.

Etzioni, A. (1997). *The new golden rule: Community and morality in a democratic society.* New York: Basic Books.

Ezrahi, Y. (1985). *Burnout in military officers ranks: A construct validation.* Unpublished dissertation, Tel Aviv, Tel Aviv University.

Fagenson, E. (1993). *Women in management: Trends, issues and challenges in managerial diversity* (Vol. 4). Newbury Park, CA: Sage.

Felner, R. D., Ginter, M. A., & Primavera, J. (1982). Primary prevention during school transitions: Social support and environmental structure. *American Journal of Community Psychology, 10,* 227–290.

Feng, G. F., & English, J. (Trans.). (1972). *Tao Te Ching.* New York: Random House.

Figley, C. R. (Ed.). (1978). *Stress disorders among Vietnam veterans: Theory, research and treatment.* New York: Brunner/Mazel.

Figley, C. R., & Leventman, S. (Eds.) (1980). *Strangers at home: Vietnam veterans since the war.* New York: Praeger.

Fisher, J. D., Nadler, A., & Whitcher-Alagna, S. (1982). Recipient reactions to aid. *Psychological Bulletin, 91,* 27–54.

Fisher, S. (1984). *Stress and the perception of control.* London: Erlbaum.

Folkman, S., & Lazarus, R. S. (1980). An analysis of coping in a middle-aged community sample. *Journal of Health and Social Behavior, 21,* 219–239.

Foucault, M. (1965). *Madness and civilization: A history of insanity in the age of reason* (Trans. Richard Howard). New York: Random House.

Foucault, M. (1970). *The order of things: an archaeology of the human sciences.* New York: Random House.

Foucault, M. (1980). *Power/knowledge: Selected interviews and other writings, 1972–1977.* New York: Pantheon.

Francis, C. E. (1955). *The Tuskegee airmen: The story of the Negro in the U.S. Air Force.* Boston: Bruce Humphries.

Frankl, V. E. (1963). *Man's search for meaning.* Boston: Beacon.

Frantz, J. B., & Choate, J. E. (1955). *The American cowboy: Myth and reality.* Norman: University of Oklahoma Press.

Freedy, J. R., & Hobfoll, S. E. (1994). Stress inoculation for reduction of burnout: A conservation of resources approach. *Anxiety, Stress and Coping: An International Journal, 6,* 311–325.

Freedy, J. R., & Hobfoll, S. E. (Eds.). (1994). *Traumatic stress: From theory to practice.* New York: Plenum Press.

Freedy, J. R., Resnick, H. S., & Kilpatrick, D. G. (1992). Conceptual framework for evaluating disaster impact: Implications for clinical intervention. In L. S. Austin (Ed.), *Responding to disaster: A guide for mental health professionals* (pp. 3–23. Washington, DC: American Psychiatric Association Press.

Freedy, J. R., Saladin, M. E., Kilpatrick, D. G., Resnick, H. S., & Saunders, B. E. (1994). Understanding acute psychological distress following natural disaster. *Journal of Traumatic Stress, 7,* 257–273.

French, J. R. P., Jr., Caplan, R. D., & Van Harrison, R. V. (1982). *The mechanisms of job stress and strain.* Chichester, UK: Wiley.

French, J. R. P., Jr.,, Rodgers, W. L., & Cobb, S. (1974). Adjustment as person–environment fit. In B. V. Coelho, D. A. Hamburg, & J. E. Adams (Eds.), *Coping and adaptation.* New York: Basic Books.

Freud, A. (1958). Adolescence. *Psychoanalytic Study of the Child, 13,* 255–278.

Freud, S. (1961). The unconscious. In J. Strachey (Ed.), *The standard edition of the complete psychological works of Sigmund Freud* (Vol. 14). London: Hogarth Press. (Original published 1915)

Freud S. (1963). Introductory lectures on psychoanalysis. In J. Strachey (Ed.), *The standard edition of the complete psychological works of Sigmund Freud* (Vols. 15 and 16). London: Hogarth Press. (First German edition, 1917)

Friedland, N., Keinan, G., & Regev, Y. (1992). Controlling the uncontrollable: Effects of stress on illusory perceptions of controllability. *Journal of Personality and Social Psychology, 63,* 923–931.

Fukuyama, F. (1992). *The end of history and the last man.* New York: Avon Books.

Fukuyama, F. (1995). *Trust: The social virtues and the creation of prosperity.* New York: Free Press.

Gallant, S. J., & Derry, P. S. (1995). Menarche, menstruation, and menopause: Psychosocial research and future directions. In A. L. Stanton & S. J. Gallant (Eds.), *The psychology of women's health.* Washington, DC: American Psychological Association.

Gambino, W. M. (1968). *Introduction to Nietzsche the thinker: A study.* New York: Frederick Ungar.

Garrison, M. (1994). The economic consequences of divorce. *Family and Conciliation Courts Review, 32,* 10–26.

Geertz, C. (1973). *Interpretation of cultures.* New York: Basic Books.

Geller, P., & Hobfoll, S. E. (1993). Gender differences in pregerence to offer social support to assertive men and women. *Sex Roles, 28,* 419–432.

Geller, P., & Hobfoll, S. E. (1994). Gender differences in job stress, tedium and social support in the workplace. *Journal of Social and Personal Relationships, 11,* 555–572.

Gerth, H. H., & Mills, C. W. (1946). *From Max Weber: Essays in sociology.* New York: Oxford University Press.

Giel, R. (1990). Psychosocial processes in disasters. *International Journal of Mental Health, 19*, 7–20.

Gilligan, C. (1982). *In a different voice: Psychological theory and women's development.* Cambridge, MA: Harvard University Press.

Glidewell, J. C. (1987). Induced change and stability in psychological and social systems. *American Journal of Community Psychology, 15*, 741–772.

Goffman, E. (1963). *Stigma.* Englewood Cliffs, NJ: Prentice-Hall.

Golembiewski, R., Scherb, K., & Boudreau, R. (1993). Burnout in cross-national settings: Generic and model-specific perspectives. In W. Schaefeli, C. Maslach, & T. Marek (Eds.), *Professional burnout: Recent developments in theory and research.* Washington, DC: Taylor & Francis.

Golovine, N. N. (1931). *The Russian army in the World War.* New Haven, CT: Yale University Press.

Goode, W. J. (1974). A theory of role strain. *American Sociological Review, 25*, 483–496.

Gotlib, I. H., & Hooley, J. M. (1988). Depression and marital distress: Current status and future direction. In Steve Duck (Ed.), *Handbook of personal relationships: Theory, research and interventions.* Chichester, UK: Wiley.

Gotlib, I. H., & Whiffen, V. E. (1989). Depression and marital functioning: An examination of specificity and gender differences. *Journal of Abnormal Psychology, 98*, 23–30.

Gottman, J. M. (1979). *Marital interaction: Experimental investigations.* New York: Academic Press.

Grant, J. (1988). Women as managers: What they can offer to organizations. *Organizational Dynamics, 16*, 56–63.

Green, B. C., Lindy, J. D., Grace, M. C., Gleser, G. C., Leonard, A. C., Korse, M., & Winget, C. (1990). Buffalo Creek survivors in the second decade: Stability of stress symptoms. *American Journal of Orthopsychiatry, 60*, 43–54.

Green, B. L. (1995). Long-term consequences of disasters. In S. E. Hobfoll & M. W. deVries (Eds.), *Extreme stress and communities: Impact and intervention.* Dordrecht, The Netherlands: Kluwer Academic Publishers.

Greenberg, A. (1979). *Artists and revolution: Dada and the bauhaus, 1917–1925.* Ann Arbor, MI: University Microfilms International.

Greenglass, E. (1985). Psychological implications of sex bias in the workplace. *Academic Psychology Bulletin, 7*, 227–240.

Greenglass, E. (1987). Anger in type A women: Implications for coronary heart disease. *Personality and Individual Differences, 8*, 639–650.

Greenglass, E. (1993). Social support and coping of employed women. In B. C. Long & S. E. Kahn (Eds.), *Women, work and coping: A multidisciplinary approach to workplace stress.* Montreal: McGill–Queen's University Press.

Grinker, R. R., & Spiegel, J. P. (1945). *Men under stress.* Philadelphia: McGraw-Hill.

Guisinger, S., & Blatt, S. J. (1994). Individuality and relatedness: Evolution of a fundamental dialectic. *American Psychologist, 49*, 104–111.

Haan, N. (1993). The assessment of coping defense and stress. In L. Goldberger & S. Breznitz (Eds.), *Handbook of stress: Theoretical and clinical aspects* (2nd ed., pp. 258–273). New York: Free Press.

Hall, G. C., & Barongan, C. (1997). Prevention of sexual aggression: Sociocultural risk and protective factors. *American Psychologist, 52*, 5–14.

Hamaguchi, E. (1977). Nihonrashisa no saihakken [A rediscovery of Japaneseness]. Tokyo: Nihon Keizai Shinbunsha.

Hardin, G. (1968). The tragedy of the commons. In J. L. Coleman (Ed.), *Private law theory* (Vol. 5). New York: Garland.

Harmon, D. K., Masuda, M., & Holmes, T. H. (1970). The social readjustment rating scale: A cross-cultural study of Western Europeans and Americans. *Journal of Psychosomatic Research, 14*, 391–400.

Hayes, H. R., & Emshoff, J. G. (1993). Substance abuse and family violence. In R. L. Hampton,

T. P. Gullotta, G. R. Adams, E. H. Potter, & R. P. Weissberg (Eds.), *Family violence: Prevention and treatment* (pp. 281–310). Newbury Park, CA: Sage.

Hazan, C., & Shaver, P. (1987). Romantic love conceptualized as an attachment process. *Journal of Personality and Social Psychology, 52,* 511–524.

Hazan, C., & Shaver, P. (1994). Attachment as an organizational framework for research on close relationships. *Psychological Inquiry, 5,* 1–22.

Herman, J. L. (1981). *Father–daughter incest.* Cambridge, MA: Harvard University Press.

Hertz, J. H. (Ed.). (1958). *The Pentateach and haftorahs.* London: Soncino Press.

Herzog, C. (1984). *The Arab–Israeli wars: War and peace in the Middle East from the War of Independence to Lebanon.* London: Arms & Armour Press.

Hinkle, L. E., Jr. (1977). The concept of "stress" in the biological and social sciences. In Z. J. Lipowski, D. R. Lipsitt, & P. C. Whybrow (Eds.), *Psychosomatic medicine: Current trends and clinical implications.* New York: Oxford University Press.

Hinkle, L. E., Jr. (1977). Measurement of the effects of the environment upon the health of behavior of people. In L. E. Hinkle, Jr., & W. C. Loring (Eds.), *The effect of the man-made environment of health and behavior.* Atlanta: Center for Disease Control, Public Health Service.

Hirsch, B. J. (1980). Natural support systems and coping with major life changes. *American Journal of Community Psychology, 8,* 159–172.

Hobfoll, S. E. (1985a). The limitations of social support in the stress process. In I. G. Sarason & B. R. Sarason (Eds.), *Social support: Theory, research and application* (pp. 391–414). The Hague, The Netherlands: Martinus Nijhoff.

Hobfoll, S. E. (1985b). Personal and social resources and the ecology of stress resistance. In P. Shaver (Ed.), *Review of personality and social psychology* (Vol. 6, pp. 265–290). Beverly Hills, CA: Sage.

Hobfoll, S. E. (1986). *Stress, social support and women.* Washington, DC: Hemisphere.

Hobfoll, S. E. (1988). *The ecology of stress.* New York: Hemisphere.

Hobfoll, S. E. (1989). Conservation of resources: A new attempt at conceptualizing stress. *American Psychologist, 44,* 513–524.

Hobfoll, S. E. (1991). Traumatic stress: A theory based on rapid loss of resources. *Anxiety Research: An International Journal, 4,* 187–197.

Hobfoll, S. E., Briggs, S., & Wells, J. (1995). Community stress and resources: Actions and reactions. In S. E. Hobfoll & M. W. deVries (Eds.), *Extreme stress and communities: Impact and intervention.* Dordrecht: The Netherlands: Kluwer Academic Publishers.

Hobfoll, S. E., Dunahoo, C. L., Ben-Porath, Y., & Monnier, J. (1994). Gender and coping: The dual-axis model of coping. *American Journal of Community Psychology, 22,* 49–82.

Hobfoll, S. E., & Hobfoll, I. H. (1994). *Work won't love you back.* New York: W. H. Freeman.

Hobfoll, S. E., & Lerman, M. (1989). Personal relationships, personal attitudes, and stress resistance: Mother's reactions to their child's illness. *American Journal of Community Psychology, 16,* 565–589.

Hobfoll, S. E., & Lilly, R. S. (1993). Resource conservation as a strategy for community psychology *Journal of Community Psychology, 21,* 128–148.

Hobfoll, S. E., Lilly, R. S., & Jackson, A. P. (1992). Conservation of social resources and the self. In H. O. F. Veiel & U. Baumann (Eds.), *The meaning and measurement of social support.* Washington, DC: Hemisphere.

Hobfoll, S. E., & London, P. (1986). The relationship of self-concept and social support to emotional distress among women during war. *Journal of Social and Clinical Psychology, 4,* 189–203.

Hobfoll, S. E., Morgan, R., & Lehrman, R. (1980). Development of a training center in an Eskimor village. *Journal of Community Development, 15,* 146–148.

Hobfoll, S. E., & Shirom, A. (1993). Stress and burnout in the workplace: Conservation of resources. In R. T. Golembiewski (Ed.), *Handbook of organizational behavior.* New York: Marcel Dekker.

Hobfoll, S. E., Shoham, S. B., & Ritter, C. (1991). Women's satisfaction with social support and their receipt of aid. *Journal of Personality and Social Psychology, 61,* 332–341.

Hobfoll, S. E., & Spielberger, C. D. (1992). Family stress: Integrating theory and measurement. *Journal of Family Psychology, 6,* 99–112.

Hobfoll, S. E., & Stokes, J. P. (1988). The process and mechanics of social support. In S. Duck, D. F. Hay, S. E. Hobfoll, W. Ickes, & B. M. Montgomery (Eds.), *Handbook of personal relationships: Theory, research and interventions.* Chichester, UK: Wiley.

Hobfoll, S. E., & Walfisch, S. (1984). Coping with a threat to life: A longitudinal study of self-concept, social support, and psychological stress. *American Journal of Community Psychology, 12,* 87–100.

Hochschild, A. (1989). *The second shift: Working parents and the revolution at home.* New York: Viking.

Holahan, C. H., & Moos, R. H. (1986). Personality, coping and family resources in stress resistance: A longitudinal analysis. *Journal of Personality and Social Psychology, 51,* 389–395.

Holahan, C. J., & Moos, R. H. (1987). Personal and contextual determinants of coping strategies. *Journal of Personality and Social Psychology, 52,* 946–955.

Holahan, C. J., & Moos, R. H. (1991). Life stressors, personal and social resources and depression: A four-year structural model. *Journal of Abnormal Psychology, 100,* 31–38.

Holahan, C. J., Moos, R. H., Holahan, C. K., & Brennan, P. L. (1997). Social context, coping strategies and depressive symptoms: An expanded model with cardiac patients. *Journal of Personality and Social Psychology, 72,* 918–928.

Holmes, T. H. (1989). Quantifying social experiences. In T. H. Holmes & E. M. David (Eds.), *Life change, life events and illness.* New York: Praeger.

Holmes, T. H., & Rahe, R. H. (1967). The social readjustment rating scale. *Journal of Psychosomatic Research, 11,* 213–218.

Horney, K. (1937). *The neurotic personality of our time.* New York: Norton.

Horney, K. (1950). *Neurosis and human growth: The struggle toward self-realization.* New York: Norton.

Hsu, F. (1963). *Clan, caste and club.* New York: Van Nostrand.

Hsu, F. (1971). *Under the ancestors' shadow: Kinship, personality and social mobility in China.* Stanford, CA: Stanford University Press.

International Federation of Red Cross and Red Crescent Societies. (1993). *World disaster report, 1993.* The Hague: The Netherlands: Martinus Nijhoff.

Ironson, G., Wynings, C., Schneiderman, N., Baum, A., Rodriguez, M., Greenwood, D., Benight, C., Antoni, M., La Perriere, A., Huang, H. S., Klimas, N., & Fletcher, M. A. (1997). Posttraumatic stress symptoms, intrusive thoughts, loss, and immune function following Hurricane Andrew. *Psychosomatic Medicine, 59,* 128–141.

Iscoe, I. (1974). Community psychology and the competent community. *American Psychologist, 29,* 607–613.

Janoff-Bulman, R. (1992). *Shattered assumptions.* New York: Free Press.

Jason, L. A., Anes, M. D., & Birkhead, S. H. (1991). Active enforcement of cigarette control laws in the prevention of cigarette smoking. *Journal of the American Medical Association, 266,* 3159–3161.

Jason, L. A., & Bogat, G. A. (1983). Preventive behavioral interventions. In R. D. Felner, L. A. Jason, J. N. Moritsugu, & S. S. Farber (Eds.), *Preventive psychology: Theory, research and practice.* New York: Pergamon Press.

Jason, L. A., McMahon, S. D., Salina, P., & Hedeker, D. (1995). Assessing a smoking cessation intervention involving groups, incentives and self-help manuals. *Behavior Therapy, 26,* 393–408.

Jenner, W. (1992). *The tyranny of history: The roots of China's crisis.* London: Allen Lane.

Jerusalem, M. (1993). Personal resources, environmental constraints and adaptational processes: The predictive power of a theoretical stress model. *Personality and Individual Differences, 14,* 15–24.

Johnson, R., Hobfoll, S. E., & Zalcberg-Linetzy, A. (1993). Social support knowledge and behavior and relations intimacy: A dyadic study. *Journal of Family Psychology, 6,* 266–277.

Kahneman, E. (1973). *Attention and effort.* Englewood Cliffs, NJ: Prentice-Hall.

Kahneman, D., & Tversky, A. (1979). Prospect theory: An analysis of decision under risk. *Econometrica, 47,* 263–291.

Kamin, L. J. (1974). *The science and politics of I.Q..* Potomac, MD: Erlbaum.

Kaniasty, K., & Norris, F. (1993). A test of the social support deterioration model in the context of natural disaster. *Journal of Personality and Social Psychology, 64,* 395–408.

Kaniasty, K., & Norris, F. (1997). The experience of disaster: Individuals and communities sharing trauma. In R. Gist & B. Lubin (Eds.), *Response to disaster: Psychosocial, ecological and community approaches.* Washington, DC: Taylor & Francis.

Kaniasty, K., Norris, F., & Murrell, S. A. (1990). Received and perceived social support following natural disaster. *Journal of Applied Social Psychology, 20,* 85–114.

Kanter, R. M. (1968). Commitment and social organization. *American Sociological Review, 33,* 499–517.

Kaplan, H. B. (1983). Psychological distress in sociological context: Toward a general theory of psychosocial stress. In H. B. Kaplan (Ed.), *Psychosocial stress: Trends in theory and research* (pp. 195–264). New York: Academic Press.

Kaplan, H. (1996). *Psychosocial stress: Perspective on structure, theory, life course and methods,* San Diego, CA: Academic Press.

Kashima, Y., Yamaguchi, S., Kim, U., Choi, S., Gelfand, M. J., & Yuhi, M. (1995). Culture, gender and self: A perspective from individualism–collectivism research. *Journal of Personality and Social Psychology, 69,* 925–937.

Kasl, S. V. (1978). Epidemiological contributions to the study of work stress. In C. L. Cooper & R. Payne (Eds.), *Stress at work.* Chichester, UK: Wiley.

Kaufmann, G. M., & Beehr, T. A. (1989). Occupational stressors, individual strains, and social supports among police officers. *Human Relations, 42,* 185–197.

Kearns, J. (1986). Stress at work: The challenge of change. BUPA Series. *The Management of Health, I: Stress and the city.* London: BUPA.

Keinan, G. (1987). Decision making under stress: Scanning of alternatives under controllable and uncontrollable threats. *Journal of Personality and Social Psychology, 152,* 639–644.

Keinan, G. (1994). Effects of stress and tolerance of ambiguity on magical thinking. *Journal of Personality and Social Psychology, 67,* 48–55.

Kellett, A. (1982). *Combat motivation: The behavior of soldiers in combat.* Boston: Kluwer Nijhoff.

Kelley, H. H. (1979). *Personal relationships: Their structures and processes.* Hillsdale, NJ: Erlbaum.

Kelley, H. H., & Thibaut, W. (1978). *Interpersonal relations: A theory of independence.* New York: Wiley–Interscience.

Kelly, J. G. (1966). Ecological constraints on mental health services. *American Psychologist, 21,* 535–539.

Kelly, J. G. (1988). *A guide to conducting prevention research in the community: First steps.* New York: Haworth.

Kessler, R. C., McLeod, J. D., & Wethington, E. (1985). The costs of caring: A perspective on the relationship between sex and psychological distress. In I. G. Sarason & C. R. Sarason (Eds.), *Social support: Theory, research and application.* The Hague, The Netherlands: Martinus Nijhoff.

Kessler, R. C., Turner, J. B., Blake, J., & House, J. S. (1988). Effects of unemployment on health in a community survey: Mai, Modifying and mediating effects. *Journal of Social Issues, 44*, 69–85.

Kidd, M. (1991). The children of Chernobyl. *Medical Journal of Australia, 155*, 764–767.

King, T. (1993). The experiences of midlife daughters who are caregivers for their mothers. *Health Care for Women International, 14*, 419–426.

Klein, G. S. (1964). Need and regulation. In M. R. Jones (Ed.), *Nebraska Symposium on Motivation*. Lincoln: University of Nebraska Press.

Kobasa, S. C., & Puccetti, M. C. (1983). Personality and social resources in stress resistance. *Journal of Personality and Social Psychology, 45*, 839–850.

Koestler, A. (1971). *The case of the midwife toad*. London: Hutchinson.

Konvitz, J. (1985). *The urban millennium: The city-building process from the early middle ages to the present*. Carbondale: Southern Illinois University Press.

Korman, A. (1988). *The outsiders: Jews and corporate America*. Lexington, MA: Lexington Books.

Kowalik, D. L., & Gotlib, I. H. (1987). Depression and marital interaction: Concordance between intent and perception of communication. *Journal of Abnormal Psychology, 96*, 127–134.

Krause, N., Liang, J., & Yatomi, N. (1989). Satisfaction with social support and depressive symptoms: A panel analysis. *Psychology and Aging, 4*, 88–97.

Kuhn, T. S. (1962). *The structure of scientific revolutions*. Chicago: University of Chicago Press.

Laing, R. D. (Ed.). (1969). *The politics of the family and other essays*. New York: Vintage Books.

Lane, C., & Hobfoll, S. E. (1992). How loss affects anger and alienates potential supporters. *Journal of Consulting and Clinical Psychology, 60*, 935–942.

Lazarus, A. A. (1968). Learning theory and the treatment of depression. *Behaviour Research and Therapy, 6*, 83–89.

Lazarus, A. A. (1972). Some reactions to costello's paper on depression. *Behavior Therapy, 3*, 248–250.

Lazarus, R. S. (1966). *Psychological stress and the coping process*. New York: McGraw-Hill.

Lazarus, R. S. (1991). *Emotion and adaptation*. New York: Oxford University Press.

Lazarus, R. S., & Folkman, S. (1984). *Stress, appraisal and coping*. New York: Springer.

Lee, S. C. (1953). China's traditional family, its characteristics and disintegration. *American Sociological Review, 18*, 272–280.

Lepore, S. J., Evans, G. W., & Schneider, M. L. (1991). Dynamic role of social support in the link between chronic stress and psychological distress. *Journal of Personality and Social Psychology, 61*, 899–909.

Lepore, S. J., Wortman, C. B., Silver, R. C., & Wayment, H. A. (1996). Social constraints, intrusive thoughts and depressive symptoms among bereaved mothers. *Journal of Personality and Social Psychology, 70*, 271–282.

Leventhal, H., Leventhal, E. A., & Schaefer, P. M. (1991). Vigilant coping and health behavior: A life span problem. In M. Ory & R. Abeles (Eds.), *Aging, health and behavior*. Baltimore: Johns Hopkins University Press.

Levine, M., & Perkins, D. (1987). *Principles of community psychology: Perspectives and applications*. New York: Oxford University Press.

Levine, M., & Perkins, D. (1997). *Principles of community psychology: Perspectives and applications* (2nd ed.). New York: Oxford University Press.

Lewis, W. K. (1996). Bias in drug sentences. *National Law Journal, 18*, A19–A20.

Light, P. C. (1988). *Baby Boomers*. New York: Norton.

Lindemann, E. (1944). Symptomatology and management of acute grief. *American Journal of Psychiatry, 101*, 141–148.

Litvin, S., Albert, S., Brody, E., & Hoffman, C. (1995). Marital status, competing demands, and role priorities of parent-caring daughters. *Journal of Applied Gerontology, 14*, 372–390.

Lloyd, W. F. (1833). *Two lectures on the checks on population*. Oxford, UK: Oxford University Press.

Locke, J. (1952). *The second treatise of government.* Indianapolis: Bobbs-Merrill.

Lomranz, J. (1990). Long-term adaptation to traumatic stress in light of adult development and aging perspectives. In M. A. Stephens, J. H. Crowther, S. E. Hobfoll, & D. L. Tennenbaum (Eds.), *Stress and coping in later-life families.* New York: Hemisphere.

Lomranz, J. (1995). Endurance and living: Long-term effects of the Holocaust. In S. E. Hobfoll & M. W. deVries (Eds.), *Extreme stress and communities: Impact and intervention.* Dordrecht, The Netherlands: Kluwer Academic Publishers.

London, P. (1964). *The modes and morals of psychotherapy.* New York: Holt, Rinehart and Winston.

London, P. (1974). The psychotherapy boom. *Psychology Today, 8,* 62–68.

London, P. (1986). *The modes and morals of psychotherapy* (2nd ed.). Washington: Hemisphere.

Lopez, D., & Little, T. (1996). Children's action–control beliefs and emotional regulation in the social domain. *Developmental Psychology, 32,* 299–312.

Luce, R. D., & Raiffa, H. (1957). *Games and decisions: Introduction and critical survey.* London: Wiley.

Lurie, S. G. (1994). Ethical dilemmas and professional roles in occupational medicine. *Social Science Medicine, 38,* 1367–1374.

Lyons, R. F., Mickelson, K. D., Sullivan, M. J. L., & Coyne, J. C. (1998). Coping as a communal process. *Journal of Social and Personal Relationships, 15,* 579–605.

Maes, S., Kittel, F., Scholten, H., & Verhoeven, C. (1996). *Health promotion in the worksite: A European perspective.* Paper presented at the July meeting of the Conference on Health Psychology, Montreal, Canada.

Malinowski, B. (1944). *A scientific theory of culture and other essays.* New York: Oxford University Press.

Mandelbaum, M. (1979). Subjective, objective, and conceptual relativisms. *Monist, 62,* 405.

Marks, S. R. (1977). Multiple roles and role strain: Some notes on human energy, time and commitment. *American Sociological Review, 41,* 921–936.

Markus, H., & Nurius, R. (1986). Possible selves. *American Psychologist, 41,* 954–969.

Marlowe, D. H. (1984). *Cohesion, anticipated breakdown and endurance in battle: Considerations for severe and high intensity combat.* Washington, DC: Walter Reed Army Institute of Research.

Martin, P. Y. (1993). Feminist practice in organizations: Implications for management. In E. A. Fagenson (Ed.), *Women in management: Trends, issues and challenges in managerial diversity.* London: Sage.

Masatsugu, M. (1982). *The modern Samurai society: Duty and dependence in contemporary Japan.* New York: AMACOM Book Division.

Maslach, M. (1993). Burnout: A multidimensional perspective. In W. Schaefeli, C. Maslach, & T. Marek (Eds.), *Professional burnout: Recent developments in theory and research.* Washington, DC: Taylor & Francis.

Maslach, M., & Jackson, S. E. (1986). *The Maslach Burnout Inventory Manual* (2nd ed.). Palo Alto, CA: Consulting Psychologists Press.

Maslow, A. H. (1962). *Toward a psychology of being.* Princeton, NJ: Van Nostrand.

Maslow, A. H. (1987). *Motivation and personality* (3rd ed., rev. by R. Frager, J. Fadiman, C. McReynolds, & R. Cox). New York: Harper & Row. (Original published 1954)

May, R. (1953). *Man's search for himself.* New York: Norton.

May, R. (Ed.). (1969). *Existential psychology* (2nd ed.). New York: Random House.

McCree Bryan, M. & Davis, A. (Eds.). (1990). *100 years at Hull House.* Bloomington: Indiana University Press.

McFarlane, A. C. (1987). Life events and psychiatric disorder: The role of natural disaster. *British Journal of Psychiatry, 151,* 362–367.

McFarlane, A. C. (1992). *Quantification of traumatic stressors.* Amsterdam, The Netherlands: World Conference of the International Society for Traumatic Stress Studies.

McFarlane, A. C. (1995). Stress and disaster. In S. E. Hobfoll, & M. W. deVries (Eds.), *Extreme stress and communities: Impact and intervention.* Dordrecht, The Netherlands: Kluwer Academic Publishers.

McFarlane, A. C., & deGirolamo, G. (1996). The nature of traumatic stressors and the epidemiology of posttraumatic reactions. In B. A. van der Kolk, A. C. McFarlane, & L. Weisaeth (Eds.), *Traumatic stress: The effects of overwhelming experience on mind, body and society.* New York: Guilford.

McGrath, J. E. (1970). *Social and psychological factors in stress.* New York: Holt, Rinehart & Winston.

McIntosh, P. (1988). White privilege and male privilege: A personal account of coming to see correspondences through work in women's studies. In M. L. Anderson, & P. H. Collins (Eds.), *Race, class and gender: American anthology* (2nd ed.). Belmont: Wadsworth.

Meichenbaum, D. (1977). *Cognitive-behavior modification: An integrative approach.* New York: Plenum Press.

Meichenbaum, D. (1994). *A clinical handbook: Practical therapist manual for assessing and treating adults with post-traumatic stress disorder.* Ontario: Institute Press.

Meichenbaum, D., & Cameron, R. (1983). Stress inoculation training: Toward a general paradigm for training coping skills. In D. Meichenbaum & M. E. Jaremko (Eds.), *Stress reduction and prevention.* New York: Plenum Press.

Meichenbaum, D. & Fitzpatrick, D. (1993). A constructivist narrative perspective on stress and coping: Stress inoculation applications. In L. Goldberger & S. Breznitz (Eds.), *Handbook of stress: Theoretical and clinical aspects* (2nd ed.). New York: Free Press.

Merton, R. K. (1968). *Social theory and social structure* (expanded edition). New York: Free Press.

Mill, T. S. (1848). *Principles of political economy.* Boston: Charles C. Little and James Brown.

Mills, K., & Clark, M. S. (1982). Communal and exchange relationships. In L. Wheeler, (Ed.), *Review of personality and social psychology* (Vol. 3.). Beverly Hills, CA: Sage.

Minuchin, S. (1974). *Families and family therapy.* Cambridge, MA: Harvard University Press.

Monnier, J., Hobfoll, S. E., & Stone, B. K. (1996). Coping resources and social context. In W. Battman & S. Dutke (Eds.), *Processes of the molar regulation of behavior.* Lengerich, Germany: Pabst Science Publishers.

Monnier, J., & Hobfoll, S. E. (1977). Crossover effects of communal coping. *Journal of Social and Personal Relationships, 14,* 263–270.

Monnier, J., Stone, B. K., Hobfoll, S. E., & Johnson, R. J. (in press) How antisocial and communal coping influences the support process among male and female postal employees. *Sex Roles.*

Monnier, J., Hobfoll, S. E., Dunahoo, C. L., Hulsiger, M. R., and Johnson, R. J. (in press). There is more than rugged individualism in coping: Part 2. Construct validity and further model testing. *Anxiety, Stress, and Coping.*

Montesquieu, C.-L. (1752). *The spirit of laws.* London: Printed for J. Nourse & P. Vaillant.

Moos, R. H. (1984). The crisis of illness: Chronic conditions. In R. H. Moos (Ed.), *Coping with physical illness: 2. New perspectives* (pp. 139–143). New York: Plenum Press.

Moos, R. H., & Schaefer, J. A. (1993). Coping resources and processes: Current concepts and measures. In L. Goldberger & S. Breznitz (Eds.), *Handbook of stress: Theoretical and clinical aspects* (2nd ed., pp. 234–257). New York: Free Press.

Moos, R. H., & Tsu, V. D. (1977). The crisis of physical illness: An overview. In R. H. Moos (Ed.), *Coping with physical illness.* New York: Plenum Medical Book Company.

Moran, R. T., & Riesenberger, J. R. (1994). *The global challenge: Building the new worldwide enterprise.* London: McGraw-Hill.

Moritsugu, J., & Sue, S. (1983). Minority status as a stressor. In R. Gelner, L. Jason, J. Moritsugu, and S. Farber (Eds.), *Preventive psychology: Theory, research and practice.* New York: Pergamon Press.

Mumford, L. (1961). *The city in history: Its origins, its transformations, and its prospects.* New York: Harcourt, Brace & World.

Myers, S. L., Jr., & Chan, T. (1995). Racial discrimination in housing markets: Accounting for credit risk. *Social Science Quarterly, 76,* 543–561.

Nathanson, C. (1976). *American pop art and the culture of the sixties.* Cleveland, OH: New Gallery of Contemporary Art.

National Association for the Advancement of Colored People. (1969). *Thirty years of lynching in the United States.* New York: Negro Universities Press.

Nelson, G., & Beach, S. (1990). Sequential interaction in depression: Effects of depressive behavior on spousal aggression. *Behavior Therapy, 21,* 167–182.

Nesselroade, J., & Baltes, P. (1974). Adolescent personality development and historical change: 1970–1972. *Monographs of the Society for Research in Child Development, 39,* 1–79.

Nietzsche, F. W. (1896). *Thus spake Zarathustra* (Trans. Alexander Tille). New York: Macmillan.

Nisbett, R. E. (Ed.) (1993). *Rules for reasoning.* Hillsdale, NJ: Erlbaum.

Nitobe, I. (1905a). Bushido: The feudal ethic. In R. Downs (Ed.), *Japan yesterday and today.* New York: Praeger.

Nitobe, I. (1905b). The soul of Japan. In R. Downs (Ed.), *Japan yesterday and today.* New York: Praeger.

Nollen, S. D., Eddy, B. B., & Martin, V. H. (1978). *Permanent part-time employment: The manager's perspective.* New York: Praeger.

Norris, F. H. (1992). Epidemiology of trauma: Frequency and impact of different potentially traumatic events on different demographic groups. *Journal of Consulting and Clinical Psychology, 60,* 409–418.

Norris, F. H., & Kaniasty, K. (1996). Received and perceived social support in times of stress: A test of the social support deterioration deterrence model. *Journal of Personality and Social Psychology, 71,* 498–511.

Olson, D. (1989). Circumplex model of family systems: VIII. Family assessment and intervention. In D. Olson, C. Russell, & D. Sprenkle (Eds.), *Circumplex model: Systemic assessment and treatment of families.* New York: Haworth Press.

Ozer, E. M., & Bandura, A. (1990). Mechanisms governing empowerment effects: A self-efficacy analysis. *Journal of Personality and Social Psychology, 58,* 472–486.

Palinkas, L. A., Downs, M. A., Petterson, J. S., & Russell, J. (1993). Social, cultural and psychological impacts of the Exxon Valdez oil spill. *Human Organization, 51,* 1–13.

Palinkas, L. A., Russell, J., Downs, M. A., Petterson, J. S. (1992). Ethnic differences in stress, coping, and depressive symptoms after the Exxon Valdez oil spill. *Journal of Nervous and Mental Disease, 180,* 287–295.

Parham, T. A. (1989). Cycles of psychological nigrescence. *Counseling Psychologist, 17,* 187–226.

Parham, T. A., & McDavis, R. J. (1987). Black men, an endangered species: Who's really pulling the trigger? *Journal of Counseling and Development, 66,* 24–27.

Park, R. E., Burgess, E. W., & McKenzie, R. D. (1926). *The city.* Chicago: University of Chicago Press.

Parkes, C. M. (1972). *Bereavement.* New York: International Universities Press.

Parsons, T. (1951). *The social system.* New York: Free Press.

Paykel, E. S. (1985). Life events, social support and clinical psychiatric disorder. In I. G. Sarason & B. R. Sarason (Eds.), *Social support: Theory, research and applications* (pp. 321–348). Dordrecht, The Netherlands: Martinus Nijhoff.

Payne, B. (1988). Religious patterns and participation of older adults: A sociological perspective. *Educational Gerontology, 14,* 255–267.

Pearlin, L. I. (1993). The social contexts of stress. In L. Goldberger & S. Breznitz (Eds.), *Handbook of stress: Theoretical and clinical aspects* (2nd ed.). New York: Free Press.

Pearlin, L. I., Lieberman, M. A., Menaghan, E. G., & Mullan, J. T. (1981). The stress process. *Journal of Health and Social Behavior, 22,* 337–356.

Pearlin, L. I., & McCall, M. E. (1990). Occupational stress and marital support: A description of microprocesses. In J. Eckenrode & S. Gore (Eds.), *Stress between work and family.* New York: Plenum Press.

Pearlin, L., & Schooler, C. (1978). The structure of coping. *Journal of Health and Social Behavior, 19,* 2–21.

Pearlman, T. (1992). *The threatened medical identity of psychiatry: The winds of change.* Springfield, IL: Charles C. Thomas.

Pennebaker, J. W., & Harber, K. D. (1993). A social state model of collective coping: The Loma Prieta earthquake and the Persian Gulf war. *Journal of Social Issues, 49,* 125–145.

Perloff, R. (1987). Self-interest and personal responsibility redux. *American Psychologist, 42,* 3–11.

Perls, F. S. (1969). *Gestalt therapy verbatim.* Lafayette, CA: Real People Press.

Pierce, G. R., Sarason, I. G., & Sarason, B. R. (1996). Coping and social support. In M. Zeidner & N. S. Endler (Eds.), *Handbook of coping: Theory, research, applications.* New York: Wiley.

Pinel, P. (1806). *A treatise on insanity* (Trans. by D. D. Davis). Sheffield, UK: W. Todd.

Pines, A., Aronson, E., & Kafry, D. (1981). *Burnout: From tedium to personal growth.* New York: Free Press.

Popper, K. R. (1959) *The logic of scientific discovery.* New York: Basic Books.

Popper, K. R. (1972). *Objective knowledge: An evolutionary approach.* Oxford, UK: Clarendon Press.

Powell, G. N. (1988). *Women and men in management.* Newbury Park, CA: Sage.

Powell, R. M. (1969). *Race, religion and the promotion of the American executive.* Columbus: Ohio State University Press.

Pynoos, R. S., Goenjian, A., Steinberg, A. M. (1995). Strategies of disaster intervention for children and adolescents. In S. E. Hobfoll & M. W. deVries (Eds.), *Extreme stress and communities: Impact and intervention.* Dordrecht, The Netherlands: Kluwer Academic Publishers.

Rabkin, J. G., & Struening, E. L. (1976). Life events, stress and illness. *Science, 194,* 1013–1020.

Raphael, B. (1986). *When disaster strikes.* London: Hutchinson.

Rappaport, J. (1977). *Community psychology: Values, research and action.* New York: Holt, Rinehart & Winston.

Rappaport, J. (1981). In praise of paradox: A social policy of empowerment over prevention. *American Journal of Community Psychology, 9,* 1–25.

Raviv, A., Keinan, G., Abazon, Y., & Raviv, A. (1990). Moving as a stressful life event for adolescents. *Journal of Community Psychology, 18,* 130–140.

Reis, H. T., & Shaver, P. (1988) Intimacy as an interpersonal process. In S. Duck, D. F. Hay, S. E. Hobfoll, W. Ickes, & B. M. Montgomery (Eds.), *Handbook of personal relationships: Theory, research and interventions* (pp. 367–389). Chichester, UK: Wiley.

Riger, S. (1993). What's wrong with empowerment. *American Journal of Community Psychology, 21,* 279–292.

Riley, D., & Eckenrode, J. (1986). Social ties: Subgroup differences in costs and benefits. *Journal of Personality and Social Psychology, 51,* 770–778.

Rizzo, T., & Corsaro, W. (1995). Social support processes in early childhood friendship: A comparative study of ecological congruences in enacted support. *Americas Journal of Community Psychology, 23,* 389–417.

Roberts, B. W., & Helson, R. (1997). Changes in culture, changes in personality: The influence of individualism in a longitudinal study of women. *Journal of Personality and Social Psychology, 72,* 641–651.

Roberts, J. E., Gotlib, I. H., & Kassel, J. D. (1996). Adult attachment security and symptoms of depression: The mediating roles of dysfunctional attitudes and low self-esteem. *Journal of Personality and Social Psychology, 70,* 310–320.

Rochefort, D. A. (Ed.) (1989). *Handbook on mental health policy in the United States.* New York: Greenwood Press.

Rogers, C. R. (1951). *Client-centered therapy.* Boston: Houghton Mifflin.

Rogers, C. R. (1961). *On becoming a person: A therapist's view of psychotherapy.* Boston: Houghton Mifflin.

Rodgers, W. (1969). *Think: A biography of the Watsons and IBM.* New York: Stein & Day.

Rogers, C. R. (1956). Intellectual psychotherapy. *Contemporary Psychology, 1,* 357–358.

Rogers, C. R. (1980). *A way of being.* Boston: Houghton Mifflin.

Rogers, S. (1982). *The shaman: His symbols and his healing power.* Springfield, IL: Charles C Thomas.

Rook, K. S. (1984). The negative side of social interaction: Impact on psychological well-being. *Journal of Personality and Social Psychology, 46,* 1097–1108.

Rook, K.S., & Dooley, D. (1985). Applying social support research: Theoretical problems and future directions. *Journal of Social Issues, 41,* 5–28.

Rorty, R. (1986). Foucault and epistemology. In D. Couzens Hoy (Ed.), *Foucault: A critical reader.* Oxford, UK: Blackwell.

Rosenbaum, M. (1998). Opening versus closing stategies in controlling one's responses to experience. In M. Kofta, G. Weary, & G. Sedek (Eds.), *Personal control in action: Cognitive and Motivational Mechanisms.* New York: Plenum Press.

Rosenberg, M. (1965). *Society and adolescent self-image.* Princeton, NJ: Princeton University Press.

Ross, C. E., & Mirowsky, J. (1989). Explaining the social patterns of depression: Control and problem solving—or support and talking? *Journal of Health and Social Behavior, 30,* 206–219.

Rostand, E. (1980). *Cyrano de Bergerac.* Danbury, CT: Grolier. (Original published 1897)

Roth, S., & Cohen, L. J. (1989). Approach, avoidance and coping with stress. *American Psychologist, 41,* 813–819.

Rubins, J. L. (1978). *Karen Horney: Gentle rebel of psychoanalysis.* New York: Dial.

Rush, B. (1812). *Diseases of the mind.* Philadelphia: Kimber & Richardson.

Rush, B. (1812). *Medical inquiries and observations on the diseases of the mind.* Philadelphia: Kimber & Richardson.

Salmon, T. (1929). In medical department of the U.S. Army. *Neuropsychiatry in the World War, 10.* Washington, DC: U.S. Government Printing Office.

Salthouse, T. (1984). Effects of age and skill in typing. *Journal of Experimental Psychology: General, 113,* 345–371.

Sampson, E. E. (1988). The debate on individualism: Indigenous psychologies of the individual and their role in personal and societal functioning. *American Psychologist, 43,* 15–22.

Sandler, I. N., West, S. G., Baca, L., Pillow, D. R., Gersten, J. C., Rogosch, F., Virdin, L., Beals, J., Reynolds, K., Kallgren, C., Tein, J., Kriege, G., Cole, E., & Ramirez, R. (1992). Linking empirically based theory and evaluation: The family bereavement program. *American Journal of Community Psychology, 20,* 491–521.

Sarason, B. R., Pierce, G. R., & Sarason, I. G. (1990). Social support, the sense of acceptance, and the role of relationships. In B. R. Sarason, I. G. Sarason, & G. R. Pierce (Eds.). *Social support: An interactional view.* New York: Wiley.

Sarason, I. G., Sarason, B. R., & Shearin, E. N. (1986). Social support as an individual difference variable: Its stability, origins, and relational aspects. *Journal of Personality and Social Psychology, 5,* 845–855.

Sarason, S. B. (1974). *The psychological sense of community: Prospects for a community psychology.* San Francisco: Jossey-Bass.

Sarason, S. B. (1977). A cultural limitation of system approaches to educational reform. *American Journal of Community Psychology, 5,* 277–289.

Savage, W., Jr. (1979). *The cowboy hero: His image in American history and culture.* Norman: University of Oklahoma Press.

Schacter, D. (1987). Implicit memory: History and current status. *Journal of Experimental Psychology: Learning, Memory and Cognition, 13,* 501–518.

Schönpflug, W. (1985). Goal-directed behavior as a source of stress: Psychological origins and consequences of inefficiency. In M. Frese & J. Sabini (Eds.), *The concept of action in psychology* (pp. 172–188). Hillsdale, NJ: Erlbaum.

Schulz, R., & Tompkins, C. A. (1990). Life events and changes in social relationships: Examples, mechanisms and measurement [Special issue: Social support in social and clinical psychology]. *Journal of Social and Clinical Psychology, 9,* 69–77.

Schwab, R. L., Jackson, S. E., & Schuler, R. S. (1986). Educator burnout: Sources and consequences. *Educational Research Quarterly, 10,* 15–30.

Schwartz, S. H., & Bilsky, W. (1990). Toward a theory of the universal content and structure of values: Extensions and cross-cultural replications. *Journal of Personality and Social Psychology, 58,* 878–891.

Schwarzer, C., & Starke, D. (1996, July). *Towards a theory-based questionnaire of coping.* Paper presented in the 17th International Conference of the Stress and Anxiety Research Society, Graz, Austria.

Schwarzer, R., Hahn, A., & Schröeder, H. (1994a). Social integration and social support in a life crisis: Effects of macrosocial change in East Germany. *American Journal of Community Psychology, 22,* 685–706.

Schwarzer, R., Jerusalem, W., & Hahn, A. (1994b). Unemployment, social support and health complaints: A longitudinal study of stress in East German refugees. *Journal of Community and Applied Social Psychology, 4,* 31–45.

Schwarzer, R., & Leppin, A. (1989). Social support and health: A meta-analysis. *Psychology and Health, 3,* 1–15.

Seligman, M. E. P. (1975). *Helplessness.* San Francisco: W. H. Freeman.

Selye, H. (1950). The physiology and pathology of exposure to stress. Montreal: Acta.

Selye, H. (1951–1956). *Annual report of stress.* Montreal: Acta.

Sepielli, P. J., & Palumbo, T. J. (1997). U. S. Census Bureau: The official statistics [on-line]. Available: http://www.census.gov/population/www/pop-profile/lfoccu.html

Shadish, W. R., Jr. (1984). Policy research: Lessons from the implementation of deinstitutionalization. *American Psychologist, 39,* 725–738.

Shalev, A. (1996). Stress versus traumatic stress: From acute homeostatic reactions to chronic psychopathology. In B. A. van der Kolk, A. C. McFarlane, & L. Weisaeth (Eds.), *Traumatic stress: The effects of overwhelming experience on mind, body and society.* New York: Guilford.

Shelley, R. (1993). *Culture shock! Japan.* Portland, Oregon: Graphic Arts Center Publishing Company.

Shinn, M., Lehman, S., Wong, N. W. (1984). Social interaction and social support. *Journal of Social Issues, 40,* 55–76.

Shirom, A. (1989). Burnout in work organizations. In C. L. Cooper & I. T. Robertson (Eds.), *International review of industrial and organizational psychology.* Chichester, UK: Wiley.

Shore, B. (1996). *Culture in mind: Cognition, culture, and the problem of meaning.* New York: Oxford University Press.

Shweder, R. A. & LeVine, R. A. (1984). *Culture theory: Essays on mind, self, and emotion.* Cambridge, UK: Cambridge University Press.

Siegel, J. P. (1986). Marital dynamics of women with premenstrual tension syndrome. *Family System Medicine, 4,* 358–365.

Siegrist, J. (1986). Adverse health effects of high-effort/low-reward conditions. *Journal of Occupational Health Psychology, 1*, 27–41.

Siegrist, J. (1996). Stressful work, self-experience and cardiovascular disease prevention. In K. Orth-Gomer & N. Schneiderman (Eds.), *Behavioral medicine approaches to cardiovascular disease prevention*. Mahwah, NJ: Erlbaum.

Siegrist, J., Peter, R., Junge, A., & Cremer, P. (1990). Low status control, high effort at work, and ischemic heart disease: Prospective evidence from blue collar men. *Social Science and Medicine, 31*, 1127–1134.

Sinclair, U. (1878). *The jungle*. New York: Penguin Books.

Skagen, A. (1992). The incredible shrinking organization: What does it mean for middle managers? *Supervisory Management, 37*, 1–3.

Skinner, B. F. (1938). *The behavior of organisms: An experimental analysis*. Englewood Cliffs, NJ: Prentice-Hall.

Skinner, B. F. (1948). *Walden two*. New York: Macmillan.

Skinner, B. F. (1953). *Science and human behavior*. New York: Macmillan.

Skinner, B. F. (1978). *Reflections on behaviorism and society*. Englewood Cliffs, NJ: Prentice-Hall.

Snyder, T. D., & Hoffman, C. M. (1995). *National center for education statistics: Digest of education statistics, 1995*. Washington, DC: U. S. Department of Education Office of Educational Research and Improvement.

Solomon, Z. (1995). The pathogenic effects of war stress: The Israeli experience. In S. E. Hobfoll & M. W. deVries (Eds.), *Impact and intervention*. Dordrecht, The Netherlands: Kluwer Academic Publishers.

Solomon, Z., Milkulincer, M., & Hobfoll, S. E. (1987). The effects of social support and battle intensity on loneliness and breakdown during combat. *Journal of Personality and Social Psychology, 51*, 1269–1276.

Solomon, Z., Waysman, M., Avitzur, E., & Enoch, D. (1991). Psychiatric symptomatology among wives of soldiers following combat stress reaction: The role of the social network and marital relations. *Anxiety Research, 4*, 213–223.

Sowell, T. (1981). *Ethnic America: A history*. New York: Basic Books.

Spence, J. T. (1985). Achievement American style: The rewards and costs of individualism. *American Psychologist, 40*, 1285–1295.

Spence, J. T., & Spence, K. W. (1966). The motivational components of manifest anxiety: Drive and drive stimuli. In C. D. Spielberger (Ed.), *Anxiety and behavior* (pp. 291–326). New York: Academic Press.

Spielberger, C. D. (Ed.). (1966). *Anxiety and behavior*. New York: Academic Press.

Spielberger, C. D. (Ed.). (1972). *Anxiety: Current trends in theory and research*. New York: Academic Press.

Spielberger, C. D., Gorsuch, R. L., & Lusbene, R. E. (1970). *Manual for the state–trait anxiety inventory (self-evaluation questionnaire)*. Palo Alto, CA: Consultant Psychologists Press.

Spielberger, C. D., Jacobs, G., Russell, S., & Crane, R. S. (1983). Assessment of anger: The state-trait anger scale. In J. N. Butcher & C. D. Spielberger (Eds.), *Advances in personality assessment* (Vol. 2). Hillsdale, NJ: Erlbaum.

Spielberger, C. D., & Sarason, I. G: (1975–1986). *Stress and anxiety, (Vols. 1–10)*. New York: Hemisphere.

Stanton, A. L., & Danoff-Burg, S. (1995). Selected issues in women's reproductive health: Psychological perspectives. In A. L. Stanton & S. J. Gallant (Eds.), *The psychology of women's health*. Washington, DC: American Psychological Association Press.

Starke, D., & Schwartzer, C. (in press). Towards a theory-based assessment of coping. *European Journal of Psychological Assessment*.

Stephens, M. A. P., & Franks, M. M. (1995). Spillover between daughters' roles as caregiver and wife: Interference or enhancement? *Journal of Gerontology, 50B*, 9–17.

Stock, W. A., Okun, M. A., Haring, M. J., & Witter, R. A. (1983). Age and subjective well-being: A meta-analysis. In R. J. Light (Ed.), *Evaluation studies: Review Annual* (Vol 8). Beverly Hills, CA: Sage.

Stoll, O. (1997). *Coping among competitive athletes.* Paper presented at the 1997 meeting of Stress Anxiety Research Society, Dusseldorf, Germany.

Stone, A., Greenberg, M., Kennedy-Moore, E., & Newman, M. (1991). Self-report, situation-specific coping questionnaires: What are they measuring? *Journal of Personality and Social Psychology, 61,* 648–658.

Stone, A. A., & Neale, J. M. (1984). New measure of daily coping: Development and preliminary results). *Journal of Personality and Social Psychology, 46,* 892–906.

Straus, M. A., & Gelles, R. J. (1986). Societal change and change in family violence from 1975 to 1986 as revealed in two national surveys. *Journal of Marriage and the Family, 48,* 465–479.

Strelau, J. (1995). Temperament risk factor: The contribution of temperament to the consequences of the state of stress. In S. E. Hobfoll & M. W. deVries (Eds,), *Extreme stress and communities: Impact and intervention* (pp. 63–82). Dordrecht, The Netherlands: Kluwer Academic Publishers.

Suh, E., Diener, E., & Fujita, F. (1996). Events and subjective well-being: Only recent events matter. *Journal of Personality and Social Psychology, 70,* 1091–1102.

Sun-Tzu (6th Century B.C.). *Art of war* (Trans. Ralph Sawyer, 1994). Boulder, CO: Westview Press.

Swann, W. B., & Read, S. J. (1981). Self-verification processes: How we sustain our self-conceptions. *Journal of Experimental Social Psychology, 17,* 351–372.

Swann, W. B., Stein-Seroussi, A., & Giesler, R. B. (1992). Why people self-verify. *Journal of Personality and Social Psychology, 62,* 392–401.

Taylor, F. (1911). *The principles of scientific management.* New York: Harper.

Taylor, R. B., & Shumaker, S. A. (1990). Local crime as a natural hazard: Implications for understanding the relationship between disorder and fear of crime. *American Journal of Community Psychology, 18,* 619–641.

Taylor, S. E. (1983). Adjustment to threatening events: A theory of cognitive adaptation. *American Psychologist, 38,* 1161–1173.

Taylor, S. E. (1991). Asymmetric effects of positive and negative events: The mobilization–minimization hypothesis. *Psychological Bulletin, 110,* 67–85.

Taylor, S. E. (1995). *Health psychology* (3rd ed.). New York: McGraw-Hill.

Taylor, S. E., & Aspinwall, L. G. (1996). Mediating and moderating processes in psychosocial stress: Appraisal, coping, resistance, and vulnerability. In H. B. Kaplan (Ed.), *Psychosocial stress: Perspectives on structure, theory, life-course and methods.* San Diego, CA: Academic Press.

Taylor, J., & Spence, K. W. (1952). The relationship of anxiety level to performance in serial learning. *Journal of Experimental Psychology, 44,* 61–64.

Taylor, S. E., & Brown, J. D. (1994). Positive illusions and well-being revisited: Separating fact from fiction. *Psychological Bulletin, 116,* 21–27.

Thoits, P. (1983). Multiple identities and psychological well-being: A reformulation and test of the social isolation hypothesis. *American Sociological Review, 48,* 174–187.

Thoits, P. (1994). Stressors and problem-solving: The individual as psychological activist. *Journal of Health and Social Behavior, 35,* 143–160.

Thoits, P. A. (1991). Gender differences in coping with emotional stress. In J. Eckenrode (Ed.), *The social context of coping.* New York: Plenum Press.

Tocqueville, Alexis de (1945). *Democracy in America.* New York: Vintage Books.

Triandis, H. C. (1994). *Culture and social behavior.* New York: McGraw-Hill.

Triandis, H. C. (1995a). *Individualism and collectivism.* Boulder, CO: Westview Press.

Triandis, H. C. (1995b). The self and social behavior in differing cultural contexts. In N. R. Goldberger & J. B. Veroff (Eds.), *The culture and psychology reader.* New York: New York University Press.

Trickett, E. J. (1978). Toward a social ecological conception of adolescent socialization: Normative data on contrasting types of public school classrooms. *Child Development, 49,* 408–414.

Trickett, E. J. (1995). The community context of disaster and traumatic stress: An ecological perspective from community psychology. In S. E. Hobfoll, & M. W. deVries (Eds.), *Extreme stress and communities: Impact and intervention.* Dordrecht, The Netherlands: Kluwer Academic Publishers.

Trickett, E. J., Watts, R. J., & Briman, D. (Eds.). (1994). *Human diversity: Perspectives on people in context.* San Francisco: Jossey-Bass.

Truax, C. B., & Mitchell, K. M. (1971). Research on certain therapist interpersonal skills in relation to process and outcome. In A. E. Bergin & S. L. Garfield (Eds.), *Handbook of psychotherapy and behavior change.* New York: Wiley.

Tuan, Yi-Fu (1982). *Segmented worlds and self: Group life and individual consciousness.* Minneapolis: University of Minnesota Press.

Tversky, A., & Kahneman, D. (1974). Judgement under uncertainty: Heuristics and biases. *Science, 185,* 1124–1131.

Van Lange, P., Otten, W., De Bruin, E., & Joireman, J. A. (1997). Development of prosocial, individualistic, and competitive orientations: Theory and preliminary evidence. *Journal of Personality and Social Psychology, 73,* 733–746.

Vanderhart, P. G. (1993). The binomial profit analysis of the home equity decisions of elderly homeowners. *Research on Aging, 15,* 299–323.

Van Yperen, N. W., Buunk, B. P., & Schaufeli, W. B. (1992). Communal orientation and the burnout syndrome among nurses. *Journal of Applied Social Psychology, 22,* 173–189.

Vaux, A. (1988). *Social support: Theory, research and intervention.* New York: Praeger.

Verkauf, W. (Ed.) (1975). *Dada: Monograph of a movement.* New York: St. Martin's Press.

Vinokur, A., Schul, Y., & Caplan, R. D. (1987). Determinants of perceived social support: Interpersonal transactions, personal outlook and transient affective states [Special issue: Integrating personality and social psychology]. *Journal of Personality and Social Psychology, 53,* 1137–1145.

Vinokur, A. D., Price, R. H., & Caplan, R. D. (1996). Hard times and hurtful partners: How financial strain affects depression and relationship satisfaction of unemployed persons and their spouses. *Journal of Personality and Social Psychology, 71,* 166–179.

Vinokur, A. D., & van Ryn, M. (1993). Social support and undermining in close relationships: Their independent effects on the mental health of unemployed persons. *Journal of Personality and Social Psychology, 65,* 350–359.

Vitaliano, P., DeWolfe, D., Maiuro, R., Russo, J., & Kayton, W. (1990). Appraised changeability of a stressor as a modifier of the relationship between coping and depression: A test of the hypothesis of fit. *Journal of Personality and Social Psychology, 59,* 582–592.

Vitaliano, P., Russo, J., & Maiuro, R. (1987). Locus of control, type of stressor, and appraisal within a cognitive-phenomenological model of stress. *Journal of Research in Personality, 21,* 224–237.

Vodopyanova, N. E., & Starchenkova, E. S. (1997, July 14–16). Burnout, coping strategies, and professional efficiency. Paper presented at the 18th Annual Conference of the Stress and Anxiety Research Society, Gies, Austria.

Von Neuman, J., & Morgenstern, O. (1947). *Theory of games and economic behavior.* Princeton, NJ: Princeton University Press.

Waldron, I., & Jacobs, J. (1989). Effects of multiple roles on women's health: Evidence from a national longitudinal study. *Women and Health, 15,* 3–19.

Weiss, R. (1990). Bringing work stress home. In J. Eckenrode & S. Gore (Eds.), *Stress between work and family.* New York: Plenum Press.

Weitzman, L. (1988). Women and children last: The social and economic consequences of

Author Index

Subject Index